CANCER ETIOLOGY, DIAGNOSIS AND TREATMENTS

ACUTE LYMPHOBLASTIC LEUKEMIA: ETIOLOGY, PATHOGENESIS AND TREATMENTS

CANCER ETIOLOGY, DIAGNOSIS AND TREATMENTS

Additional books in this series can be found on Nova's website under the Series tab.

Additional E-books in this series can be found on Nova's website under the E-books tab.

CANCER ETIOLOGY, DIAGNOSIS AND TREATMENTS

ACUTE LYMPHOBLASTIC LEUKEMIA: ETIOLOGY, PATHOGENESIS AND TREATMENTS

SEVERO VECCHIONE
AND
LUIGI TEDESCO
EDITORS

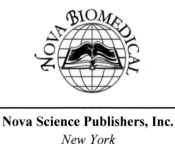

Nova Science Publishers, Inc.
New York

Copyright © 2012 by Nova Science Publishers, Inc.

All rights reserved. No part of this book may be reproduced, stored in a retrieval system or transmitted in any form or by any means: electronic, electrostatic, magnetic, tape, mechanical photocopying, recording or otherwise without the written permission of the Publisher.

For permission to use material from this book please contact us:
Telephone 631-231-7269; Fax 631-231-8175
Web Site: http://www.novapublishers.com

NOTICE TO THE READER

The Publisher has taken reasonable care in the preparation of this book, but makes no expressed or implied warranty of any kind and assumes no responsibility for any errors or omissions. No liability is assumed for incidental or consequential damages in connection with or arising out of information contained in this book. The Publisher shall not be liable for any special, consequential, or exemplary damages resulting, in whole or in part, from the readers' use of, or reliance upon, this material. Any parts of this book based on government reports are so indicated and copyright is claimed for those parts to the extent applicable to compilations of such works.

Independent verification should be sought for any data, advice or recommendations contained in this book. In addition, no responsibility is assumed by the publisher for any injury and/or damage to persons or property arising from any methods, products, instructions, ideas or otherwise contained in this publication.

This publication is designed to provide accurate and authoritative information with regard to the subject matter covered herein. It is sold with the clear understanding that the Publisher is not engaged in rendering legal or any other professional services. If legal or any other expert assistance is required, the services of a competent person should be sought. FROM A DECLARATION OF PARTICIPANTS JOINTLY ADOPTED BY A COMMITTEE OF THE AMERICAN BAR ASSOCIATION AND A COMMITTEE OF PUBLISHERS.

Additional color graphics may be available in the e-book version of this book.

Library of Congress Cataloging-in-Publication Data

Acute lymphoblastic leukemia : etiology, pathogenesis, and treatments / editors, Severo Vecchione and Luigi Tedesco.
    p. ; cm.
 Includes bibliographical references and index.
 ISBN 978-1-61470-872-8 (hardcover)
 I. Vecchione, Severo. II. Tedesco, Luigi.
 [DNLM: 1. Precursor Cell Lymphoblastic Leukemia-Lymphoma. WH 250]

 616.99'419071--dc23
                             2011041383

Published by Nova Science Publishers, Inc. ✦ New York

Contents

Preface		vii
Chapter I	Genome Wide Association Studies in Pediatric Acute Lymphoblastic Leukemia: Pathogenesis and Therapy *Kyriaki Hatziagapiou, Maria Braoudaki,* *Katerina Katsibardi, George I. Lambrou,* *Fotini Tzortzatou-Stathopoulou*	1
Chapter II	Mice Deficient for the Slp65 Signaling Protein: A Model for Pre-B Cell Acute Lymphoblastic Leukemia *Van B. T. Ta and Rudi W. Hendriks*	53
Chapter III	Childhood Acute Lymphoblastic Leukemia *Adriana Zámečníkova*	85
Chapter IV	Systems Approaches to Childhood Leukemogenesis *George I. Lambrou, Maria Braoudaki,* *Kyriaki Hatziagapiou, Katerina Katsibardi,* *Fotini Tzortzatou-Stathopoulou*	119
Chapter V	Histone Deacetylase Inhibitors: Pre-clinical and Clinical Evidence in Treating Acute Lymphoblastic Leukemia *Ana Lucia Abujamra*	135
Chapter VI	A Therapeutic Target in Leukemia: The NK-1 Receptor *Miguel Muñoz, Ana González-Ortega and* *Rafael Coveñas*	153
Chapter VII	Minimal Residual Disease Monitoring in Childhood Acute Lymphoblastic Leukemia *Katerina Katsibardi, Maria Braoudaki,* *George I. Lambrou, Kyriaki Hatziagapiou,* *Fotini Tzortzatou-Stathopoulou*	169

Chapter VIII	Clinical Relevance and Application of Cytogenetic Approaches in Pediatric Acute Lymphoblastic Leukaemia *Maria Braoudaki, Katerina Katsibardi, George I. Lambrou, Kyriaki Hatziagapiou, Fotini Tzortzatou-Stathopoulou*	**183**
Chapter IX	Maintenance Therapy in Ph Negative Adult Acute Lymphoblastic Leukemia *Michael Doubek and Jiří Mayer*	**197**
Chapter X	The Role of Innate and Adaptive Immunity in Childhood Acute Lymphoblastic Leukemia *Maria Hatzistilianou*	**205**
Index		**223**

Preface

Acute lymphoblastic leukemia (ALL) is a malignant disorder of the bone marrow in which a lymphoid precursor cell becomes genetically altered resulting in dysregulated proliferation and clonal expansion of neoplastic cells. It is the most common malignancy in children, representing nearly one third of all pediatric cancers. In this book, the authors present topical research in the study of acute lymphoblastic leukemia including genome wide association studies in pediatric acute lymphoblastic leukemia; mice deficient for the Slp65 signaling protein which is a model for ALL; histone deacetylase inhibitors and maintenance therapy in Ph negative adult acute lymphoblastic leukemia.

Chapter I - Acute lymphoblastic leukemia (ALL) remains an imperative cause of mortality among cancer pediatric patients, who carry a dismal prognosis. Ongoing genome wide profiling research has offered an alternative approach in understanding the biology underlying the etiology, pathogenesis and targeted treatment of childhood ALL. More specifically, such studies have detected certain gene mutations and polymorphisms that play known or potential roles in leading cellular pathways. Subsequently their mutational or polymorphism patterns might be associated with the risk of leukemogenesis by altering cell cycle regulation, lymphoid development and differentiation. Several current high through-put genome mutational analysis efforts have been employed to identify such submicroscopic genetic lesions, including micro-array based assays; single nucleotide polymorphism arrays, loss of heterozygocity, gene-expression profiling and potential gene mutation screening. Collectively, these molecular approaches attempt to increase the knowledge of ALL pathogenesis, enable diagnosis, advance the efficacy of current treatments by leading to the development of personalized ALL therapy and subsequently improve patients' clinical outcomes.

Chapter II - Acute lymphoblastic leukemia (ALL) is characterized by oncogenic transformation of progenitors of the B-cell lineage in the bone marrow. Extensive molecular characterization of genetic abnormalities, in particular chromosomal translocations, have allowed the development of sensitive assays for the identification of underlying molecular defects that are applicable to ALL diagnosis and to monitor response to treatment. The need for further improvement of therapy requires in-depth understanding of the fundamental nature of the disease process and of mechanisms by which lymphoid cells undergo malignant transformation and progression. Research in this area is strongly facilitated by the availability of animal models. Mice deficient for the signaling molecule Slp65 spontaneously develop pre-B cell leukemia. Importantly, deficiency of SLP65 has been reported in a fraction of childhood precursor-B cell ALL cases. Moreover, in precursor-B ALL positive for the BCR-ABL translocation the activity of the BCR-ABL1 kinase fusion protein was linked to expression of the same aberrant SLP65 transcripts. In the B-cell lineage, diversity of the antibody repertoire is generated by recombination of various gene segments at the immunoglobulin (Ig) heavy (H) and light (L) chain loci, which occurs in an ordered manner. Signaling by membrane Ig governs a number of distinct checkpoints in B cell differentiation that shape the antibody repertoire. A central checkpoint is the pre-B cell receptor (pre-BCR), which monitors successful expression of the Ig H chain and signals for proliferation, differentiation and Ig L chain recombination. In pre-B cells cooperative signals initiated from the pre-BCR and the interleukin-7 receptor (IL-7R) govern pre-B cell proliferation. The adapter protein Slp65 and the cytoplasmic tyrosine kinase Btk are key components of signaling pathways downstream of the pre-BCR and cooperate as tumor suppressors. Slp65 is essential for cell cycle exit and developmental progression of large, cycling into small, resting pre-B cells in which Ig L chain recombination is initiated. At this transition, IL-7 responsiveness and expression of the c-myc oncogene is downregulated and the Bcl6 transcriptional repressor is activated, thereby protecting pre-B cells from DNA damage-induced apoptosis during Ig L chain gene recombination. In this review, authors discuss recent findings that define the role of Slp65 in pre-B cell differentiation and give insight into molecular mechanisms by which Slp65-deficient pre-B cells undergo oncogenic transformation in the mouse.

Chapter III - Acute lymphoblastic leukemia (ALL) is a malignant disorder of the bone marrow in which a lymphoid precursor cell becomes genetically altered resulting in dysregulated proliferation and clonal expansion of neoplastic cells. It is the most common malignancy in children, representing nearly one third of all pediatric cancers. The disease has a bimodal distribution; there is an early incidence peak at 2 to 5 years of age, where they represent about 80% of the childhood leukemias and with a second incidence peak at around 50 years old. Although there are some identified factors associated with increased risk of developing the disease, the etiology of acute lymphoblastic leukemia remains largely unknown. A small percentage of cases are associated with inherited genetic abnormalities, with the best characterized being Down's syndrome and congenital immunodeficiencies. In addition to genetics, parental and environmental factors have been suggested to contribute to susceptibility, supported by the observation that the type and frequency of childhood ALL vary by geographic region and ethnicity. Improvement in molecular biology research as well as better cytogenetic techniques revealed that childhood acute lymphoblastic leukemia is a highly heterogeneous disease, comprising many entities. A number of genetic subtypes has been and continue to be discovered in pediatric ALL and it has been repeatedly shown that recurrent genetic abnormalities are present in the majority of successfully karyotyped patients with ALL. In addition, several new cryptic abnormalities have been discovered recently using genome-wide surveys, leading to identification of previously unrecognized diversity among individual patients. More importantly, recurrent chromosomal abnormalities observed in leukemia cells have shown correlations between specific genomic alterations and clinical-biological features of patients with diagnostic and prognostic significance. The recognition of these anomalies has contributed greatly to the authors' understanding of disease pathogenesis, leading to the concept of risk-adapted treatment strategies and intensive therapy approaches for patients. Due to the exponential growth in the authors' understanding, the treatment of childhood acute lymphoblastic leukemia is a success story in modern oncology with the potential to change the medicine fundamentally. This review provides insight into clinical and biological characteristics of ALL in children, as well as highlights some of the recently described prognostic markers that might serve as new and potential therapeutic targets for future drug development.

Chapter IV - The mechanisms underlying leukemogenesis in lymphocytes are hitherto poorly elucidated. Understanding those mechanisms is crucial for treatment, quality of life purposes and ethical reasons, since neoplasms in children could prove devastating. In the advent of the 21st century, the trend in research has taken an interesting turn, looking for global patterns in biological systems in a holistic approach. Although this concept is not novel, it has been nowadays *baptized* as systems approach, borrowing its name from engineers. Meanwhile, additional biological principles have emerged, such as systems biology, computational biology and more lately physical biology. These disciplines aim the assistance of explaining biological phenomena with the attribution of general rules, similar to older natural sciences such as chemistry and physics. Hence, it would not be an exaggeration to state that the maturity of biological sciences would endure their "mating" with other disciplines such as mathematics and physics.

Chapter V - Acute lymphoblastic leukemia is the most common type of cancer in the pediatric population. In spite of recent reports stating that standard treatment may yield 5-year event-free survival rates of approximately 80%, and 5-year survival rates approaching 90%, a significant subset of pediatric leukemia patients either relapse or fail to ever achieve a complete remission. Moreover, there have been increasing incidences of late therapy-related effects, warranting a need for new therapies which prove to be effective for high-risk patients, all the while decreasing the incidence of long-term sequelae. Histone deacetylase inhibitors (HDIs) promote or enhance several different anticancer mechanisms and therefore are in evidence as potential antileukemia agents. Studies on leukemia have provided examples for their functional implications in cancer development and progression, as well as their relevance for therapeutic targeting. A number of HDIs have been tested in clinical trials, and most studies have shown that they are safe, all the while demonstrating significant clinical activity. The use of HDIs in association with other molecules, such as classical chemotherapeutic drugs and DNA demethylating agents, has been implied as a promising treatment alternative for leukemia patients. Taking into consideration the process of leukemogenesis and the clinical course of acute lymphoblastic leukemia, this chapter will focus on the pre-clinical and clinical results of histone deacetylase inhibitors as single-agent or in combination with other drugs for the treatment of this disease.

Chapter VI - Acute lymphoblastic leukemia (ALL) is the most common malignancy in children and represents approximately 75% of all leukemias. Despite the advances in the treatment of the disease achieved over the past years, the five-year event-free survival rate is nearly 80% for children with ALL and approximately 40% for adults. Thus, there is an urgent need to improve therapy in leukemia patients. In recent years, the expression and secretion of peptides by tumors has attracted increasing interest and, in particular, it is known that the substance P (SP)/neurokinin (NK)-1 receptor system plays an important role in the development of cancer (SP, after binding to the NK-1 receptor, induces mitogenesis in tumor cells). It is also known that after binding to NK-1 receptors NK-1 receptor antagonists (aprepitant, L-733,060, L-732,138) inhibit cancer cell proliferation and that tumor cells die by apoptosis and that NK-1 receptor expression is significantly increased in cancer cells in comparison with normal cells. This means that the NK-1 receptor is a promising new target in human cancer treatment. Here, authors review the data currently available concerning the involvement of the SP/NK-1 receptor system in human ALL: 1) SP is expressed in blast cells; 2) SP induces the proliferation of ALL cells; 3) NK-1 receptors are expressed in such cells; 4) Isoforms of the NK-1 receptor of about 33, 58 and 75 kDa have been reported in ALL cells; 5) ALL cells express mRNA for the tachykinin NK-1 receptor; 6) The tachykinin 1 (*TAC1*) gene is overexpressed in ALL cells; 7) NK-1 receptors are involved in the viability of ALL cells; 8) NK-1 receptor antagonists elicit the inhibition of ALL cell growth; 9) The specific antitumor action of NK-1 receptor antagonists on ALL cells occurs through the NK-1 receptor; and 10) ALL cell death is due to apoptosis. These findings suggest that NK-1 receptor antagonists could be considered as new antitumor drugs for the treatment of human ALL.

Chapter VII - Minimal residual disease (MRD) is a powerful prognostic indicator which might be used to adjust treatment intensity in childhood acute lymphoblastic leukemia (ALL). Assays measuring MRD are capable to determine the treatment response in children with ALL much more precisely than morphologic screening of bone marrow. Minimal residual disease monitoring is performed through cytogenetic, immunologic and molecular information obtained from fluorescence in situ hybridization (FISH), flow cytometry (FC) and polymerase chain reaction (PCR) techniques, respectively. Specifically, PCR techniques use either patient specific junctional regions of immunoglobulin and T-cell receptor genes or chromosome aberrations which result in fusion genes or aberrant expression of transcripts. These techniques illustrate particular advantages and disadvantages while considering specificity, sensitivity, applicability, feasibility and precise MRD quantification. The incorporation of modern applications of PCR techniques, such as real time quantitative PCR (RQ-PCR), permits the accurate quantification of MRD levels. The clinical significance of MRD detected either by FC or PCR-based methods in childhood ALL has been evaluated during the last years. Both techniques have been incorporated in multicenter treatment protocols. However, it still remains open to discussion which is the appropriate and whether there is a universal technique to investigate MRD among different diagnostic laboratories. Issues related to MRD techniques and the evidence supporting the use of MRD for risk assignment in childhood ALL will be discussed in this chapter.

Chapter VIII - Childhood acute lymphoblastic leukaemia (ALL) is commonly characterized by specific and non-random chromosomal abnormalities, which might play a vital role in the etiology and pathogenesis of the disease. The majority of patients with ALL demonstrate an abnormal karyotype, either in chromosome number (ploidy) or as structural changes often translocations, inversions, or deletions. Translocations fuse oncogenes with other gene loci leading to the production of chimeric fusion genes and the activation of oncogenes under specific regulatory genes that are responsible for malignant transformation. A number of these cytogenetic abnormalities are associated with distinct immunologic phenotypes of ALL and characteristic outcomes. The detection of precise prognostic cytogenetic markers in ALL is necessitated to guide diagnosis and the choice of treatment. For this purpose, several molecular approaches have been described, which can provide high through-put including conventional cytogenetics, real-time quantitative polymerase chain reaction (RQ-PCR), fluorescence in situ hybridization (FISH), comparative genome hybridization (CGH) and array-based CGH. These techniques, although useful, include several limitations. In the current review the application of major cytogenetic aberrations as prognostic, diagnostic and therapeutic markers and the clinical relevance of current approaches were recapitulated.

Chapter IX - Maintenance therapy means long-term administration of low-dose chemotherapy or other drugs. Despite extensive study involving many types of leukemia, maintenance therapy has clinically proven efficacy for only two diseases: acute lymphoblastic leukemia (ALL) and acute promyelocytic leukemia (APL). This section focuses on maintenance therapy in Ph negative ALL. Maintenance therapy in Ph positive ALL is discussed in a separate section.

Chapter X - Acute lymphoblastic leukemia (ALL) accounts for about 30–50 new cases per million children and represents 25–30% of all childhood malignancies. ALL is the most common subtype of leukemia in childhood (approximately 80%). The pathogenesis of ALL is unknown. The development of leukemias requires the concerted action of different agents. Patients with ALL demonstrate alteration of normal immune function. Several investigators have demonstrated poor *in vivo* anti-leukemia immune responses in ALL patients, even in the bone marrow as the primary site of disease. The central problem is to determine the effector mechanisms responsible for resistance of the host against tumor growth.

In: Acute Lymphoblastic Leukemia
Editors: Severo Vecchione and Luigi Tedesco

ISBN: 978-1-61470-872-8
©2012 Nova Science Publishers, Inc.

Chapter I

Genome Wide Association Studies in Pediatric Acute Lymphoblastic Leukemia: Pathogenesis and Therapy

Kyriaki Hatziagapiou[1], Maria Braoudaki[1,2], Katerina Katsibardi[1], George I. Lambrou[1], Fotini Tzortzatou-Stathopoulou[1,2]

[1]Hematology/Oncology Unit, First Department of Pediatrics, University of Athens, «Aghia Sophia» Children's Hospital, Athens, Greece

[2]University Research Institute for the Study and Treatment of Childhood Genetic and Malignant Diseases, University of Athens, «Aghia Sophia» Children's Hospital, Athens, Greece

Abstract

Acute lymphoblastic leukemia (ALL) remains an imperative cause of mortality among cancer pediatric patients, who carry a dismal prognosis. Ongoing genome wide profiling research has offered an alternative approach in understanding the biology underlying the etiology, pathogenesis and targeted treatment of childhood ALL. More specifically, such studies have detected certain gene mutations and polymorphisms that play known or potential roles in leading cellular pathways. Subsequently their mutational or polymorphism patterns might be associated with the risk of leukemogenesis by altering cell cycle regulation, lymphoid development and differentiation. Several current high through-put genome mutational analysis efforts have been employed to identify such submicroscopic genetic lesions, including micro-array based assays; single nucleotide polymorphism arrays, loss of heterozygocity, gene-expression profiling and potential gene mutation screening. Collectively, these molecular approaches attempt to increase the knowledge of ALL pathogenesis, enable diagnosis, advance the efficacy of current treatments by leading to the development of personalized ALL therapy and subsequently improve patients' clinical outcomes.

Abbreviations

ABL1:	V-abl Abelson murine leukemia viral oncogene homolog 1
ALL:	*Acute lymphoblastic* leukemia
AML:	Acute myeloid leukemia
BCR:	B-cell receptor
BCP-ALL:	B-cell precursor acute lymphoblastic leukemia
CLL:	*Chronic lymphocytic leukemia*
CML:	Chronic myelogenous (or myeloid) leukemia
DHPLC:	Denaturing high-performance liquid chromatography
DN:	Double negative
DP:	Double positive
ERK:	Extracellular-signal regulated kinase
FLT3:	Fms-related tyrosine kinase 3
FLT3L:	Fms-related tyrosine kinase 3 ligand
GAPs:	GTPase activating proteins
GDP:	Guanosine diphosphate
GEFs:	Guanine Nucleotide Exchange Factors
GPCRs:	G protein-coupled receptors
GSIs:	γ-secretase inhibitors
GTP:	Guanosine-5'-triphosphate
HSCs:	Hematopoietic stem cells
ICN:	Notch-1 intracellular domain
ITD:	Internal tandem duplication
JM:	Juxtamembrane domain
JME:	Extracellular juxtamembrane domain
JMML:	Juvenile myelomonocytic leukemias
LNRs:	Notch-1/Lin-12 repeats
MAPK:	Mitogen-activated protein (MAP) kinases
MDS:	Myelodysplastic syndromes
MLL:	Mixed-lineage leukemia
MNCs:	Mononuclear cells
MRD:	Minimal residual disease
MuLV:	Moloney murine leukemia virus
NEC:	Notch-1 extracellular domain
NHL:	Non-Hodgkin's lymphoma
NK cells:	*Natural killer cells*
NTM:	Notch-1 transmembrane domain
PCR:	polymerase chain reaction
PI3K:	Phosphatidylinositol 3-kinase
RQ-PCR:	Real-time quantitative PCR
RT-PCR:	Reverse transcriptase PCR
STAT5:	Signal transducer and activator of transcription-5
TAD:	tTranscriptional activation domain

TAL-1/SCL: T-cell *acute lymphoblastic* leukemia/Stem cell factor
TAN-1:   Translocation-associated Notch-1 homologue
TCR: *T cell receptor*
TKDs: Tyrosine kinase domains
TKIs: Tyrosine kinase inhibitors
WBC: White blood cell counts
WT1:   Wilms' tumor gene 1

Introduction

Acute lymphoblastic leukemia (ALL) remains one of the most challenging malignancies in children with respect to therapy. ALL represents a highly heterogenous disease with dissimilar clinical manifestations and prognostic and therapeutic implications. Despite the breakthroughs in therapy that have been achieved resulting in more than 80% of children cured, a subset of pediatric patients is being overtreated, while the survival rates for others remain inferior.

The molecular pathogenesis of leukemia involves a stepwise accumulation of mutations affecting both cellular oncogenes and tumor suppressor genes. To improve outcome, it is vital to tailor therapy towards the potential genetic markers underlying the disease and predict the likelihood of relapse. Subsequently, there is a need to identify clinical and molecular genetic markers that distinguish patients who require less intensive therapy from those requiring aggressive or novel therapeutic regimens.

Gene mutations may affect the activity of corresponding proteins and might be associated with the progression of the disease. Hitherto, with the use of high throughput procedures a range of gene mutations with variable frequency have been identified in pediatric ALL including *IKZF1, NOTCH, RAS, PTEN, HOX, FLT3, WNT, WT1* among others. Ongoing efforts are necessitated to fully characterize all gene mutations potentially present in pediatric ALL, in order to identify novel targets for therapeutic intervention.

In this chapter we will attempt to address the commonest gene mutations identified in pediatric ALL and we will analyze their potential role in leukemogenesis, diagnosis, prognosis and therapeutic outcome of the disease.

Ikaros

Ikaros is a member of the Kruppel family of lymphoid-restricted zinc finger transcription factors that also include Helios, Aiolos, Eos and Pegasus and are central regulators lymphocyte differentiation. It is encoded by the IKZF1 gene which is located at 7p12 locus and comprises 8 exons. Alternative splicing can generate at least 8 alternatively spliced transcripts of the IKZF1, which share a common C-terminal domain, but differ in their N-terminal domain. The isoforms have distinct DNA-binding capabilities and specificities and therefore different functions [1,2].The C-terminal domain contains a bipartite transcription activation motif and two zinc finger motifs, encoded by exon 7, which are required for protein-protein interactions. The N-terminus contains 4 DNA-binding zinc fingers, encoded by exons 3-5. At least three N-terminal zinc fingers are required for high affinity DNA-binding to the GGGGA or AGGAA motif, whereas isoforms lacking most or all N-terminal zinc fingers have attenuated DNA-binding capacity, although retaining their ability to homo- or heterodimerize. [2]. Long isoforms (Ik1-Ik3) contain at least three NH2-terminal zinc fingers, localize to the nucleus and exhibit an efficient DNA-binding capacity. DNA-binding affinity of long isoforms increases when they form homo- and heterodimers. On the other hand short isoforms (Ik4 -Ik8) have fewer than three NH2-terminal zinc fingers, localize to the cytoplasm and act as dominant negative regulators of Ikaros, by interfering with the ability of DNA-binding Ikaros isoforms to form homo- and heterodimers or complexes with Aiolos and Helios, rendering the DNA-binding isoforms transcriptionally inactive [2-5]. Ikaros has been shown to have multiple functions, such as transcriptional activation or repression and chromatin remodeling. During fetal development, it is required at the earliest stage of T- and B-cell specification, whereas in adulthood is implicated in very early stages of B-cell development, as demonstrated in mice with attenuated Ikaros expression which show defects in normal B-cell differentiation and function. Mice with homozygous deletion of the IKZF1 exons 3 and 4 are characterized by complete arrest in the development of all lymphoid lineages and therefore are devoid of B, T, NK and dendritic cells and their earliest progenitors, whereas mice, lacking exon 7 lack B, NK, most of the thymic dendritic cells and fetal T cells, but thymocytes and T cells gradually appear, displaying lower thresholds of activation [6-11]. Apart from normal lymphocyte development IKZF1 functions as tumour suppressor, as its down-regulation in murine models leads to leukemias and lymphomas [8,11,12]. Mice with heterozygous deletion of the IKZF1 exons 3 and 4 express higher than normal levels of Ik-6, Ik-7 and Ik-8 isoforms and a few months after birth develop a highly aggressive form of T-cell leukemia, due to a lower TCR stimulation threshold with a concomitant loss of heterozygosity [11]. The previous are in line with other studies, where a decrease in Ikaros activity within developing and mature T lymphocytes led to T- cell clonal expansion and its absence was associated with neoplastic transformation [8,12]. Prior to development of leukemia, DNA-binding affinity of Ikaros was diminished in lymphocyte precursors, along with a change in compartmentalization of Ikaros from nucleus to cytoplasm [4]. Moreover, Fas expression was down-regulated in the thymus of the mutant mice, probably explaining the failure of T lymphocytes to undergo apoptosis [12].

Based on observations in murine models, concerning the central role played by Ikaros in the normal lymphoid development and the development of T-cell leukemia in germ-line mutant mice, expressing dominant-negative isoforms of Ikaros, several researchers attempted to elucidate whether specific mutations in IKZF1 may be implicated in human leukemogenesis. Whilst the composition of the patient groups and the assays used varied considerably, a common finding was the expression of dysfunctional dominant-negative Ikaros isoforms. In humans impaired Ikaros activity has been associated with the development of infant T-ALL, adult B-ALL, AML, adult and juvenile CML and myelodysplastic syndromes [4,13-16]. Deletion of IKZF1 is frequent in BCR-ABL1 (+) positive ALL and during the progression of CML to blast crisis [17]. Sun et al., sought to determine whether abnormal IKZF1 expression and function could be implicated in childhood T-ALL. Using Western blot analysis, they found that normal thymocytes and bone marrow cells expressed isoforms Ik-1 and Ik-2, whereas leukemic cells from children with T-ALL and T-ALL cell lines MOLT-321 and JK-E6-1 expressed the dominant-negative isoforms Ik-4- 8, lacking critical for DNA binding NH2-terminal zinc fingers. Ik-1 and Ik-2 in normal thymocytes and bone marrow MNCs were localized in the nuclei. JK-E6–1 and MOLT-3 T-ALL cell lines and 64% of samples from children with T-ALL expressed Ikaros truncated isoforms in the cytoplasm. However, in 36% of patients an abnormal "patchy" nuclear staining with or without cytoplasmic staining was found. RT-PCR and sequence analysis in leukemic T-cells from 60% T-ALL patients and MOLT-3 cell lines revealed an inframe deletion of 30 bp at the 3' end of exon 6, leading to the loss of a 10-amino acid peptide (D KSSMPQKFLG) upstream to the transcription activation domain and adjacent to the COOH-terminal zinc finger dimerization domain of Ik-2, Ik-4, Ik-7 and Ik-8 isoforms. The structural changes caused by this mutation could interfere with the accessibility of the mutant Ikaros with the transcription machinery or interfere with its ability to form homo- or heterodimers, altering its DNA binding affinity or subcellular localization. One T-ALL patient demonstrated a unique 21-amino acid insertion (VTYGADDFRDFHAIIPKSFSR), due to a 60-bp insertion at 5' end of exon 4 of Ik-2. The insertion altered the DNA-binding activity of Ik-2 and its subcellular compartmentalization [4]. However, later studies failed to detect dominant-negative Ikaros isoforms in T-ALL patients, using RT-PCR and Western blot analysis, whereas other researchers demonstrated low frequencies of Ikaros deletions in T-ALL, using high resolution CGH-arrays [14,18-21]. For example, Maser et al., identified by RT-PCR and high resolution CGH-arrays a mono-allelic genomic deletion at the 5' region of IKZF1 only in one sample of 25 patients with T-ALL, thus supporting the notion that inactivation of Ikaros by mutation is rare in human T-ALL [21]. Sun et al., attempted to clarify the involvement of abnormal IKZF1 expression in infant ALL. Using Western blot analysis they found that leukemic cells from all infants with ALL showed high levels of dominant-negative isoforms Ik-4, Ik-5, Ik-6, Ik-7 and Ik-8. These isoforms were expressed predominantly in the cytoplasm. On the contrary, wild-type Ik-1 and Ik-2 isoforms with normal nuclear localization were found in normal infant bone marrow cells and thymocytes. Cloned RT-PCR products with coding sequences of Ik-2, Ik-4, Ik-7 and Ik-8 were subjected to nucleotide sequencing and revealed an in-frame 30-bp deletion at the 3' end of exon 6, resulting in deletion of 10 amino acids (Δ KSSMPQKFLG). The deleted peptide was located within the first 81 amino acids of exon 7, adjacent to the C-terminal zinc finger motifs. The mutation resulted in abrogation of both transactivation and dimerization domains of Ikaros [2]. In line with the previous is another study, involving children with T- or B-ALL, T- or B-lineage ALL cell lines [22]. Normal human bone marrow cells, thymocytes and fetal liver-derived human lymphocyte precursor cell lines expressed DNA-binding *Ikaros* isoforms *Ik-1* and *Ik-2* with normal subcellular localization. Leukemic cells expressed the alternatively spliced isoforms Ik-4, Ik-6, Ik-7 and Ik-8, which localized predominantly in the cytoplasm, although some cells exhibited an abnormal, diffuse, patchy nuclear staining with or without cytoplasmic staining. RT-PCR and genomic sequence analysis identified the specific Ikaros isoforms and the in-frame 30-bp deletion at the 3' end of exon 6, which resulted in the 10-amino acid deletion Δ KSSMPQKFLG, upstream of the transcription activation domain. The mutation was identified in 15 of 21 ALL samples sequenced and involved the Ik-2, Ik-4, Ik-7 and Ik-8 coding sequences. In leukemic cells bi-allelic expression pattern of aberrant and/or non–DNA-binding isoforms *along with wild-type isoforms was observed, suggesting that trans-acting factor(s), possibly affect splice-site recognition [22]. Nishii et al., using RT-PCR analysis failed to detect* Ik-6 *expression in adult pre-T ALL samples, whereas predominant expression of* Ik-6 *was detected in pre-B ALL samples. The* Ik-6 *acts as a dominant inhibitor of Ikaros, as it* lacks all N-terminal, DNA-binding zinc fingers. Ik1-3, *isoforms were not detected in* Ik-6 *expressing cells.* Ik-6 *was frequently expressed in stages II and III of pre-B ALL, whereas* Ik-6 *was not detected in CD19+CD10- stage I pre-B ALL cells [23]. The researchers did not observe any correlation between* Ik-6 *expression and karyotype abnormalities, as it was observed in another study, implying that leukemogenesis might differ between adults and infants [22]. Kano et al., demonstrated that* Ik-6 prolonged the survival of murine pro-B cell lines in IL-3 deprived condition, through activation of the JAK2-STAT5 pathway and thus upregulation of the Bcl-xl, an anti-apoptotic molecule. The Ik-6 expressing cell lines did not express CD45R, B-cell differentiation surface marker [24]. *Mullighan* et al., *attempted to elucidate the* association between alterations of IKZF1 and the clinical outcome in B-cell–progenitor ALL in childhood. They identified more than 50 recurring copy-number abnormalities, most of which involved genes regulating B-cell development, e.g deletions in PAX5 and IKZF1. Genomic sequencing of IKZF1 revealed alterations; deletions of the entire IKZF1 locus, sets of exons or the genomic region immediately upstream of IKZF1. The mutations were identified in a substantial proportion of patients with BCR-ABL1 negative B-cell-progenitor ALL, and without other common recurrent cytogenetic abnormalities. More specifically, they identified a deletion of coding exons 3-6, resulting in the expression of Ik-6 and novel missense (G158S), frameshift (L117fs, H224fs, S402fs, E504fs) and nonsense (R111) IKZF1 mutations which impaired Ikaros' function or resulted in the expression of dominant-negative isoforms (G158S) [25].

High-resolution, genomewide copy number analysis of the genetic alterations revealed significant association between deletions or mutations of IKZF1 and an increased risk of relapse or poor outcome. The association was independent of age, WBC at presentation, cytogenetic subtype and levels of minimal residual disease, thus rendering identification of IKZF1 mutations an important tool in identifying patients with a high risk of treatment failure. Gene-set enrichment analysis validated that gene-expression signatures of patients bearing IKZF1 mutations and thus have a poor prognosis were similar to each other and to the signature of BCR/ABL1(+) ALL, an aggressive leukemia with poor outcome which constitutes 5% of pediatric B-progenitor ALL and approximately 40% of adult ALL. In BCR/ABL1(+) CML BCR/ABL1 tyrosine kinase plays a central role, whereas in BCR/ABL1(+) ALL cooperating oncogenic lesions are essential for the generation of blastic leukemia, as demonstrated in murine models [26,27]. In BCR/ABL1 (+)-ALL IKZF1 deletions are very common, suggesting their implication in the pathogenesis of both BCR/ABL1 (+)-ALL and BCR/ABL1 (-)-ALL. Gene-set enrichment analysis also revealed up-regulation of hematopoietic stem-cell and progenitor genes and under-expression of B lymphoid development genes in patients with poor prognosis disease. This finding suggested that IKZF1 mutations impaired B-cell development and differentiation, while rendering leukemic cells chemoresistant [17]. Implication of IKZF1 in ALL relapse and chemoresistance was already supported in another study [28]. Genome-wide analysis of DNA copy number abnormalities (CNAs) and loss-of heterozygosity assays on matched diagnostic and relapse bone marrow samples from pediatric B-progenitor- ALL and T-ALL patients revealed that IKZF1 mutations emerge as new genomic alterations at relapse, along with a diversity of mutations in other genes controlling cell cycle, lymphoid/B-cell development and tumor suppression [28]. Negative prognostic implication of genomic aberrations of IKZF1 in the pathogenesis of BCR/ABL1-ALL was also demonstrated in other studies, suggesting that IKZF1 deletions should be considered as a routine screening assay for BCR/ABL1-ALL [25,29-31]. Mullighan et al., using genome-wide analysis demonstrated that IKZF1 was deleted in 84% of BCR/ABL1 (+)-ALL and during the transformation of CML to ALL, along with other genomic alterations (deletions of CDKN2A and PAX5), suggesting that attenuated Ikaros activity may contribute to leukaemogenesis in additional ways. The IKZF1 deletions identified in BCR/ABL1 (+)-ALL were predominantly mono-allelic and frequently confined to exons 3-6, encoding the Ik-6 isoform. RT–PCR analysis also revealed two previously unknown Ikaros isoforms in cases harboring larger deletions (Ik-9 in deletion of exons 2-6 and Ik-10 in deletion of exons 1-6). Iacobucci et al., apart from validating the previous results, attempted to determine whether the different Ikaros isoforms expressed in BCR/ABL1 (+)-ALL patients were correlated with BCR/ABL transcript levels and resistance to tyrosine kinase inhibitors. RT-PCR and sequencing analysis revealed that in the majority of samples the Ik-6 isoform was expressed, predominantly in the cytoplasm of leukemic cells, alone or along with isoforms Ik-1, Ik-2 and Ik-4. Ik-6 expression was correlated with the percentage of blast cells and BCR/ABL1 transcript levels, irrespective of BCR/ABL arrangement, as Ik-6 was detected in patients carrying both a p210 and a p190 oncoprotein. They also linked the expression of Ik-6 and the resistance to tyrosine kinase inhibitors (TKIs) imatinib and dasatinib in BCR/ABL1 (+)-ALL, as at the time of resistance the major isoform expressed was the Ik-6, whereas it was not expressed during the response to the drugs. Amplification and genomic sequence analysis of the exon splice junction regions in BCR/ABL1 (+)-ALL patients who expressed the Ik-6 revealed two mutations: a G →A substitution in the exon 2/3 splice junction and a G →A substitution in the exon 3/4 splice junction. Computational analysis on the IKZF1 gene revealed that some mutations could function as splicing enhancer or silencers [29]. Klein et al., have previously shown that BCR/ABL1 kinase induced derangement of Ikaros pre-mRNA splicing, resulting in aberrant expression of the Ik-6 isoform. Inhibition of BCR/ABL1 corrected splicing and nuclear localization of Ikaros in pre-B ALL cells. Also, silencing Ik-6 expression by RNA interference in BCR/ABL1 leukemia cells partially restored B lymphoid lineage commitment. The latter implied that Ik-6 probably was implicated in lineage infidelity, interfering with lineage determination of pre-B ALL and inducing the expression of myeloid lineage-specific genes [30]. Given the pleiotropic activity of Ikaros and its aberrant isoforms in normal hematopoiesis and leukemogenesis, understanding its role in the pathogenesis of ALL might enable the development of new therapeutic approaches.

HOX

Homeodomain or homeobox genes (HOX) have a markedly conserved 61-amino acid sequence, encoding DNA-binding domain. The HOX genes encode a family of transcription factors thought to be involved in embryonic development as well as in the regulation and differentiation of primitive hematopoietic cells, including stem cells (HSCs) and early committed progenitors [32,33]. Several homeobox genes, located in four clusters are designated HOX A, B, C and D, while others are described as divergent homeobox genes [34]. More specifically, *HOX* genes are located in two main clusters, the primordial cluster and the ParaHox cluster, which are thought to originate from the duplication of a hypothetical ProtoHox cluster of four genes early in evolution; Anterior, PG3, Central, and Posterior groups based on sequence similarity [35,36]. The primordial *HOX* cluster consists of 13 paralogous groups of genes that exist as distinct, unlinked complexes on human chromosomes 7p15 (*HOXA*), 17q21 (*HOXB*), 12q13 (*HOXC*), and 2q31 (*HOXD*). During hematopoiesis, *HOX* genes are expressed in lineage- and stage-specific combinations; however, cell commitment to myeloid or erythroid lineages is accompanied by global downregulation of *HOX* gene expression.

HOX genes have been commonly dysregulated in ALL [32,33]. Direct evidence for HOX involvement in leukemic transformation came from mice transplanted with bone marrow cells engineered to overexpress HOXB8 and IL-3 simultaneously [37]. These mice succumbed to an aggressive acute leukemia. It has also been shown that a high proportion of mice transplanted with bone marrow cells, which overexpress HOXB8 and HOXA10 but not HOXB4, eventually develop AML after a long latency, suggesting the requirement for secondary genetic events in HOX-induced leukemic transformation [38,39]. Of note, upregulation of HOXB4 o induces a unique expansion of hematopoietic stem cells both in vivo and in vitro without causing leukemia [40]. Previous studies also proposed that in vivo, HOXB6 expression promotes the expansion of HSCs and myeloid precursors but inhibits erythropoiesis and lymphopoiesis [41].

HOXA9 is considered the most commonly upregulated HOX gene in acute leukemia. MLL dependent T- and B- cell ALL revealed an elevated expression of HOXA9. Overexpression of HOXA9 has also been shown to perturb normal hematopoiesis in mice resulting in the progression of leukemia [33]. Nevertheless, HOXA9 is upregulated in a subset of human myeloid leukemias in the form of a fusion with a sub-domain of nucleoporin (NUP98), as the result of a reciprocal translocation between chromosomes 7 and 11 [42].

The dysregulation of specific HOX genes appears to be a dominant mechanism of leukemic transformation. Recently, Soulier et al. (2011) reported that HOXA dysregulation might be critical in T-ALL oncogenesis [43]. In addition, HOX cofactor myeloid ecotropic viral integration site 1 (MEIS1), HOXA5 and HOXA7 have been reported to be correlated with acute leukemia and the occurrence of MLL gene rearrangements [44,45].

FLT3 (fms-Related Tyrosine Kinase 3)

The FLT3 gene encodes a class III membrane-bound receptor tyrosine kinase (RTKIII) which is mainly expressed in early myeloid and lymphoid progenitor cells and is implicated in the proliferation, differentiation and apoptosis of haematopoietic cells [46]. FLT3 comprises of 24 exons, rather than the previously reported 21 exons, which range from 83 bp-562 bp and span approximately 100 kb [47]. The genes encoding the transmembrane and intracellular regions of RTKIII receptors are conserved in exon size, number and sequence and exon/intron boundary positions, suggesting that they have arisen from a common ancestral gene. The receptor has the same overall structure as other members of RTKIII (c-kit, c-fms, PDGF a and b) and consists of an extracellular domain composed of five immunoglobulin-like domains, a transmembrane domain, a juxtamembrane domain (JM) and two intracellular tyrosine kinase domains (TKDs), linked by a kinase-insert domain. Ligand binding of the fms-related tyrosine kinase 3 ligand (FLT3L) to the extracellular domain of FLT3 leads to conformational changes that induce and stabilize receptor homodimerization. The dimerization brings the kinase domains into close proximity inducing autophosphorylation of tyrosine residues and activation of tyrosine kinases. The latter subsequently bind adaptor-proteins and/or phosphorylate downstream effector molecules of the phosphatidylinositol 3-kinase (PI3K) and RAS signal-transduction cascades, leading to activation of Akt, STAT5 (signal transducer and activator of transcription-5) and ERK-1,2 (extracellular-signal regulated kinase- 1 and -2) [48-55]. FLT3L is expressed, as membrane-bound or soluble form, in various tissues, including organs of the haematopoietic system (spleen, thymus, peripheral blood, bone marrow), with the highest expression levels observed in peripheral MNCs [56,57]. FLT3L exerts a stimulatory effect on primitive haematopoietic cells, leading to the growth of primitive and more committed myeloid progenitor cells, an action which is potentiated by other growth factors such as IL-3, G-CSF, GM-CSF, erythropoietin and KIT ligand. FLT3-FLT3L interaction is also important in lymphoid clonal expansion and differentiation, in conjunction with IL-7 and IL-11, whereas it has no significant effect on erythropoiesis or megakaryopoiesis, as these cell lineages do not express FLT3L [58-63]. Incubation of leukaemic blasts with FLT3L enhanced DNA synthesis and in some, but not all, cases led to AML [64-66]. The importance of FLT3 in hematopoiesis has been depicted in FLT3 knockout mice. Mutants developed into healthy adults with relatively normal mature hematopoietic populations, but possessed deficiencies in pro-B-cell and pre-B-cell compartments. Bone marrow transplantation of a mixture of early haematopoietic progenitor cells expressing wild-type functional FLT3 revealed inadequate reconstitution in T cell and myeloid compartments by mutant stem cells [67]. Subsequent studies in murine models have depicted that transfection of FLT3L cDNA into their bone marrow led to increased WBC, progressive splenic fibrosis, infiltration by abnormal lymphoreticular cells of the spleen, bone marrow and liver and a predisposition to B-lymphoid, myeloid and biphenotypic leukemias [68-70].

FLT3 is highly expressed at high levels in most cases of AML and ALL, as well as in leukemia and lymphoma cell lines [57,71-74]. FLT3 is expressed in most B-ALL samples, but less frequently in T-ALL. Its ligand FLT3L is also expressed, creating autocrine and paracrine signalling loops that may have a key role in survival and proliferation of malignant clones. The most common FLT3 mutation is an internal tandem duplication (ITD) in exons 11 and 12 (later known as exons 14 and 15) which occurs in approximately 15-35% of adult AML- with the highest frequency reported in the M3 subtype and the lowest in the M2 subtype-, 5-10% of myelodysplastic syndromes and 1-3% of ALL, whereas it has not been detected in CML, CLL, JMML, adult T-ALL, non-Hodgkin lymphoma or multiple myeloma [75-80]. There is also evidence that FLT3/ITD is associated with leukemic transformation of myelodysplasia [81]. Nakao et al., were the first to describe FLT3/ITD mutations in AML

[82]. Using RT-PCR they demonstrated FLT3 expression in 73% of patients with AML and 78% with ALL. Sequence analyses of the abnormal RT-PCR products identified in 16% of patients with AML a FLT3 internal duplication. In FLT3/ITD a fragment of the JM domain-coding sequence (exons 11 and 12) was duplicated in direct head-to-tail orientation and the duplicated sequence was always in-frame. However, their position and length varied in different samples. A subsequent study on various hematopoietic malignancies confirmed the presence of FLT3/ITD with or without insertions of nucleotides in samples from AML and MDS patients. The duplication took place within the JM and 5' TK-1 domains, resulting in an elongated product [76]. In different studies the length of the duplicated DNA sequences varied significantly from 3-400bp and in most patients, the duplicated sequence included those from exon 11 and in rare cases from intron 11 or exon 12 [82,83]. The reading frame of the transcript was always retained, either by faithful in-frame duplication or by the insertion of nucleotides at the ITD junction to maintain the original reading frame. Thus, the abnormal FLT3 had a dominant function and favored the growth of leukemic cells by stimulating proliferation, promoting viability or/and inhibiting apoptosis [84]. In vitro studies in AML blasts have shown that mutant FLT3/ITD receptors dimerized in a ligand-independent manner, thus underwent autophosphorylation on tyrosine residues and constitutive activation [79,85]. The way FLT3/ITDs promote constitutive activation of the receptor has been elucidated in various studies [86]. It has been proposed that elongation of the JM domain probably disrupts a negative regulatory domain which abrogates the receptor dimerization and autoactivation in the absence of ligand. Amino-acid residues Y597 and Y599 of FLT3 may be involved in the negative regulatory activity. Another explanation is that FLT3/ITDs possibly disrupt the intrinsic negative regulatory effects of the JM domain on its own TKDs, due to conformational changes which lead to exposure of phosphorylation sites in the TKDs. Once these sites are exposed, the receptor can lay intracellular signals, without ligand stimulation and dimerization. Studies in mutant FLT3/ITD-transfected IL-3-dependent hematopoietic progenitors (32D and BA/F3) exhibited constitutive activation of STAT5 and MAPK and thus autonomous growth, whereas full-length wild type FLT3-transfected cells in the presence of FLT3L exhibited activation only of MAPK and thus a minimal cell growth. In the same study FLT3/ITD caused sustained autophosporylation of the receptor and activation of downstream effector molecules, even in the absence of IL-3. Similar activation was observed in clinical samples of AML patients with FLT3/ITD mutation [70]. The implication of FLT3 JM domain in receptor activation and the ligand-independent FLT3 activation in the presence of length-mutated JM domain were elucidated in another study [86]. They also suggested that JM domain had a negative role in the autophosphorylation of wild type FLT3 and that the tyrosine residues within the JM domain were not essential for signal transduction. They found that both elongating and shortening mutations of FLT3 and FLT3/ITDs were able to transform murine IL3-dependent myeloid progenitor cell line 32D, regardless of the tyrosine residues in the JM domain. The mutant FLT3s remained constitutively tyrosine phosphorylated and thus activated signal-transduction molecules such as SHC, MAPKand STAT5a, without the presence of IL3 or FLT3L. Also, they demonstrated that co-transfection of the truncated FLT3/ITD receptor, lacking kinase and C-terminal domains with the wild type-FLT3 in the same cell line led to autonomous proliferation, as truncated FLT3/ITD dimerized with wild type-FLT3 in a trans-manner [86]. The oncogenic

potential of FLT3/ITD mutations was demonstrated in another study, where injection of 32D cells transfected with FLT3/ITD into syngeneic murine models led to the rapid development of a disease resembling leukemia [87]. In AML the FLT3/ITD was not found in diagnosis, but during relapse, suggesting that the mutation was implicated in leukemia progression and not initiation. The FLT3/ITD in acute promyelocytic leukemia has been positively correlated to peripheral blast and WBC counts, indicating that the mutation was closely related with proliferation of leukemic cells [75]. Although FLT3/ITDs have been also observed in childhood AML, their frequency was significantly lower when compared to adult AML, ranging from 5-15% in pediatric patients. Most studies in pediatric patients with AML have found that FLT3/ITDs were strong, independent predictors of poor prognosis [78,88]. However, there is inconsistency concerning the prognostic impact of FLT3/ITD in adult AML cohorts, probably due to differences in the cohort size and therapeutic strategies followed. Besides, the impact of FLT3 mutations may depend on intracellular conditions, as determined by cell lineage and the co-existence of other genetic alterations. FLT3/ITDs have been associated with other prognostic abnormalities, e.g. t(15;17)(q24;q21)/PML-RARA, t(6;9)/ DEK-CAN, MLL (mixed lineage leukemia) intragenic abnormalities or MLL translocation. Some of these abnormalities have been related with favorable outcome, such as t(15;17) and others with poor prognosis, e.g. t(6;9). In several studies FLT3/ITD was proposed as a significant and independent prognostic factor for poor outcome in adult and pediatric AML, regardless of diagnostic WBCs, induction regimen, or cytogenetic markers. More specifically, patients with FLT3/ITD were found be refractory to induction chemotherapy, whereas those who achieved remission were in danger of relapse [77-79,83,89,90]. Schnittger et al., also suggested that FLT3/ITD could provide a new PCR target for detection of minimal residual disease during AML monitoring, especially in patients who do not carry fusion genes.

Xu et al. were among the first to have identified FLT3/ITD in ALL in addition to AML [91]. The tandem duplication was identified in 3.3% of ALL samples and 13.8% of AML, with the highest frequency being observed in M4 AML subtype. Sequence analysis revealed a simple duplication within exon 11, a duplication with insertion within exon 11 and duplications extending from exon 11 to intron 11 and exon 12. In most patients the numbers of duplicated sequences were multiples of three, thus no insertion of nucleotides occurred. Although the duplications varied in size and location, they always either involved amino acid residue Y591 or Y597. ALL patients with FLT3/ITD had also myeloid antigens, suggesting the mutation occured mainly in cells of myeloid origin and partly in lymphoid cells with the potential of myeloid differentiation. As in previous studies, the prognosis of AML patients with FLT3/ITD was extremely poor, as patients were resistant to initial chemotherapy and did not enter complete remission, whereas the results in ALL were inconclusive due to the small number of ALL patients with FLT3/ITD. In the same study the researchers, using RT-PCR demonstrated higher expression of FLT3 in T- and B-ALL cell lines, than a previous report, where FLT3 mRNA was detected with Northern blot analysis [57]. Interestingly, the expression of FLT3 was higher in B-precursor ALL, myeloid and monocytic cell lines, in accordance with previous studies suggesting that FLT3 was expressed more frequently in undifferentiated cells [91]. Van Vlierberghe et al., confirmed the low incidence of FLT3/ITDs mutations in pediatric T-ALL samples. More specifically they detected only two mutations, a 51 bp and a 57 bp insertion, along with high expression of LYL1 and LMO2 and a HOX11L2 translocation. Patients presented with an early T-cell differentiation stage, but the maturation stage was more advanced compared with the FLT3- mutated adult T-ALLs. One of the two patients relapsed and the FLT3/ITD mutation was not found in the relapse sample, probably due to eradication of the mutated allele during chemotherapy [92]. Karabacak et al., confirmed the low frequency of FLT3/ITD mutations among patients with ALL. FLT3/ITD mutations were found in 7.5% of ALL patients and 22.5% of AML. In contrasts with previous studies on AML they did not observe any association of FLT3/ITD mutations and overall prognosis (overall survival, event free survival, disease free survival) in the group of ALL patients. In AML there was a statistically significant difference in overall survival, but not in event free survival and disease free survival. An interesting finding was that FLT3/ITD positivity increased as age advanced in childhood acute leukemias [93].

The second most common type of FLT3 mutation is a missense point mutation in exon 20 (previously known as exon 17) of the TKD. TKD mutations are found in AML (5-10%), MDS (2-5%) and ALL (1-3%). FLT3 D835 occur more commonly in AML samples with MLL intragenic abnormalities or MLL translocation suggesting that FLT3 and MLL loci have similar susceptibility to DNA damage and/or DNA repair defects [94,95]. Usually it is a nucleotide substitution (GAT →TAT) which changes an aspartic acid to tyrosine (D835Y). Deletions in the same locus have rarely been identified, as well as point mutations, deletions and insertions in the surrounding codons 840, 841 and 842. Similarly to the FLT3/ITDs the previous mutations maintain the same open reading frame. Observations of the reported effects of homologous mutations in the closely related receptors c-kit and c-fms, suggest that Asp835 is probably an important part of the TKD and its mutation may lead to sustained activation of FLT3 receptor [96,97]. Based on the model proposed by Morley et al., concerning the transforming activity of c-fmsD802V mutation in haemopoietic cells, it has been suggested that hydrophobic amino acid substitutions result in the formation of b-sheets, which in turn lead to conformational changes within the activating loop and stabilize the interaction of the A helix and the activating loop. Thus, in the presence of FLT3 TKD mutations FLT3 adopts an active configuration. The mutations increase the level of intrinsic tyrosine-kinase activity, rather than interfere with repressive domains. When D835 mutation was transfected into Cos7 cells led FLT3L-independent tyrosine phosphorylation, similar to the activity of FLT3/ITD mutation. Similar were the results in the D835 mutant-expressing 32D cells, which proliferated without the presence of FLT3L or IL-3. The previous confirmed that D835 mutations were gain-of-function mutations [98]. Yamamoto et al., identified several missense mutations of D835 in 7% of AML patients, 3.4% of MDS and 2.8% of B-cell precursor ALL in a large cohort of patients with different hematopoietic malignancies. The mutation was not found in samples derived from healthy volunteers. Sequence analysis revealed mainly G→T nucleotide substitution in D835, resulting in an Asp to Tyr amino acid change (D835Y). Rare mutations were D835V, D835H, D835E and D835N. Contrary to FLT3/ITD mutations, D835 mutations did not significantly affect the prognosis [98].

Activating mutations in FLT3 have also been identified in the A-loop of the catalytic domain. Sequence analysis in AML samples revealed an insertion between the codons S840 and N841 just 5 amino acids downstream of D835. The mutation resulted in the insertion of a glycine and a serine between amino acids 840 - 841 of FLT3 (840GS). The 840GS mutation induced a conformational change of the A-loop, resulting in the opening of the catalytic pocket and activation of tyrosine kinases. In vitro studies in Ba/F3 cells indicated that FLT3840-GS mutants were hyper-phosphorylated on tyrosine residues and underwent IL-3-independent growth. However, the cell growth rate was significantly slower than cells with FLT3/ITD mutation [99]. Other activating mutations within the TKD have been identified, such as I836L+D, I836Del, Y842C, N841I and N841Y [90,96,100,101]. In one study, point mutations in the TKD of FLT3 at D835 or I836 were found in 5.4% ALL samples from children older than 1 and in 16% of infant samples. All mutations were heterozygous and mainly missense (Asp835Tyr, Asp835His, Asp835Glu, Ile836Met). Also, they observed deletions of 3 base pairs (Ile836del) and a deletion along with an insertion mutation [4-amino acid (Asp835-Ser838) deletion in 1 allele and 3-amino acid (Ala835, Leu836, and Gly837) insertion in another allele]. In all cases the open reading frame remained the same. The mutations were correlated with sustained activation and highly phosphorylation of the receptor, leading to the constitutive activation of downstream signals, as STAT5, as demonstrated in 32Dcl3 cells. Sustained activation of FLT3 was associated with the proliferation of leukemic cells. FLT3-D835/I836 mutations in infants with ALL were associated with MLL rearrangements [t(4;11)(q21;q23)/MLL-AF4, t(11;19)(q23;p13)/MLL-ENL] and with hyperdiploidy. Infants with ALL and MLL rearrangements had inferior prognosis, whereas ALL patients older than 1 year or hyperdiploid ALL had good prognosis. However, the results concerning the clinical outcome were not statistically significant, suggesting the need for further prospective studies [102]. The high frequency of FLT3 TKD mutations in hyperdiploid ALL was also confirmed in another study [95]. FLT3 mutations were also found in patients with relapsed ALL. In one study, 3 of 16 children who had relapsed ALL bore FLT3 mutations- one FLT3/ITD and two FLT3-TKD mutations, one I836M and one D835Y - at first relapse, which were not identified in pre-treatment samples [103]. In this research FLT3-TKD mutations were not associated with hyperdiploidy, which was in agreement with the observation of Taketani et al., that hyperdiploidy was associated with favorable outcome and thus not relapse. The high prevalence of FLT3/D835 mutations in ALL patients with hyperdiploidy was also confirmed by Braoudaki et al. [104]. However, they did not observe any FLT3/D835 mutation in ALLs with MLL rearrangement t(4;11) (q21;q23). In line with previous studies they detected a low incidence of FLT3/D835 mutation in the cohort of ALL pediatric patients (2.3%) [104].

FLT3 mutations and their downstream pathways are attractive targets for directed inhibition, even though their prevalence in ALL is low and are not sufficient to initiate leukemogenesis, but cooperate with other genetic alterations. Thus FLT3 represents a potential therapeutic target in pediatric acute leukemias, as in vitro studies and clinical trials have provided promising data.

Notch-1 and FBXW7 (F-Box andWD Repeat Domain Containing) Mutations

T. H. Morgan first described a Drosophila melanogaster mutant strain with 'notched' wings in 1917. The gene that is responsible for this phenotype was identified almost 70 years later as Drosophila Notch (dNotch) [105,106]. Notch1 signaling is an evolutionarily ancient mechanism of cell interactions in multicellular organisms. Notch gene family encodes single pass transmembrane receptors that are expressed broadly in several tissues and in different life periods. They are involved in a wide variety of cellular processes, including the maintenance of stem cells, specification of cell fate, differentiation, proliferation, survival and apoptosis [106,107]. Notch-1 signal is triggered by the Delta/Serrate/ Lag2 (DSL) family of ligands (Delta-like 1, 3 and 4; Jagged 1 and 2). Aberrant Notch-1 signaling has been implicated in the development of various cancers, including breast, ovarian, lung, pancreatic and prostatic cancer, melanoma, gliomas anaplastic large cell lymphoma, Hodgkin disease and leukemias.

Notch-1 signals have a fundamental role in the commitment of pluripotent hematopoietic progenitors to the T-cell fate and promote their proliferation, differentiation and survival. Notch-1 signaling might also be involved in self-renewal of haematopoietic stem cells, through Jagged-1-Notch-1 interactions between stromal cells and haematopoietic stem cells in stem-cell niches. Inactivation of Notch-1 signaling in bone-marrow precursors or early lymphoid progenitors results in the development of cells towards the B-lineage, preventing the generation of T cells. Conversely, constitutive activation of Notch-1 inhibits B-cell development and results in extrathymic T-cell differentiation, within the bone marrow at the expense of B-cell differentiation. T-cell precursors formed in the bone marrow migrate to the thymus to become double-negative (DN) thymocytes, proliferate and differentiate. Notch-1 might have a dual function in further T-cell lineage commitment, as it participates in the regulation of TCRB gene rearrangement, usually together with TCRG and TCRD genes and regulates lineage decisions between TCRγ/δ or α/β and between CD4+ or CD8 +. Activated Notch-1 signaling within a small developmental window in early thymocyte populations favors $\gamma\delta$-lineage, whereas inhibition of Notch-1 in slightly later stages (DN3) blocks $\alpha\beta$-development [105,108,109]. Later in T-cell development its expression is physiologically down-regulated to permit successful T-cell maturation by interfering with TCR signal strength. Therefore, Notch-1 expression is high in early CD4-CD8-double negative (DN) thymocytes, low in CD4+CD8+ double positive (DP) cells and intermediate in CD4+ and CD8+ single positive (SP) thymocytes [107]. Also, Notch-1 affects cell proliferation by accelerating progression through G1 phase and rescuing cells from apoptosis [105,109-113].

The Notch-1 is a heterodimeric class I transmembrane glycoprotein which is generated from the precursor proNotch1 by proteolysis. A furin protease cuts the proNotch1 approximately 70 amino acids external to the transmembrane domain (S1 site) to generate the extracellular (NEC) and the transmembrane-intracellular (NTM) Notch1 subunits. The two subunits remain noncovalently associated through the C-terminus of NEC (103-amino acids) and N-terminus of NTM (65-amino acids), forming the heterodimerization domain (HD). The NEC subunit contains 36 EGF-like repeats that bind DSL ligands and 3 Notch/Lin-12 repeats (LNRs) which stabilize the interaction between the extracellular and transmembrane subunits and help keep the receptor in a resting state in the absence of ligand. NTM subunit contains a RAM domain [RBP-Jκ (recombination-signal-sequencebinding protein for Jκ genes) associated molecule], 7 ankyrin repeats, a proline-rich and glutamine-rich transcriptional activation domain (TAD) and a carboxyterminal PEST domain (rich in the amino acids proline [P], glutamic acid [E], serine [S], and threonine [T]). The latter regulates protein turnover, as it is implicated in the cleavage of the ICN1 (Intracellular Notch1 fragment). Binding of ligands to the EGF repeats in the NEC leads to a conformational change in the LNR repeats-HD domain complex initiating a cascade of proteolytic cleavages of the NTM. The first cleavage is mediated by an ADAM metalloprotease which cuts the extracellular juxtamembrane just 12 amino acids proximal to the membrane (S2 site). Subsequently, γ-secretase, an aspartyl multiprotein protease complex cuts the receptor at at position Val1744 (S3 site), releasing the intracellular ICN1. ICN1 translocates to the nucleus, interacts and displaces the co-repressors from the transcription factor CSL and recruits transcriptional co-activators, including mastermind-like protein 1 (MAML1) and histone acetyltransferases, forming a transcriptional activation complex which results in up-regulation of target genes, e.g. Relb, Nfkb2, c-Myc, DELTEX1, mammalian target of rapamycin/mTor, Hairy and Enhancer of Split/ HES, HERP/ HES-related protein, p21, Ptcra, cyclin D1 and the proapoptotic receptor NUR. [106,108,110,114-120].

In human leukemias, Notch-1 activation was first demonstrated in T-ALL cases harboring the t(7;9)(q34;q34.3), a rare chromosomal translocation that juxtaposes the C-terminal region of Notch-1 gene downstream TCR-b regulative sequence (TCRB), leading to the aberrant expression of a truncated and constitutively active intracellular domain (TAN-1/translocation-associated Notch homologue) [113,121]. The translocation occurs only in a relatively small subset of T-cells, undergoing V-D-J recombination at the TCRB locus. This form has been proved to be neoplastic in vivo in rare patients (<1%) and when over expressed in the bone marrow of murine models, induced selectively T-ALL. The oncogenic activity of TAN-1 could be due to its inability to down-regulate T lineage development at the DP stage, while inhibiting B-cell development, leading to a differentiation block at intermediate stages, contributing to genomic instability at these stages of differentiation and facilitating secondary genetic events that result in malignant transformation. In the presence of TAN-1 the DP cells are polyclonal and not cycling initially, but subsequently become monoclonal and rapidly cycling tumor cells, indicating that additional mutations are essential in the development of T-ALL [122-125]. Recent evidences further support the hypothesis that several oncogenes, as IKFZ1 dominant negative form, BMP2, the bHLH transcriptional regulators, TAL1, TAL2, LYL1, BHLHB1 and LMO may play a role in T-ALL genesis by acting upstream Notch-1 pathway. Moreover, Notch-1 aberrant activation is a common event in T-cell cancers, induced by retroviral mutagenesis in murine models, e.g. proviral integration of the Moloney murine leukaemia virus (MuLV) or feline leukaemia virus into Notch -1 or Notch-2, respectively caused T-ALL [126]. Also, the Notch pathway was implicated in preserving leukemia stem cells (T-ALL initiating cells/ T-LiC) that could be insensitive to treatments.

In the early days of Notch1-dependent T-ALL, a murine model was developed to confirm that Notch-1 mediated leukemogenesis required T-cell-specific cooperative signals to facilitate cell expansion and leukemic transformation. Mice transplanted with hematopoietic stem cells from Rag2 $^{-/-}$ or Slp76$^{-/-}$ mice, both of which lack pre-TCR signaling did not develop T-ALL. On the contrary, reconstitution of pre-TCR signaling in Rag2 $^{-/-}$ mice by introduction of a TCRβ transgene restored oncogenic function of Notch-1 [122,127]. Notch-1 is directly involved in upregulation of the pre-TCR (Ptcra), but is not required to maintain its expression [105,128,129]. However, there is a study suggesting that Notch-1 might exert its oncogenic activity also through pre-TCR-independent pathways [130]. ChIP-on-chip analysis of Notch-1 targets has identified many genes that are directly controlled by oncogenic Notch-1 [117]. One of the most important effectors of pre-TCR signaling is the transcription factor E2A, which is downregulated by pre-TCR signaling, whereas high levels of E2A impose a developmental and proliferative block in thymocytes at the pre-TCR checkpoint [105]. The E2A gene, which is also a Notch-regulated gene, produces two helix loop-helix transcription factors, E12 and E47, implicated in normal B and T lymphopoiesis and leukemogenesis. Notch-1 induces E2A ubiquitination and degradation through ERK (extracellular signal-regulated kinase)/ MAPK (mitogen-activated protein kinase) signaling, while Notch-1 and the Notch-interacting protein Deltex-1 inhibit the E2A protein E47 by inhibiting signaling through Ras [111,131-138]. TAL-1/SCL (T-cell acute lymphocytic leukemia 1/ stem cell factor), a member of the basic helix-loop-helix family of transcription factors, is the second most commonly activated oncogene in human T-ALL and is implicated in leukemogenesis by the transcriptional activity of the E2A proteins E47 and HEB. TAL1-induced leukemias accumulate Notch-1 mutations rapidly, suggesting that both TAL-1 and Notch are important in cell malignant transformation, possibly by completely down-regulating E2A activity [111,139-142]. Ras can induce Notch-1, Dll1 (Delta1) and Psen1 (Presenilin1) transcription, resulting in Notch-pathway activation, and Notch activity is required for maintenance of the malignant properties of Ras-transformed cells [105]. Sharma et al. identified c-myc as a novel direct target gene of Notch1, using mouse T-cell leukemic lines that expressed ICN in a doxycycline-dependent manner [115,143]. The presence of conserved CSL binding sites (TTCCCAA) in the regulatory regions of human and mouse c-myc suggested that Notch-1 may directly regulate c-myc. Similarly, Weng et al. demonstrated the Notch-1/c-myc signaling axis in a murine T-ALL cell line, as Notch-1 increased c-myc RNA in T-ALL cells by directly stimulating its transcription [144]. Inhibition of Notch-1 decreased c-myc mRNA and inhibited leukemic cell growth. Notch-1 has a direct proliferative effect on T-cell precursors by the upregulation of c-myc and cyclin D1, while it protects against apoptosis through downregulation of the glucocorticoid receptor and the PI3K/Akt pathway. In a study it was found that Notch-1 signaling protected against diverse stimuli that triggered apoptotic cell death, by up-regulating the expression of the anti-apoptotic genes IAP-2, Bcl-xL and FLIP. They demonstrated that Notch-1 activated the PI3K/Akt signaling pathway, through the non-receptor tyrosine kinase p56^{lck}, which in turn mediated expression of anti-apoptotic molecules. On the other hand, Notch-1 antagonist Numb compromised PI3K/Akt signaling, attenuating the expression of anti-apoptotic molecules [145]. In another study, attenuation of Notch signaling resulted in a dramatic increase of p53 levels, leading to tumor regression by an apoptotic death program [146-148]. There is another study, in which Notch1 signaling was implicated in chemoresistance by inhibiting p53 pathway through mTOR-dependent PI3K-Akt/PKB pathway [146,147]. PI3K-Akt/mTOR pathway is an important effector downstream of Notch-1, as indicated in a phosphoproteomic microarray analysis of T-ALL cell lines treated with Notch-1 inhibitors. This finding further supported a prominent role of Notch-1 in cell growth, as PI3K-AKT-mTOR signal transduction pathway mediates multiple cellular responses, including increased cell growth, proliferation and survival, whereas its function is antagonized by the PTEN tumor suppressor gene. The researchers suggested a model in which Notch-1 sent permissive signals to mTOR, enabling responsiveness to signals from PI3K/Akt pathway, as mTOR activity was inhibited in GSI-sensitive cell lines. They also suggested that c-Myc, a direct transcriptional target of Notch-1, may integrate Notch-1 signaling and mTOR activation, as c-Myc could rescue growth arrest produced by Notch withdrawal in a subset of human T-ALL cell lines. An important finding of this study with clinical application is that T-ALL cell growth was suppressed in a highly synergistic manner by simultaneous treatment with the mTOR inhibitor and g-secretase inhibitors (GSIs) [149]. Recent studies have identified NF-kB signaling pathway as a new major downstream target of Notch-1 in T-ALL. NF-kB induction by Notch-1 was independent of pre-TCR, but resulted from direct transcriptional activation of NF-kB subunits Relb and Nfkb2 or direct stimulation of the activity of the IKK complex, resulting in increased transcription of genes in lymphocyte progenitors. However, the NF-kB pathway was insufficient to generate alone T-ALL, in the absence of activating Notch-1 mutations. Suppression of the NF-kB pathway by bortezomib or BMS-345541 (inhibitor of IKKa kinase) induced apoptosis in Notch1-dependent T-ALL cell lines and restricted tumor growth both in vitro and in vivo. Therefore, the NF-kB pathway can be a promising molecular target in T-ALL therapeutic strategies [150]. Several studies have suggested that increased expression of non DNA-binding Ikaros isoforms and aberrant Notch signaling cooperate in leukemogenesis and pre-TCR was a prerequisite to sustain a Notch-induced altered expression of spliced Ikaros isoforms [107]. Proviral insertional mutagenesis with Moloney murine leukemia virus in N_{ic} transgenic mice, expressing aberrantly the ICN, demonstrated that the Ikaros locus was a common target of proviral integration in 40% of tumors. The insertional mutagenesis of Ikaros locus led to the production of dominant negative Ikaros isoforms, which inhibited repression maintained by the DNA-binding isoforms of Ikaros on Notch dependent genes [151].

There are reports addressing the way deregulated Notch-1 signaling is implicated in alterations in cell cycle progression in ALL. More specifically, there is a study suggesting that Notch-1 signaling promoted S and G1/S cell phase transition in hematopoietic progenitors, through direct gene targeting of SKP2 (S phase kinase-associated protein 2), a component in the $SCF^{Skp}2$ E3 ubiquitin ligase complex and the proteasome-mediated degradation of CDKN1B (p27/Kip1) and CDKN1A (p21/Cip1), target substrates for ubiquitinylation. Notch-1 signaling in T-ALL cell lines was related with elevated levels of SKP2, in parallel with low levels of p27Kip1, situation that was reversed by blocking Notch-1 signaling with GSIs, resulting in G0/G1 cell cycle arrest [152-154]. Also, Notch-1 activation promotes progression to G1/S phase of both peripheral and leukemic T cells, by mediating upregulation of CCND3, CDK4, and CDK6 in T-ALL, an effect abrogated with GSI treatment. In a study it was demonstrated that cyclin D3 is a direct target of Notch1, as Notch-1and CSL associate with the cyclin D3 promoter. Also, they showed that NF-kB subunit p50 enhanced Notch1-dependent activity on cyclin D3 promoter by binding to the promoter. The previous were confirmed by the observation that expression of cyclin D3 could partially rescue T-ALL cell lines from GSI-induced G_1 arrest. CDK4 and CDK6 were also identified as direct targets of Notch-1 in leukemic T cells and are highly overexpressed in Notch-dependent T-cell lymphomas. On the contrary, inhibition of Notch-1 signaling led to exit from the cell cycle, by up-regulating the cyclin-dependent kinase inhibitors CDKN2D (p19/INK4d) and CDKN1B (p27/Kip1) [152-154]. Another cell-cycle regulator and Notch target in T-ALL is the tumor suppressor p53. In the transgenic mice Top-Notch[ic] the researchers showed that initiation and maintenance of lymphomagenesis and leukemogenesis required Notch-1 induced p53 suppression through increased activity of MDM2, an E3 ubiquitin ligase that targets p53 for degradation. MDM2 activity was increased because of decrease in ARF expression, encoded by CDKN2A.

Activating Notch-1 mutations have been found as a frequent occurrence in both pediatric and adult T-ALL, being detected in >50% of patients at disease presentation and result in aberrant up-regulation of Notch-1 -dependent signal transduction, effect that could be abrogated by inhibition of γ-secretase. However, frequency of Notch-1 mutations differed in different studies, reflecting differences in sequencing analysis and the unique features of T-ALL cohorts. Notch-1 mutations affect critical domains, responsible for preventing the spontaneous, ligand-independent receptor or for terminating Notch-1 signaling in the nucleus [117]. The mutations disappeared after patients with T-ALL achieved complete remission, which indicated their relation to the disease. An increase in Notch-1 signaling caused atypical T-cell differentiation and expanded the pool of immature T-cell progenitors [109-111,122,130,155]. However, Notch-1 mutations conferred different levels of oncogenic activation and thus had marked differences in their potential to induce T-cell transformation in murine models. For example, Notch-1 mutations which generated strong activation of Notch signaling, e.g. Notch-1 HD1-ΔPEST and Notch-1 HD2, induced ectopic T cell development and T-ALL. On the other hand, weaker alleles, e.g. HD1 or ΔPEST mutations inhibited myeloid and B cell development and forced differentiation of hematopoietic progenitors to the T-cell lineage and proliferation in preleukemic cells, but were insufficient to initiate leukemogenesis. Importantly, weak Notch-1 alleles accelerated T-cell malignant transformation in hematopoietic progenitors expressing the k-ras oncogene, whereas these leukemias were dependent to Notch-1 signaling for cell growth and survival and thus sensitive to Notch-1 inhibition [156]. There also other studies which have demonstrated that T-ALL development is accelerated by Notch-1 cooperation with c-Myc, Bcr/Abl and E2a/Pbx [157-159].

Weng et al. proposed that Notch-1 mutations clustered in two hotspots: the heterodimerization domain HD [N-terminal region of the heterodimerization domain/HD-N (exon 26) and the C-terminal region of the heterodimerization domain/HD-C (exon 27)] and the PEST domain (exon 34). They also identified mutations in the transcriptional activation domain (TAD) (exon 34). Mutations of HD-N and HD-C probably destabilized the noncovalent intersubunit association of NEC and NTM, enhancing the ligand independent cleavage of the active ICN. In most HD domain mutations Pro-residues were introduced into the protein, disrupting α-helical structures and the 3-dimensional structure of the protein. The disrupted structure facilitated the S3 cleavage, resulting in increased ICN1 liberation and translocation to the nucleus in a ligand-independent manner. Alternatively, some of the Notch-1 mutations might convey ligand-hypersensitivity and increase S3 cleavage in the absence of any destabilization or conformational change of heterodimerization. Most of the

HD domain mutations were located within the HD-N region, spanning amino acid residues 1574 to 1602 and 1606 to 1638. The HD-C domain mutations were located in a region spanning amino acid residues 1674 to 1723. HD-domain mutations were mostly short in-frame insertions or deletions of up to 6 residues. Mutations of the PEST domain led to a COOH-terminally truncated ICN, without the negative regulatory domain. PEST domain mutations were nonsense or frame-shift mutations, creating premature termination codons (PTCs) in the last exon of the Notch-1. The mutated ICN escaped from FBXW7-mediated degradation, therefore having prolonged half-life [105,108,110,114,116,160,161]. HD and ΔPEST mutations have been found in cis in the same Notch-1 transcript in 15% of T-ALLs. These HD-PEST double-mutant alleles resulted in synergistic activation of Notch-1 signaling and were 10 times more active than Notch-1 alleles containing an HD or a PEST mutation alone [117,162,163]. Malecki et al. attempted to elucidate how T-ALL-associated HD domain mutations caused pathophysiologic increases in Notch-1 function. They chose 14 representative point mutations (L1575P, V1577E, F1593S, L1594P, L1597H, R1599P, L1601P, I1617T, I1617N, V1677D, L1679P, I1681N, A1702P, I1719T) and one insertional mutation (P12). These mutations in U2OS cells stimulated the activity of a Notch-1 responsive luciferase reporter gene containing multiple CSL-binding sites, independent of stimulation by canonical ligands. The stimulation was completely abolished by GSIs, confirming the key role of γ-secretase in Notch-1 pathway. They also noted qualitative differences among mutations, with respect to their relative strength and their effects on Notch-1 heterodimer stability. Most HD domain mutations were typically single amino acid substitutions and small in-frame deletions and insertions, resulting, as previously reported, in ligand hypersensitivity or ligand-independent Notch-1 activation, due to destabilization of Notch-1 heterodimers. These mutations were further subdivided into mutations that enhanced subunit dissociation of NEC from NTM under native conditions (class 1A) or in the presence of mildly denaturing conditions, e.g. urea (class 1B). A second group of HD domain mutations (class 2) were longer insertions of at least 12 residues located at the C-terminal region of HD domain, adjacent to the S2 cleavage site. These insertions enhanced proteolytic activation by positioning an exposed, mutation-associated S2 cleavage site away from protective residues that normally prevented metalloprotease access prior to ligand binding. Thus, they correlated with high levels of ligand-independent Notch-1 activation, without affecting the stability of the heterodimer [116,117]. Sulis et al. demonstrated high levels of ICN1 in Jurkat T-ALL cell line which lacked mutations in exons 26, 27 and 34 of the Notch-1, suggesting the presence of an as-yet-unidentified oncogenic mutation, responsible for constitutively active Notch-1 signaling in T-ALL. Sequence analysis of RT-PCR products revealed an in-frame insertion of the CAGG tetranucleotide, followed by an internal tandem duplication of 47 bp in the 3' end of intron 27 and/or in the proximal region of exon 28 of Notch-1, resulting in the insertion of 17 amino acids (QAVEPPPPAQLHFMYVA) at position 1740 in the extracellular juxtamembrane region of the Notch-1 receptor, without altering the primary structure of any of LNR-HD complex components. Sequencing of exon 28 from genomic DNA of primary T-ALL samples identified few patients with internal tandem duplications, ranging from 33 -108 bp in the region extending from the distal part of intron 27 to the proximal segment of exon 28. The duplication resulted in an in-frame insertion of 11 - 36 amino acids in the extracellular juxtamembrane (JME) segment of Notch-

1, around amino acid 1740. JME mutant alleles encoded Notch-1 receptors with significantly extended extracellular juxtamembrane regions, leading to the displacement of the S2 site and the LNR repeats-HD domain complex away from the membrane, without altering the primary structure of any of these elements. The displacement of the LNR-HD complex facilitated aberrant metalloprotease S2 cleavage of the Notch-1 receptor. Moreover the mutant Notch-1 receptors all shared a common tetrapeptide sequence (QLHF) in each peptide inserted in the extracellular juxtamembrane region of the receptor. Notch-1 JME mutations might lead to aberrant proteolytic processing of the JME by creating an alternative S2-like cleavage site, possibly located within their common QLHF sequence. Alternatively, aberrant activation of Notch-1 might result from conformational changes in the HD-LNR complex upon its displacement away from the membrane. Activation of Notch-1 in JME mutants depended on the number of amino acid residues inserted between the HD-LNR repeat complex and the membrane, while it was independent of the specific amino acid sequence introduced in the JME region of the receptor by these mutations. Thus, artificially generated JME insertions of 5, 8, and 11 amino acids in position 1740 failed to induce significant activation of the Notch-1 receptor, while the insertion of 12-14 amino acids induced marked increase in Notch-1 signaling, ranging from 200- to 700-fold over baseline [110]. Sulis et al. also evaluated the levels of activated ICN1 in cells transfected with wild-type Notch-1, -the JME mutation isolated from Jurkat cells and a series of prototypical mutant forms of Notch-1- HD (L1600P), ΔPEST and HD (L1600P)/ΔPEST mutant alleles- in order to elucidate the function of Notch-1 JME mutants. ICN1 levels were markedly increased in cells expressing mutant Notch-1 alleles compared with control wild-type Notch-1 transfected cells, while both wild-type Notch-1 and each Notch-1 mutant alleles resulted in high levels of pro Notch-1. Notably, the Notch-1 Jurkat JME mutant allele induced ICN1 levels higher than the other mutations [110]. Recently, a novel mutation located in a loop of the third LNR (LNR-C) repeat of Notch-1 has been identified. The H1545P substitution triggered ligand-independent Notch-1 activation, while it modestly affected the stability of the LNR-HD complex, similarly to the class Ib mutations [161].

Eguchi et al. in an attempt to elucidate the prenatal occurrence of Notch-1 mutations, they screened diagnostic, leukemic DNA from patients with T-ALL and their archived neonatal blood spots from Guthrie cards. They identified Notch-1 mutations in either HD or PEST domains in four patients. The mutations involved insertions of unrelated short sequences [HD; 4894ins (-TCTTACCGAGAAACGAAGACAAG-), HD; 4894ins (-TCT TTGTCGCCAAG-), PEST; 7403ins (-AGACTGCACTGCA-)] and a duplication of a relatively long sequence from within Notch-1 [PEST; 7123ins (-GCCCTCCCTGCAGCAT GGTAGGTGAGGCCCTCCC-)]. The patient harboring the 4894ins (-TCTTACCGAG AAACGAAGACAAG-) mutation had a SIL-TAL1 fusion gene. For the latter patient the mutation was present in blood spots of the Guthrie card. Although they could not draw general conclusion about the usual timing of Notch-1 mutations in T-ALL, they suggested that the mutations can occur prenatally as an early or possibly initiating event in T-cell leukemogenesis [164].

Lin et al. identified activating Notch1 mutations in pre-T LBL(precursor T-cell lymphoblastic leukemia/lymphoma) cell lines (SCL/LMO1, OLIG2/LMO1, LMO1 and NHD13) and SCL/LMO1, OLIG2, OLIG2/LMO1, LMO1 and NUP98/HOXD13 (NHD13) transgenic mice and p27$^{-/-}$/SMAD3$^{-/+}$mice. Using sequence analysis of Notch-1 they found mutations in 11 of 13 SCL/LMO1 cell lines, of which 10 were mutations in the PEST domain (all insertions or deletions) and only one was found in the HD domain. The mutations in OLIG2/LMO1 and LMO1 cell lines were both insertion mutations in the PEST domain which resulted in premature stop codons. Similarly to human pre-T LBL cell lines that harbor Notch-1 mutations they found that SCL/LMO1 cell lines were sensitive to GSIs, showing a decrease in ICN1 expression and growth inhibition. Thus, Notch-1 mutations activated Notch-1 receptors, whereas ongoing signals from ICN1 were essential in the maintenance of malignant characteristics of the cells. Also, Notch-1 mutations were found in most primary pre-T LBL tumors, of which 6 missense mutations (single-base substitutions) were found in the HD domain and 23 within the PEST domain (insertions and/or deletions). In contrast to human pre-T LBL, none of the samples with Notch-1 mutations had mutations in both the HD and PEST domains. Experiments in SCL/LMO1 murine models confirmed that the mutations were acquired, as they were not identified in germ lines [165].

Analysis of the prognostic significance of Notch-1 activation in T-ALL has shown that Notch-1 mutations were not associated with unfavorable outcome and that in some series they may confer better prognosis. In the context of ALL-BFM 2000 therapy Notch-1 status was found to represent an independent prognostic factor on event-free survival, regardless of other clinical prognostic factors such as age, sex, initial WBC count or T-cell immunophenotype at the time of diagnosis. There was a highly significant correlation between the presence of activating Notch-1 mutations and a favorable early treatment response, as assessed by prednisone response and MRD kinetics (MRD after 33 days and 78 days of treatment) and long-term prognosis (follow-up ranging from 6 months-5.3 years), as assessed by favorable minimal residual disease and improved relapse-free survival. Therefore patients may benefit from a reduction of treatment intensity. The effect of Notch-1 on treatment response and relapse-free survival was independent from the type of the Notch-1 mutations. Thus, activating Notch-1 mutations could be proposed as clinically reliable genetic prognostic markers in T-ALL [108,109].

Asnafi et al. evaluated the incidence and prognostic impact of Notch-1 and FBXW7 mutations in adult T-ALLs (>15 years) from the Lymphoblastic Acute Leukemia in Adults (LALA)-94 and Group for Research on Adult Acute Lymphoblastic Leukemia (GRAALL)-2003 prospective multicenter trials. FBXW7 is a ubiquitin ligase, which targets proteins for proteosomal degradation and thus is implicated in ICN ubiquitination and turnover. Mutations in the tumor suppressor gene FBXW7 have been identified in both T-ALL cell lines and primary T-ALL samples. In total about 15% of T-ALL cases harbor deletions or mutations in FBXW7, nevertheless, their prognostic impact is unknown in both pediatric and adult T-ALL [117]. Loss-of-function mutations of FBXW7 offered an alternative mechanism of sustained Notch-1 activation by leading to inhibition of ubiquitin-mediated degradation of the activated form of Notch-1. Also, FBXW7 targets other substrates for ubiquitination, including c-Myc, Cyclin E and JUN, thus is implicated in additional oncogenic pathways. Importantly in T-ALL cell lines and primary T-ALL samples, missense FBXW7 mutations or homozygous FBW7 deletion have been associated with resistance to GSIs, due to inhibition of Myc and/or NIC degradation, causing sustained Myc transcription and Notch-1 signaling, respectively [162]. Asnafi et al. sequenced exons 26 (HD N-terminal), 27 (HD C-terminal),

28 (juxtamembrane domain) and 34 (transactivation domain TAD and the PEST domain) of Notch-1 and exons 9, 10, and 12 of WD40 domain of FBXW7, using peripheral blood or bone marrow samples. Overall, Notch-1 mutations were identified in 88 of the 141 samples. HD mutations alone (59 cases), in association with PEST (15 cases) or TAD mutations (1 case) were the most frequent Notch-1 mutations, while PEST mutations were detected in 9 cases as a unique mutation. The JME mutation was detected in 3 cases, in association with HD or TAD mutation in 2 cases. FBXW7 mutations were present in 34 cases, alone (13 cases) or in association with Notch-1 mutations (21 cases). These mutations corresponded to the 4 previously reported arginine substitutions at R479, R465, R505 and R689.21 (30 cases), while the remaining were G423V, G477S, S516G and a stop insertion. Furthermore, clinical features of patients were analyzed according to the presence or absence of Notch-1 and/or FBXW7 mutations. There was a trend for a higher WBC count and more frequent CNS involvement in patients demonstrating WT Notch-1 and FBXW7, but there was no significant correlation between Notch-1 and/or FBXW7 mutations and clinico-biologic features. Notch-1/FBXW7 mutations were more frequent in cases expressing TLX1. Median event-free survival was 22 months for patients with WT Notch-1 versus 36 months for the group with mutated Notch-1 and overall survival was 38 months for patients with WT Notch-1 but had not been reached for cases with Notch-1/FBXW7 mutations. Multivariate analysis showed that the presence of Notch-1/FBXW7 mutations was an independent good prognostic factor for both median event-free survival and overall survival, regardless of TLX1 expression [166]. The previous were in line with another study, performed in T-ALL and T-NHL patients who were treated on the Japan Association of Childhood Leukaemia Study (JACLS) protocols ALL-97 and NHL-98 [167]. FBXW7 mutations were detected in 14.6% of T-ALL patients and 21.4% of T-NHL patients, whereas Notch-1 mutations were found in 30.9% of T-ALL patients and 42.9% of T-NHL patients. Only a minor percentage of patients harbored mutations in both genes. FBXW7 mutations included one 31 bp insertion (1450_1451ins AGCTGTTGTCTCTCATCATATGCCTTCTCAC), one single nucleotide deletion (2107del), one deletion/insertion (715_718delinsGAC) and nine missense mutations (1662C > T, 1542C > T, 2029T > C, 1543G > A, 2 1585G > A, 3 1543G > A). Seven of nine missense mutations were clustered in a 'hot spot' encoding arginines 465 and 479 residues, which are highly conserved in the WD40 (tryptophan–aspartic-acid) repeat of FBXW7. Notch-1 mutations were located in the HD domain (66.7%), in PEST domain (33.3%) and in both the HD and PEST domains in one case. Notch-1 mutations included 17 short in-frame insertion or deletions, 5 missense mutations and 2 nonsense mutations. FBXW7 mutations, but not Notch1 mutations, were negatively associated with chromosome abnormalities in both T-ALL and T-NHL. An important finding of this study was that patients with FBXW7 and/or Notch-1 mutation, as well as Notch-1 mutations alone were correlated with good prognosis in T-ALL [167]. Similar, but not statistically significant were the results in another study, concerning the presence of Notch-1 and/or FBXW7 mutations and a favorable outcome [168]. The researchers identified a high incidence of activating mutations Notch-1 (60%) and FBXW7genes (18%) in T-ALL patients, treated on the Medical Research Council (MRC) United Kingdom Acute Lymphoblastic Leukaemia XII (UKALLXII)/Eastern Cooperative Oncology Group (ECOG) E2993 trial. FBXW7 mutations (R465C, R505C, R479Q, R479L, R465H, G423V) altered conserved arginine residues in the WD40 domain, which is

responsible for binding to the Notch-1 PEST domain. Notch-1 mutations were located mainly in the HD domain, but some patients had mutations in the PEST domain and in both HD and PEST domains. There was a positive association between having a mutation in the Notch-1 HD only and a FBXW7 mutation, as these mutations cooperate in signal amplification and a negative association between having a mutation in the Notch-1 PEST domain and a FBXW7 mutation. Mutations in the PEST domain probably relieve mutational pressure on FBXW7. Patients having combined Notch-1 /FBXW7 had a better prognosis, whereas mutations in Notch1 or FBXW7 alone did not confer to a favorable outcome [168]. In another cohort of adult patients with T-ALL who were registered on the GMALL 05/93 and 06/99, the prognostic impact of mutations in Notch-1 and FBXW7 did not reach statistical significance, but the high frequency of Notch-1 mutations was confirmed [169]. They identified Notch-1 mutations in 57% of T-ALL patients. The mutations involved mainly the HD domain (insertions and/or deletions), but were also located in the PEST domain (deletions and insertions) and the TAD (premature stop codon). Some patients had co-existing mutations (HD/PEST domain, HD/TAD). FBXW7 mutations were demonstrated in 12% of T-ALL patients, whereas most of these patients had co-existing Notch-1 mutations, mainly in the HD domain. FBXW7 mutations were identified in exon 8 (R465C/H) and exon 9 (R505C, G517R). Interestingly, one patient had three mutations (R465C/H, HD-N and PEST-1 domain). Notch-1-FBXW7 mutation status did not confer to a favorable outcome, with the exception of a small subgroup with low expression of ERG and BAALC, in which lack of Notch1/FBXW7 mutations was associated with unfavorable prognosis. Elevated expression of ERG and BAALC genes has been associated with poor prognosis in ALL and AML. They also observed that Notch1/FBXW7 mutations were correlated with a mature (thymic) immunophenotype, whereas absence of mutations was correlated with immature DN immunophenotype [169]. There are observations suggesting that immature immunophenotype was associated with chemoresistance and poor outcome [170]. In a subsequent study in a cohort of pediatric T-ALLs Notch1 and FBXW7 mutations were also not predictive of outcome [171]. They found Notch-1 mutations in 22% of T-ALL patients, located in the HD domain (12%), in the PEST domain (7%) or infrequently in both domains (3%). HD domain mutations were point mutations and positioned mainly at the HD-N region (L1586P, L1575P, R1599P, K1608N missense mutations) within the conserved amino acid residues 1554 and 1610. HD-C mutations (thymine insertions, point mutations) were uncommon and clustered in amino acid residues 1681 to 1737. PEST mutations were mainly premature stop codons and located in amino acid residues 2375 to 2571. FBXW7 mutations were identified in 10% of T-ALL samples and included missense mutations, duplication and synonymous mutations. Missense mutations were located in a locus encoding conserved arginine amino acid residues 465 and 479, thus altering arginine residues in the WD40 domain, are responsible for binding to the PEST domain. Only two patients had co-existing HD domain / FBXW7 mutations. They did not find any significant correlation between Notch-1 and/or FBXW7 mutations and long-term prognosis. The discrepancies among different studies concerning the prognostic impact of Notch-1 and/or FBXW7 mutations could be due to differences in the number of patients in different cohorts and short term follow up of the patients [171]. Gedman et al. assessed the prognostic significance of mutations in Notch-1 in a cohort of pediatric T-ALLs with documented treatment outcome and attempted to elucidate the implication of Notch-1 target genes in the pathogenesis of T-ALL. They found Notch-1 mutations in 34% of T-ALL patients which resulted in sustained activation of Notch-1 signaling. Notch-1 activation was higher in samples having mutations in the PEST domain and/or in combination with mutations in HD domain, than in samples with mutations in the HD domain. These mutations included single point mutations, deletions and insertions in the HD and PEST domains, resulting in amino acid substitutions and premature stop codons. Contrary to previous reports, they did not observe any significant association between Notch-1 mutations and favorable prognosis. They suggested that this discrepancy could be due to mutations in additional genes, e.g. FBW7 PTEN, leading to sustained Notch-1 signaling and Akt signaling, respectively or differences in treatment protocols. FBW7 inactivating mutations, placed in exon 11, were detected in 11% of T-ALL patients. Similarly to Notch-1 mutations they did not correlate with treatment outcome. FBW7 mutations did not co-exist with mutations in the PEST domain of Notch-1, but sometimes were accompanied with mutations in the HD domain. Notch-1 and FBW7 mutations were accompanied by increased median transcripts for Notch-1 target genes HES1, DELTEX1 and cMYC, which in turn were associated with significant transcriptional activation of genes encoding proteins of apoptosis, drug transporters, drug metabolizing enzymes and drug targets, e.g. MDR1, ABCC5, asparagine synthetase, Bcl-2, reduced folate carrier, dihydrofolate reductase and thiopurine methyl-transerase. Therefore, Notch-1 and FBW7 mutations could affect treatment outcome indirectly by increasing methotrexate sensitivity due to increased expression of human reduced folate carrier or by increasing chemoresistance, due to increased expression of MDR1 (doxorubicin, vincristine), ABCC5 (6-mercaptopurine, methotrexate), asparagine synthetase (L-asparaginase) and dihydrofolate reductase (methotrexate) [120].

The characterization of the Notch-1 pathway in T-ALL and the high prevalence of Notch-1 mutations in T-ALL will hopefully identify target molecules for novel and specific pharmacological intervention. One of the most promising targets in inactivating Notch signaling is γ-secretase complex. Small-molecule inhibitors of γ-secretase (GSIs) have been tested in T-ALL cell lines and induce cell cycle arrest [172]. However, potential adverse effects of GSIs have to be considered as these drugs affect cleavage of other substrates, such as CD44, syndecan, ErbB4 and generation of Aβ peptide which is associated with Alzheimer's disease. Furthermore, in vitro studies suggested that simultaneous treatment of T-ALL cells with GSIs and mTOR inhibitors have synergistic effect [111,117]. While the role of Notch in T-cell leukemogenesis is widely accepted, its involvement in the development of B-cell malignancies remains controversial, as both oncogenic and tumor suppressive effects of Notch activity in B cells have been suggested.

PTEN

The PTEN gene (phosphatase and tensin homologue deleted on chromosome 10) has been identified as a tumor suppressor gene located on chromosome 10q23.3 [173]. It is considered a central negative regulator of the phosphatidylinositol-3-OH kinase through serine-threonine kinase akt (PI3K/AKT) signaling cascade that influences multiple cellular functions including cell growth, survival, proliferation and migration in a context-dependent manner. Dysregulation of this signaling pathway is thought to contribute to many cancers in humans. PTEN is the most commonly altered component of the PI3K pathway in human malignancies [174].

PTEN is critically involved in maintaining hematopoietic stem cells and preventing leukemogenesis [175]. Inactivation of *PTEN* is thought to play a vital role in resistance to NOTCH inhibition in T-ALL cell lines and has been demonstrated in human T-ALL [176]. Somatic deletions or mutations have been identified in a variety of cancers, including glioblastomas, metastatic prostate cancers, lung, breast and endometrial cancers, malignant melanoma and hematological malignancies [177]. Interestingly, several T-ALL cases present with inactivating PTEN gene mutations [175,178]. According to Larson Gedman et al., (2009) there is no association between PTEN mutations in pediatric T-ALL and therapeutic outcome. However, this is not in line with the findings of Jotta et al. (2010), who suggested a negative prognostic impact of PTEN mutations in childhood T-ALL. More specifically, they reported that T-ALL patients harboring exon 7 PTEN mutations may be at increased risk of relapse [175,178].

Ras Oncogenes

The Ras subfamily are small GTPases, anchored at the cytosolic side of the plasma membrane, functioning as 'molecular switches' in cellular signal transduction, relaying proliferative stimuli from the plasma membrane to the nucleus, mainly through the MAPK/ERK pathway to promote proliferation, differentiation, survival, and apoptosis depending on cellular conditions. The Ras proteins are activated through several types of receptors, such as tyrosine kinase receptors, non-receptor tyrosine kinases and GPCRs. Ras activation and deactivation cycle between an active(GTP)-bound state and an inactive(GDP)-bound state. These conversions are facilitated by Ras GEFs (Guanine Nucleotide Exchange Factors)- Sos, GRF, and GRP- and Ras GAPs (GTPase Activating Proteins)- p120GAP and neurofibromin [179]. The ras genes were first identified as oncogenes, responsible for the cancer-causing activities of the Harvey (HRAS) and Kirsten (KRAS) sarcoma viruses. There are three human Ras genes that encode four highly homologous 188 to 189 amino acid proteins H-Ras (transforming protein p21), N-Ras (Neuroblastoma RAS viral oncogene homolog) and K-Ras4A and K-Ras4B (V-Ki-ras2 Kirsten rat sarcoma viral oncogene homolog and KRAS). Their function is unique, as well as their expression patterns. K-Ras is expressed at high levels in the gut and thymus, N-Ras in the testis and thymus and H-Ras in the skin and skeletal muscles [180]. Aberrant Ras signaling is achieved by constitute activation of other proto-oncogenes or inactivation of tumor suppressor genes. However, oncogenic *Ras* mutations, which are very common genetic aberrations in human tumors, can also be implicated in constitute activation of Ras, leading to Ras accumulation in their active GTP-bound form, by disrupting Ras GTPase activities as well as their association with Ras GAP. Deregulated Ras signaling due to Ras mutations has been identified in cancers of many different origins, e.g. pancreas, colon, lung, thyroid, bladder, ovaries, breast, skin, liver and kidney. N-Ras mutations have been identified in both lymphoid and myeloid malignancies and are 2–3 times more often than K-Ras mutations. Occurrence of N-Ras mutations in AML varied between 20-40% in different studies, whereas in JMML was 30% [181-183]. Also, 10% of T lymphoma and T leukemias harbor N-Ras or K-Ras mutations, but are rarely identified in B-cell malignancies. Ras mutations are important in the transformation from MDS to AML. The oncogenic potential of K-Ras is highly tissue-specific and many somatic tissues tolerate K-Ras mutations, without undergoing malignant transformation. Activating H-Ras mutations are rare in hematopoietic malignancies, whereas germline mutations in humans were not found to increase leukemia incidence [180]. The point mutations in N-Ras occur frequently in codons 12, 13 and 61 and in K-Ras in codon 12 [179,184,185]. Amino acid substitutions due to the previous mutations constitutively activate the Ras pathway by increasing intracellular levels of Ras-GTP, as these residues participate in GTP binding [179]. Oncogenic Ras mutations might initiate leukemogenesis by providing proliferative/survival advantages to precursor T cells, affecting T-cell differentiation or genome stability [186]. Comparison of the leukemogenic potential of mutant N-Ras, K-Ras and H-Ras in murine models demonstrated that while all isoforms have the potential to induce myeloid leukemias, they produced distinct phenotypes. N-Ras induced AML- or CMML-like disease, K-Ras CMML-like disease and H-Ras AML-like disease [187]. However, Ras hyperactivation has been also implicated in T-ALL pathogenesis in murine models [188-190]. E mu-N-Ras transgenic mice, bearing a mutant, activated N-Ras oncogene, sporadically developed T-cell lymphomas and non-lymphoid tumors [191]. Zhang et al., to address the cellular mechanism underlying oncogenic *K-Ras* induced leukemogenesis, they transplanted unfractionated bone marrow cells expressing oncogenic *K-Ras* ^{G12D} mutation from its endogenous locus into lethally irradiated mice. Depending on the donor cell dosages, the recipient mice developed hematopoietic malignancies in multiple lineages, including acute or chronic T-ALL (10%), thymic T-cell lymphoblastic lymphoma (50%) and juvenile myelomonocytic leukemia (8%). None of the recipient mice developed B-cell malignancies, whereas B-cell development was normal [186]. Previous studies have already demonstrated that mice expressing oncogenic *K-Ras* ^{G12D} in hematopoietic cells suffered from a myeloproliferative disorder, resulting to death at 3 months of age [192,193]. In a subsequent study when Mx1-Cre, *K-Ras* $^{LSL-G12D}$ mice expressed oncogenic *K-Ras* G^{12D} in hematopoietic stem cells (HSCs) they developed a myeloproliferative disorder and T-ALL. Myeloproliferative disorders were established earlier in primary *K-Ras* $^{LSL-G12D}$ mice, whereas T-ALL was observed particularly in recipients of transplanted *K-Ras* ^{G12D} HSCs. They demonstrated that oncogenic *K-Ras* G^{12D} perturbed homeostasis in the thymus, particularly in early stages of thymocyte maturation, conferring a strong growth advantage and increasing proliferation of HSCs and/or progenitor cells. However, they hypothesized that oncogenic Ras expression has a negative long term impact on self-renewal capacity [194]. In another study, when lethally irradiated mice were reconstituted with bone marrow cells, infected with a mutant Ras-containing retrovirus [murine stem cell virus (MSCV)-v-H-Ras], the mice developed pre-T-cell thymic lymphomas and/or pre-B-cell lymphoblastic leukemia/ lymphomas between 7 and 12 weeks post-transplantation [189].

Von Lintig et al., were among the first who assessed Ras activation in normal WBCs and demonstrated its implication in T-ALL. Using a nonradioactive assay which measured absolute amounts of GTP and GDP bound to Ras, they demonstrated that Ras was significantly activated in half of T-ALLs samples, but in none of the B-ALLs. There was no correlation between Ras activation levels and the peripheral WBC count of the T-ALL patients. Moreover, in most of T-ALLs Ras activation levels were extremely high, exceeding 30% [195]. In cultured cell systems Ras activation levels exceeding 30% were correlated with the presence of an activating Ras mutation, which could be responsible for malignant transformation of the cells [196]. The previous data suggested that increased Ras activation in T-ALL compared with B-ALL could be the cause of the more aggressive characteristics of T-ALL [195]. Lubbert et al. detected a 6% incidence of heterozygous point mutations at codon 12 or 13 of exon 1 of the N-Ras in a cohort of childhood ALLs, whereas no mutations were identified at exon 2 of the N-Ras or at K-Ras and H-Ras. Two of the patients bearing Ras mutations had early B-precursor-ALL, three common ALL and one T-ALL. The mutations were correlated strongly with a poor outcome, suggesting that N-Ras mutations could represent an independent prognostic variable. This notion was supported by the disappearance of the previously detected N-Ras mutations in remission samples. Nevertheless the researchers suggested that Ras mutations alone were probably insufficient to cause leukemogenesis, but must be complemented by other genetic alterations [186,197]. For example, insertion of c-myc or N-myc in E mu-N-ras transgenic mice by insertional mutagenesis with Moloney murine leukemia virus accelerated tumorigenesis in lymphoid cells expressing a mutant Ras gene [191]. Also, in a murine model with the Kras^{G12D} mutation the researchers demonstrated that IKZF1 mutations are an initiating event, which subsequently cooperate with K-Ras and Notch-1 somatically acquired mutations in T lineage leukemogenesis[198]. They hypothesized that IKZF1 and K-Ras mutations create a field of thymocytes with aberrant proliferation, survival and/or differentiation which require a Notch-1 mutation to induce full leukemic transformation [198]. In another study, K-Ras mutations cooperated with Notch-1 mutations in leukemogenesis [199]. More specifically, in Mx1-Cre, K-Ras $^{LSL-G12D}$ murine models oncogenic K-Ras expression in HSCs is responsible for T-ALL initiation, but full malignant transformation occurred with the acquisition of Notch-1 mutations in a T- lineage cell. It is possible that K-Ras mutations created a favorable environment for acquisition of cooperating mutations by expanding the size of susceptible lymphoid progenitor pools and/or by conferring resistance to apoptosis, during thymic selection. Acquisition of secondary mutations in self-renewing preleukemic population could be responsible for disease relapse [194]. However, there are other studies which have demonstrated that activating mutations in N-Ras and K-Ras are efficient in initiating myeloid leukemias in murine models, without secondary mutations [192,193,200]. Raepple et al., failed to demonstrate any N-Ras mutations in samples from ALL patients. On the contrary, they found two N-Ras mutations of six AML cases, one of two plasma cell leukemias and two of four juvenile myelomonocytic leukemias [201]. Yokota et al., in a cohort of childhood ALL patients (common-ALL, pre-B-ALL, T-ALL, B-ALL, undifferentiated ALL and unclassified ALL) found that N-Ras mutations were present in 11% of patients. Patients with undifferentiated ALL harbored an N-Ras mutation at a significantly higher rate, whereas mutations were not identified in pre-B-ALL and B-ALL. Sequence analyses revealed that the majority of the patients had an N-ras mutation of a G→A transition. They failed to demonstrate any prognostic impact of mutations, concerning event-free survival rates [202]. Similarly, Perentesis et al., did not find any association of Ras mutations with high-risk disease or adverse outcomes in a large cohort of children with ALL (early pre-B ALL, pre-B

ALL, B-ALL, T-ALL, unclassified). Ras mutations in samples with greater than 50% blasts were demonstrated by direct DNA sequencing of amplified Ras exon fragments, whereas samples with less than 50% blasts were screened by single-strand conformation polymorphism (SSCP) analysis. Ras mutations were identified in approximately 15% of patients and were located predominantly in exon 1 (codons 12/13) of N-Ras and K-Ras, while mutations at exon 2 (codon 61) of N-Ras and K-Ras were infrequent. Mutations at codons 12/13 involved a G:C to A:T transition and their frequency of were similar to the rates reviewed by Yokota et al.. The researchers proposed that mutations may be responsible of endogenous oxidant-induced genetic damage and/or defective DNA repair mechanisms in early lymphoid cells [203]. Case et al., were among the first to report a comprehensive mutational screen of key exons of genes implicated on the RAS-RAF-MEK-ERK pathway in ALL patients at diagnosis and at disease relapse. Mutational screening of N-Ras, K-Ras2, Ptpn11, FLT3 and BRAF by denaturing high-performance liquid chromatography (DHPLC) demonstrated a combined mutation incidence of 35% at diagnosis and of 26% at recurrence. The incidence of N-Ras (N-Ras G12C, N-Ras G12S, N-Ras G12D, N-Ras G13D, N-Ras Q61H, N-Ras G12V, N-Ras Q61R, K-Ras G12V, K-Ras G13D, K-Ras G12A, K-Ras G13D, K-Ras G12V, K-Ras L19F, K-Ras G12D) and K-Ras mutations at diagnosis was 31%, an incidence which was in the higher range of other studies, probably due to the increased sensitivity of DHPLC. No mutations were identified in BRAF, while some patients bared more than one mutated genes. Mutations were predominantly associated with high hyperdiploidy, suggesting that the mutations served as additional, cooperative genetic events in leukemogenesis. However, the mutations were not correlated with poor prognosis and early treatment response [204]. Paulsson et al., conducted a similar mutational analysis on N-Ras, K-Ras, PTPN11 and FLT3, but focused exclusively on hyperdiploid ALL. However, they found a lower combined incidence of 33%, which could be attributed to the different sensitivities of the mutational screening methods. More specifically, they identified six activating point mutations (Asp835/Ile836 mutation) and one internal tandem duplication of FLT3, eight codon 12, 13 or 61 N-Ras mutations, five codon 12 or 13 K-Ras mutations and six exon 3 and one exon 13 PTPN11 mutations. Mutations generally were mutually exclusive, with one exception. Similarly to the previous study, they did not demonstrate any statistically significant association between the presence of a mutation and negative prognosis [205]. Association of Ras mutations with high hyperdiploid ALL had already been demonstrated in a previous study in case series of children with ALL, AML or CML [206]. In this study identification of Ras mutations was accomplished by Restriction Endonuclease-Mediated Selective (REMS)-PCR screen. Ras mutations were present in 20% of all leukemias and their frequency was similar in B- and T-lineage leukemias. However, a higher proportion of Ras mutations were observed in hyperdiploid B-cell ALL children. Higher rates of Ras mutations in children were significantly associated with young maternal age and inversely associated with paternal pre-pregnancy smoking, suggesting that Ras mutations in ALL could be a prenatal event [206]. The same group confirmed in a larger cohort of ALL patients that high hyperdiploidy was strongly associated with Ras mutations, but failed to demonstrate any association with maternal age and parental smoking. They suggested that hyperdiploidy was a prenatal event, providing some clonal advantage, while Ras mutations appeared afterwards, conferring to leukemogenesis. They detected N-Ras and K-Ras mutations in 16% of patients, with the frequency being higher in ALL compared to AML and in hyperdiploid ALLs than in ALLs of other subtypes. Also, among ALL patients mutations were more frequent in B-ALL than in T-ALL. All point mutations were non-synomymous, identified in codons 12 or 13, except for one in codon 19 (L19F in K-Ras). Mutations were predominantly G→T transversions and rarely T→ G, G→T or G→C transitions They rarely found mutations in additional genes implicated in Ras-pathway (PTPN11, FLT3 and BRAF), as demonstrated in previous studies, probably due to differences in etiologic risk factors or genetic background of the patients [207].

Ras and its downstream effectors have been the subject of intense research, concerning their implication in the pathogenesis of malignant transformation, therefore, laying the groundwork for novel treatment strategies of childhood ALL. Therefore, multiple Ras inhibitors have been developed, e.g. farnesyl-transferase inhibitors, GGTase inhibitors, viral oncotherapeutic agents, that require an activated Ras for their cytotoxic effect and antibodies against activated Ras, which can be applied in the context of targeted therapies. Thus, assessing Ras activation could be used before initiating therapy, to determine the patients that could be good candidates of these therapeutic strategies [179,195,208-210].

Wnt

Wnt genes encode a large family of lipid modified glycoproteins that regulate cell-to-cell interactions. Signaling is initiated by Wnt proteins binding to receptors of the Frizzled family (Fzd) on the cell surface. Depending on particular Wnt/Fzd combinations, at least three signaling cascades may be activated. The canonical Wnt pathway is considered the most studied (Figure 2) and is activated by members of the Wnt1 class (including Wnt1, Wnt2, Wnt3 and Wnt8) [211]. Central to this pathway is cytoplasmic β-catenin. In the absence of Wnt signaling, β-catenin is present in a cytoplasmic 'destruction complex' and is continuously phosphorylated by the negative regulatory glycogen-synthase kinase 3β (GSK3β) and degraded. When Wnt protein binds to the receptor complex consisting of seven transmembrane proteins and an LDL-receptor related protein (LRP5 or LRP6), β-catenin is no longer phosphorylated and translocates to the nucleus, where it activates Tcf/Lef transcription factors in thymocytes predominantly Tcf-1 [212,213].

Wnt signaling pathway is involved in several aspects of cellular development including embryonic cell growth, stem cell self-renewal and cancer formation [214]. It is also required for thymocyte development and B-cell survival at the pre-B-cell stages, while it has been linked to T-ALL leukemogenesis [215]. The abnormal methylation of various Wnt genes have been associated with human T-ALL, however it remains to be elucidated whether they compose the etiology underlying T-ALL leukemogenesis, or they form a secondary outcome of the abnormal tumor state of the ALL cells [212]. It is notable though that in T-cell leukemia two types of mutations have been detected; inactivating (loss-of-function) mutations in the tumor suppressor genes Axin and adenomous polyposis coli (APC) and activating (gain-of-function) mutations in β –catenin, however their involvement in the development of T-ALL has not thus far been implicated [213]

Little is known about the role of Wnt signaling in B-cell ALL, apart from a single evidence suggesting the potential role of Wnt16B in a pre-B-leukemia cell survival [216]. Additionally, previous functional and microarray analyses suggested that Wnt3A inhibited the proliferation of several B-cell lines and identified a number of Wnt3A target genes that might give insights into the function of canonical Wnt signalling in leukemia cells, respectively [214,217].

Wilms' Tumor Gene 1 (WT1)

Wilms' tumor gene 1 (WT1) is a tumor suppressor gene, located on chromosome 11p13. It encodes a zinc-finger transcription factor which recognizes and binds the DNA sequence 5'-CGCCCCGC-3'. WT1 is a bifunctional regulator of transcription, acting as a transcriptional activator or repressor, depending on the WT1 isoform –there are at least 32 isoforms. It is implicated in the transcription of several growth factors and their receptors, e.g. EGF, TGF-β, PDGFA, CSF-1, IGF-2, IGF-1R and vitamin D receptor and genes, such as bcl-2 and c-myc [218-228]. It has also been implicated in post-transcriptional regulation, such as RNA-splicing. Normally, it is expressed during the embryogenesis of the urogenital tract. In adults, it is expressed at very low levels in the kidney, ovary, testis, spleen, and normal hematopoietic progenitor cells, controlling cell proliferation, differentiation and apoptosis. In the hematopoietic system there is biphasic WT1 expression, as it is transiently expressed in very few immature quiescent CD34+ CD38(-) progenitors, capable of producing both myeloid and lymphoid progeny, absent in lineage-committed precursors, promoting cell differentiation and finally present in a subset of the more differentiated populations [CD19(+)/ CD3(-) B lymphocytes, CD11b(+)/CD14(-) granulocytes and CD11b(+)/CD14(+) monocytes][218,229-232]. Overexpression of WT1 has been detected in various cancers, such as lung, gastric, colorectal, ovarian and breast cancer, mesothelioma, renal cell carcinoma, melanoma and glioblastoma [218,233-246].

In acute leukemia, chronic myelogenous leukemia during blast crisis and myelodysplastic syndromes high levels of wild-type WT1 are continuously expressed, irrespective of lineage, while mutations have been reported in ~10-15% of cases AML, 20% of biphenotypic leukemias and sporadic cases of T-ALL, suggesting a role for disruption of WT1 function in leukemogenesis [218,247-251]. Several studies on adult acute leukemias indicated WT1 overexpression as an independent risk factor of recurrence and an attractive marker for disease prognosis and minimal residual disease (MRD) detection and a target for antileukemic vaccines, as continuous WT1 expression characterizes leukemic blasts, while transient WT1 expression is expected only in very few physiologic hematopoietic progenitors. [218,229,252-259]. On the contrary, there are studies that have failed to demonstrate the prognostic impact of WT1 expression levels in MNCs, concerning achievement of complete remission, disease-free survival or overall survival in childhood acute leukemias [218,258,260]. Also, levels of WT1 in leukemic cells vary significantly in different studies [218]. These discrepancies probably result from differences in the assays of WT1 detection and quantification, e.g. (qualitative PCR, Northern blot analysis or real-time quantitative PCR/RQ-PCR), in control genes and control groups and in type of samples (bone marrow or peripheral blood).

Miwa et al., using Northern blot found that WT1 was expressed in MNCs from 43% of patients with ALL, 68% of patients with AML-with the lowest levels observed in more differentiated AML subtypes and 80% of patients with CML during blast crisis. They did not detect WT1 RNA in chronic leukemias, e.g CLL, CML in chronic phase, hairy cell leukemia and plasma cell leukemia [261]. Inoue et al., using semiquantitative WT1 Reverse Transcriptase-PCR (RT-PCR) were the first to examine relative levels of WT1 in bone marrow cells or blood MNCs from patients with hematopoietic malignancies (AML, ALL, AMLL, CML, NHL). The expression levels of WT1 were higher for AML than for ALL patients and for ALL patients the levels were more than 20 times higher in CD19+CD20- pro-B-cell ALL than in CD19+CD20+ pre-B-intermediate B-cell ALL, indicating that WT1 expression was associated with immature phenotypes of ALL. On the contrary, in NHL WT1 expression was almost undetectable, probably because NHL tumor cells originate from more mature lymphoid cells. In normal bone marrow and peripheral blood cells and lymph nodes WT1 was also expressed in very low levels. Moreover, the researchers found a correlation between the levels of WT1 expression and poor prognosis, as patients with low levels of WT1 had significantly higher rates of complete remission, disease-free survival and overall survival, whereas complete remission could not be induced in patients with high levels of WT1, probably because the immature leukemic cells expressing WT1 are chemoresistant. Finally, they showed the usefulness of the quantitation of WT1 expression in MRD monitoring of leukemia, as WT1 transcripts increased rapidly or gradually, even before relapse became clinically apparent. On the other hand, WT1 expression levels decreased or were undetected in patients in clinical remission. [262,263]. Menssen et al., using RT-PCR found that WT1 was expressed in MNCs of 86% of pre-pre-B-ALL patients, 80% of cALL patients, 74% of T-ALL patients and 93% of AML patients, while it was not expressed in mononuclear cells (bone marrow and peripheral blood) and peripheral CD34+ hematopoietic progenitors of healthy volunteers. The results were confirmed by immunofluorescence assays on single cell level [232]. Asgarian Omran et al., also suggested that WT1 expression levels could be employed as a reliable marker in leukemia diagnosis and prognosis of relapse or remission. The researchers, using a semi-quantitative RT-PCR assay detected WT1 mRNA in leukemic cells of 52% of the newly diagnosed Iranian ALL patients and 58% of the relapsed patients. WT1 was expressed in immature subtypes of B-ALL and was more frequently expressed in T-ALL compared with B-ALL. WT1 was not expressed in any ALL patients in remission, as well as in healthy donors [264]. The previous were in line with other studies [256,265].

There are studies where molecular monitoring of AML, ALL and CML with quantitative real-time WT1 RT-PCR gave satisfactory results, in order to evaluate the levels of WT1 expression in leukemic blast cells and to monitor MRD after chemotherapy [266-269]. Kreuzer et al., attempted to set up a sensitive real time quantitative RT-PCR approach in order to assess the expression levels of WT1 in different leukemias and tried to verify if the method could also be applied to MRD monitoring. WT1 RNA levels were detectable in MNCs from AML, ALL and CML patients, but WT1 was not expressed in samples from healthy donors. More importantly, they found that WT1 expression levels in MNCs were correlated to the disease status, while longitudinal measurements of WT1 transcripts could contribute to the evaluation of disease prognosis and treatment response, as their levels augmented in parallel with the disease course and decreased quickly after treatment initiation. Thus, quantitation of WT1 expression levels appeared to be an important tool for MRD monitoring, allowing early prediction of clinical relapse [266]. Cilloni et al., also attempted to evaluate the clinical applicability and prognostic significance of quantitative WT1 real time RQ-PCR in leukemias. WT1 was overexpressed in all AML and ALL samples and WT1 transcripts were generally higher in AML. When concerning different cytogenetic groups in ALL, translocations t(4;11) and t(9;22) were related with very high values, while translocation t(1;19) was related with lower levels of WT mRNA. This observation is in contrast to another study where levels of WT1 transcripts in samples with the previous translocations did not differ significantly [270]. The results were minimal or negative in samples obtained from patients in complete remission and healthy donors. Sequential WT1 analysis was performed in AML patients, lacking additional molecular markers. They found that WT1 levels were predictive of an impending hematological relapse, as in remission WT1 levels were constantly within the normal range, whereas in relapse the levels increased [269]..

Boublikova et al., evaluated WT1 expression and its clinical implications in childhood ALL (106 B-cell precursor-ALL, 19 T-ALL), using RQ-PCR for WT1 detection and WT1/CG (control gene) NCN (normalized copy number) approach for WT1 quantification. They evaluated WT1 expression in hematopoietic cells from healthy adult donors (peripheral blood, bone marrow, peripheral stem cells) and MRD-negative regenerating bone marrow from childhood ALL patients. They detected WT1 in all control samples, in agreement with other studies [252,255,269,271,272]. When considering MRD-negative regenerating bone marrow samples taken at different times during the induction therapy, they found median WT1 expression in early follow-up samples, tending to reach lower levels during the later phases, comparable to normal bone marrow samples. WT1 expression in bone marrow samples from BCP-ALL patients varied within a wide range (overexpression, low expression, undetectable levels), while in T-ALL patients WT1 expression was significantly higher, even though it did not reach statistical significance, when considering normal bone marrow controls. Moreover, its expression was much lower than in AML or adult ALL. In multivariate analysis including age and WBC they found WT1 both under- and over-expression to be an independent risk factor of relapse. Collectivelly, they concluded that WT1 must not be considered a marker for MRD monitoring in childhood ALL, as its expression was very variable.

King-Underwood et al., hypothesized that WT1 mutations have a role in leukemia, based on observations that leukemia occurs as a second primary tumor in Wilms' tumor patients, while hematopoietic malignancies are common in relatives of children with Wilms' tumor. Screening the DNA from 35 patients with sporadic acute leukemia for the presence of mutations in the WT1 gene, they detected five mutations in patients with acute myeloid leukemia and biphenotypic leukemia. Four of the mutations were insertions (1-5 bp), one in exon 1 and the other three in exon 7, while the fifth was a nonsense mutation in exon 9. All mutations caused truncation of the encoded protein, leading to the loss or disruption of the zinc finger region, rendering its DNA binding capacity and thus transcriptional activity [249].

Tosello et al., attempted to address the actual prevalence and potential significance of WT1 mutations in T-ALL. WT1 mutations were analyzed by PCR amplification of WT1 exons 1 to 10, followed by direct bidirectional DNA sequencing, after identifying chromosomal deletions in 11p13 locus, via SNP array and FISH analysis. The mutation analysis of WT1 which was performed in 294 primary T-ALL samples demonstrated the presence of WT1 mutations at diagnosis in 13.2% of pediatric and 11.7% of adult T-ALLs. The mutations were primarily frameshift insertions and deletions and occasional nonsense point mutations located in exons 7 and 8, which encoded prematurely truncated WT1 proteins, devoid of the C-terminal zinc finger domains. Other mutations identified were splice donor mutations in exons 1 and 7, frameshift mutations in exons 1 and 2-predicted to encode N-terminal truncations in WT1 proteins- and missense mutations in codon 462 (R462Q and R462P) located in exon 9. WT1 mutations were somatically acquired in the leukemic clone, as the WT1 mutant allele was lost during remission. They also found that the mutations were associated with aberrant expression of the TLX1, TLX3, and HOXA9 transcription factor oncogenes, suggesting an additional role of WT1 in the pathogenesis of T-ALL. Survival analysis in pediatric and adult T-ALL patients showed that WT1 mutations did not confer adverse prognosis in T-ALL [251]. Consistent with the previous are the results in another study [273]. The researchers found WT1 mutations, predominantly frameshift mutations in exon 7, in 15 out of 143 T-ALL patients. The mutations, consisting of small duplications, deletions or combined insertions/deletions, resulted in a truncated WT1 protein, missing the zinc finger domains. However the mutations were not associated with poor prognosis. They also demonstrated that in WT1 mutated T-ALL samples TLX1 and TLX3 were overexpressed [273]. Heesch et al., examined the prognostic implications of WT1 mutations and mRNA levels in a cohort of adult patients with newly diagnosed T-ALL. WT1 mutations were identified in 8% of T-ALL patients at initial diagnosis and were associated with a more immature T-ALL subtype. Mutations in exon 7 were identified in all cases, resulting in a truncated protein. Two patients had coexisting missense mutations in exon 9, resulting in single amino-acid substitutions. WT1 mutations were not predictive for poor response to chemotherapy but few patients bearing WT1 mutations showed a higher relapse rate, compared to those without WT1 mutations. Moreover, WT1 mutations were associated with WT1 overexpression and aberrant HOX11L2 expression. In line with other studies they found that altered WT1 expression -negative or high WT1 expression- was an independent negative prognostic factor. Nevertheless, they hypothesized that WT1 mutations may cooperate with coexistence mutations, e.g. in NOTCH1, FBXW7 or FLT3 in leukemogenesis [250].

Thus under-expression of WT1 function, either by mutational inactivation or lack of mRNA expression and over-expression might contribute in different ways in ALL pathogenesis and prognosis, through different downstream pathways. However, a sensitive method for absolute quantification of WT1 is a prerequisite for understanding its involvement in ALL.

Conclusion

The early identification of recurrent and novel gene mutations underlying pediatric ALL could prove vital in disease diagnosis, prognosis and therapeutic stratification. Subsequently, novel and highly sensitive technologies are required for a better understanding of the mechanisms underlying leukemogenesis, as well as treatment evaluation, early detection of relapse, before it is clinically apparent and tailored therapy.

References

[1] Klug CA, Morrison SJ, Masek M, et al. Hematopoietic stem cells and lymphoid progenitors express different Ikaros isoforms, and Ikaros is localized to heterochromatin in immature lymphocytes. *Proc Natl Acad Sci* U S A 1998;95 (2):657-62.
[2] Sun L, Heerema N, Crotty L, et al.. Expression of dominant-negative and mutant isoforms of the antileukemic transcription factor Ikaros in infant acute lymphoblastic leukemia. *Proc Natl Acad Sci* U S A 1999;96 (2):680-5.
[3] Rebollo A, Schmitt C. Ikaros, Aiolos and Helios: transcription regulators and lymphoid malignancies. *Immunol Cell Biol* 2003;81 (3):171-5.
[4] Sun L, Crotty ML, Sensel M, et al. Expression of dominant-negative Ikaros isoforms in T-cell acute lymphoblastic leukemia. *Clin Cancer Res* 1999;5 (8):2112-20.
[5] Matulic M, Paradzik M, Puskaric BJ, et al. Analysis of Ikaros family splicing variants in human hematopoietic lineages. *Coll Antropol;*34 (1):59-62.
[6] Georgopoulos K, Bigby M, Wang JH, et al. The Ikaros gene is required for the development of all lymphoid lineages. *Cell* 1994;79 (1):143-56.
[7] Kirstetter P, Thomas M, Dierich A, et al. Ikaros is critical for B cell differentiation and function. *Eur J Immunol* 2002;32 (3):720-30.
[8] Wang JH, Nichogiannopoulou A, Wu L, S et al. Selective defects in the development of the fetal and adult lymphoid system in mice with an Ikaros null mutation. *Immunity* 1996;5 (6):537-49.
[9] Nichogiannopoulou A, Trevisan M, Neben S, et al. Defects in hemopoietic stem cell activity in Ikaros mutant mice. *J Exp Med* 1999;190 (9):1201-14.
[10] Wu L, Nichogiannopoulou A, Shortman K, et al. Cell-autonomous defects in dendritic cell populations of Ikaros mutant mice point to a developmental relationship with the lymphoid lineage. *Immunity* 1997;7 (4):483-92.
[11] Avitahl N, Winandy S, Friedrich C, et al. Ikaros sets thresholds for T cell activation and regulates chromosome propagation. *Immunity* 1999;10 (3):333-43.
[12] Winandy S, Wu P, Georgopoulos K. A dominant mutation in the Ikaros gene leads to rapid development of leukemia and lymphoma. *Cell* 1995;83 (2):289-99.
[13] Crescenzi B, La Starza R, Romoli S, et al. Submicroscopic deletions in 5q- associated malignancies. *Haematologica* 2004;89 (3):281-5.

[14] Nakase K, Ishimaru F, Avitahl N, et al. Dominant negative isoform of the Ikaros gene in patients with adult B-cell acute lymphoblastic leukemia. *Cancer Res* 2000;60 (15):4062-5.

[15] Nakayama H, Ishimaru F, Avitahl N, et al. Decreases in Ikaros activity correlate with blast crisis in patients with chronic myelogenous leukemia. *Cancer Res* 1999;59 (16):3931-4.

[16] Yagi T, Hibi S, Takanashi M, Kano G, et al. High frequency of Ikaros isoform 6 expression in acute myelomonocytic and monocytic leukemias: implications for up-regulation of the antiapoptotic protein Bcl-XL in leukemogenesis. *Blood* 2002;99 (4):1350-5.

[17] Mullighan CG, Su X, Zhang J, et al. Deletion of IKZF1 and prognosis in acute lymphoblastic leukemia. *N Engl J Med* 2009;360 (5):470-80.

[18] Kuiper RP, Schoenmakers EF, van Reijmersdal SV, et al. High-resolution genomic profiling of childhood ALL reveals novel recurrent genetic lesions affecting pathways involved in lymphocyte differentiation and cell cycle progression. *Leukemia* 2007;21 (6):1258-66.

[19] Maser RS, Choudhury B, Campbell PJ, et al. Chromosomally unstable mouse tumours have genomic alterations similar to diverse human cancers. *Nature* 2007;447 (7147):966-71.

[20] Ruiz A, Jiang J, Kempski H, et al. Overexpression of the Ikaros 6 isoform is restricted to t(4;11) acute lymphoblastic leukaemia in children and infants and has a role in B-cell survival. *Br J Haematol* 2004;125 (1):31-7.

[21] Marcais A, Jeannet R, Hernandez L, et al. Genetic inactivation of Ikaros is a rare event in human T-ALL. *Leuk Res;*34 (4):426-9.

[22] Sun L, Goodman PA, Wood CM, et al. Expression of aberrantly spliced oncogenic ikaros isoforms in childhood acute lymphoblastic leukemia. *J Clin Oncol* 1999;17 (12):3753-66.

[23] Nishii K, Katayama N, Miwa H, et al. Non-DNA-binding Ikaros isoform gene expressed in adult B-precursor acute lymphoblastic leukemia. *Leukemia* 2002;16 (7):1285-92.

[24] Kano G, Morimoto A, Takanashi M, et al. Ikaros dominant negative isoform (Ik6) induces IL-3-independent survival of murine pro-B lymphocytes by activating JAK-STAT and up-regulating Bcl-xl levels. *Leuk Lymphoma* 2008;49 (5):965-73.

[25] Mullighan CG, Miller CB, Radtke I, et al. BCR-ABL1 lymphoblastic leukaemia is characterized by the deletion of Ikaros. *Nature* 2008;453 (7191):110-4.

[26] Daley GQ, Van Etten RA, Baltimore D. Blast crisis in a murine model of chronic myelogenous leukemia. *Proc Natl Acad Sci* U S A 1991;88 (24):11335-8.

[27] Williams RT, Roussel MF, Sherr CJ. Arf gene loss enhances oncogenicity and limits imatinib response in mouse models of Bcr-Abl-induced acute lymphoblastic leukemia. *Proc Natl Acad Sci* U S A 2006;103 (17):6688-93.

[28] Mullighan CG, Phillips LA, Su X, et al. Genomic analysis of the clonal origins of relapsed acute lymphoblastic leukemia. *Science* 2008;322 (5906):1377-80.

[29] Iacobucci I, Lonetti A, Messa F, et al. Expression of spliced oncogenic Ikaros isoforms in Philadelphia-positive acute lymphoblastic leukemia patients treated with tyrosine

kinase inhibitors: implications for a new mechanism of resistance. *Blood* 2008;112 (9):3847-55.

[30] Klein F, Feldhahn N, Herzog S, et al M. BCR-ABL1 induces aberrant splicing of IKAROS and lineage infidelity in pre-B lymphoblastic leukemia cells. *Oncogene* 2006;25 (7):1118-24.

[31] Martinelli G, Iacobucci I, Storlazzi CT, et al. IKZF1 (Ikaros) deletions in BCR-ABL1-positive acute lymphoblastic leukemia are associated with short disease-free survival and high rate of cumulative incidence of relapse: a GIMEMA AL WP report. *J Clin Oncol* 2009;27 (31):5202-7.

[32] van Scherpenzeel Thim V, Remacle S, Picard J, et al. Mutation analysis of the HOX paralogous 4-13 genes in children with acute lymphoid malignancies: identification of a novel germline mutation of HOXD4 leading to a partial loss-of-function. *Hum Mutat* 2005;25 (4):384-95.

[33] Whelan JT, Ludwig DL, Bertrand FE. HoxA9 induces insulin-like growth factor-1 receptor expression in B-lineage acute lymphoblastic leukemia. *Leukemia* 2008;22 (6):1161-9.

[34] Shimamoto T, Ohyashiki K, Toyama K, et al. Homeobox genes in hematopoiesis and leukemogenesis. *Int J Hematol* 1998;67 (4):339-50.

[35] Garcia-Fernandez J. Hox, ParaHox, ProtoHox: facts and guesses. *Heredity* 2005;94 (2):145-52.

[36] Rice KL, Licht JD. HOX deregulation in acute myeloid leukemia. *J Clin Invest* 2007;117 (4):865-8.

[37] Perkins A, Kongsuwan K, Visvader J, et al. Homeobox gene expression plus autocrine growth factor production elicits myeloid leukemia. *Proc Natl Acad Sci U S A* 1990;87 (21):8398-402.

[38] Sauvageau G, Thorsteinsdottir U, Hough MR, et al. Overexpression of HOXB3 in hematopoietic cells causes defective lymphoid development and progressive myeloproliferation. *Immunity* 1997;6 (1):13-22.

[39] Thorsteinsdottir U, Sauvageau G, Hough MR, et al. Overexpression of HOXA10 in murine hematopoietic cells perturbs both myeloid and lymphoid differentiation and leads to acute myeloid leukemia. *Mol Cell Biol* 1997;17 (1):495-505.

[40] Starkova J, Zamostna B, Mejstrikova E, et al. HOX gene expression in phenotypic and genotypic subgroups and low HOXA gene expression as an adverse prognostic factor in pediatric ALL. *Pediatr Blood Cancer;*55 (6):1072-82.

[41] Fischbach NA, Rozenfeld S, Shen W, et al. HOXB6 overexpression in murine bone marrow immortalizes a myelomonocytic precursor in vitro and causes hematopoietic stem cell expansion and acute myeloid leukemia in vivo. *Blood* 2005;105 (4):1456-66.

[42] Borrow J, Shearman AM, Stanton VP, Jr., et al. The t(7;11)(p15;p15) translocation in acute myeloid leukaemia fuses the genes for nucleoporin NUP98 and class I homeoprotein HOXA9. *Nat Genet* 1996;12 (2):159-67.

[43] Soulier J, Clappier E, Cayuela JM, et al. HOXA genes are included in genetic and biologic networks defining human acute T-cell leukemia (T-ALL). *Blood* 2005;106 (1):274-86.

[44] Ferrando AA, Armstrong SA, Neuberg DS, et al. Gene expression signatures in MLL-rearranged T-lineage and B-precursor acute leukemias: dominance of HOX dysregulation. *Blood* 2003;102 (1):262-8.

[45] Quentmeier H, Dirks WG, Macleod RA, et al. Expression of HOX genes in acute leukemia cell lines with and without MLL translocations. *Leuk Lymphoma* 2004;45 (3):567-74.

[46] Rosnet O, Buhring HJ, Marchetto S, et al. Human FLT3/FLK2 receptor tyrosine kinase is expressed at the surface of normal and malignant hematopoietic cells. *Leukemia* 1996;10 (2):238-48.

[47] Abu-Duhier FM, Goodeve AC, Wilson GA, et al. Genomic structure of human FLT3: implications for mutational analysis. *Br J Haematol* 2001;113 (4):1076-7.

[48] Agnes F, Shamoon B, Dina C, et al. Genomic structure of the downstream part of the human FLT3 gene: exon/intron structure conservation among genes encoding receptor tyrosine kinases (RTK) of subclass III. *Gene* 1994;145 (2):283-8.

[49] Rosnet O, Birnbaum D. Hematopoietic receptors of class III receptor-type tyrosine kinases. *Crit Rev Oncog* 1993;4 (6):595-613.

[50] Lavagna-Sevenier C, Marchetto S, Birnbaum D, et al. FLT3 signaling in hematopoietic cells involves CBL, SHC and an unknown P115 as prominent tyrosine-phosphorylated substrates. *Leukemia* 1998;12 (3):301-10.

[51] Srinivasa SP, Doshi PD. Extracellular signal-regulated kinase and p38 mitogen-activated protein kinase pathways cooperate in mediating cytokine-induced proliferation of a leukemic cell line. *Leukemia* 2002;16 (2):244-53.

[52] Zhang S, Broxmeyer HE. p85 subunit of PI3 kinase does not bind to human Flt3 receptor, but associates with SHP2, SHIP, and a tyrosine-phosphorylated 100-kDa protein in Flt3 ligand-stimulated hematopoietic cells. *Biochem Biophys Res Commun* 1999;254 (2):440-5.

[53] Zhang S, Broxmeyer HE. Flt3 ligand induces tyrosine phosphorylation of gab1 and gab2 and their association with shp-2, grb2, and PI3 kinase. *Biochem Biophys Res Commun* 2000;277 (1):195-9.

[54] Zhang S, Mantel C, Broxmeyer HE. Flt3 signaling involves tyrosyl-phosphorylation of SHP-2 and SHIP and their association with Grb2 and Shc in Baf3/Flt3 cells. *J Leukoc Biol* 1999;65 (3):372-80.

[55] Markovic A, MacKenzie KL, Lock RB. FLT-3: a new focus in the understanding of acute leukemia. *Int J Biochem Cell Biol* 2005;37 (6):1168-72.

[56] Brasel K, Escobar S, Anderberg R, et al. Expression of the flt3 receptor and its ligand on hematopoietic cells. *Leukemia* 1995;9 (7):1212-8.

[57] Meierhoff G, Dehmel U, Gruss HJ, et al. Expression of FLT3 receptor and FLT3-ligand in human leukemia-lymphoma cell lines. *Leukemia* 1995;9 (8):1368-72.

[58] Gabbianelli M, Pelosi E, Montesoro E, et al. Multi-level effects of flt3 ligand on human hematopoiesis: expansion of putative stem cells and proliferation of granulomonocytic progenitors/monocytic precursors. *Blood* 1995;86 (5):1661-70.

[59] Rusten LS, Lyman SD, Veiby OP, et al. The FLT3 ligand is a direct and potent stimulator of the growth of primitive and committed human CD34+ bone marrow progenitor cells in vitro. *Blood* 1996;87 (4):1317-25.

[60] Shah AJ, Smogorzewska EM, Hannum C, et al. Flt3 ligand induces proliferation of quiescent human bone marrow CD34+CD38- cells and maintains progenitor cells in vitro. *Blood* 1996;87 (9):3563-70.
[61] Moore TA, Zlotnik A. Differential effects of Flk-2/Flt-3 ligand and stem cell factor on murine thymic progenitor cells. *J Immunol* 1997;158 (9):4187-92.
[62] Namikawa R, Muench MO, de Vries JE, et al. The FLK2/FLT3 ligand synergizes with interleukin-7 in promoting stromal-cell-independent expansion and differentiation of human fetal pro-B cells in vitro. *Blood* 1996;87 (5):1881-90.
[63] Ray RJ, Paige CJ, Furlonger C, et al. Flt3 ligand supports the differentiation of early B cell progenitors in the presence of interleukin-11 and interleukin-7. *Eur J Immunol* 1996;26 (7):1504-10.
[64] Piacibello W, Fubini L, Sanavio F, et al. Effects of human FLT3 ligand on myeloid leukemia cell growth: heterogeneity in response and synergy with other hematopoietic growth factors. *Blood* 1995;86 (11):4105-14.
[65] Dehmel U, Zaborski M, Meierhoff G, et al. Effects of FLT3 ligand on human leukemia cells. I. Proliferative response of myeloid leukemia cells. *Leukemia* 1996;10 (2):261-70.
[66] McKenna HJ, Smith FO, Brasel K, et al. Effects of flt3 ligand on acute myeloid and lymphocytic leukemic blast cells from children. *Exp Hematol* 1996;24 (2):378-85.
[67] Mackarehtschian K, Hardin JD, Moore KA, et al. Targeted disruption of the flk2/flt3 gene leads to deficiencies in primitive hematopoietic progenitors. *Immunity* 1995;3 (1):147-61.
[68] Juan TS, McNiece IK, Van G, et al. Chronic expression of murine flt3 ligand in mice results in increased circulating white blood cell levels and abnormal cellular infiltrates associated with splenic fibrosis. *Blood* 1997;90 (1):76-84.
[69] Hawley TS, Fong AZ, Griesser H, et al. Leukemic predisposition of mice transplanted with gene-modified hematopoietic precursors expressing flt3 ligand. *Blood* 1998;92 (6):2003-11.
[70] Hayakawa F, Towatari M, Kiyoi H, et al. Tandem-duplicated Flt3 constitutively activates STAT5 and MAP kinase and introduces autonomous cell growth in IL-3-dependent cell lines. *Oncogene* 2000;19 (5):624-31.
[71] Birg F, Courcoul M, Rosnet O, et al. Expression of the FMS/KIT-like gene FLT3 in human acute leukemias of the myeloid and lymphoid lineages. *Blood* 1992;80 (10):2584-93.
[72] Birg F, Rosnet O, Carbuccia N, et al. The expression of FMS, KIT and FLT3 in hematopoietic malignancies. *Leuk Lymphoma* 1994;13 (3-4):223-7.
[73] Carow CE, Levenstein M, Kaufmann SH, et al. Expression of the hematopoietic growth factor receptor FLT3 (STK-1/Flk2) in human leukemias. *Blood* 1996;87 (3):1089-96.
[74] DaSilva N, Hu ZB, Ma W, et al. Expression of the FLT3 gene in human leukemia-lymphoma cell lines. *Leukemia* 1994;8 (5):885-8.
[75] Kiyoi H, Naoe T, Yokota S, et al. Internal tandem duplication of FLT3 associated with leukocytosis in acute promyelocytic leukemia. Leukemia Study Group of the Ministry of Health and Welfare (Kohseisho). *Leukemia* 1997;11 (9):1447-52.

[76] Yokota S, Kiyoi H, Nakao M, et al Internal tandem duplication of the FLT3 gene is preferentially seen in acute myeloid leukemia and myelodysplastic syndrome among various hematological malignancies. A study on a large series of patients and cell lines. *Leukemia* 1997;11 (10):1605-9.

[77] Kiyoi H, Naoe T, Nakano Y, et al. Prognostic implication of FLT3 and N-RAS gene mutations in acute myeloid leukemia. *Blood* 1999;93 (9):3074-80.

[78] Kondo M, Horibe K, Takahashi Y, et al. Prognostic value of internal tandem duplication of the FLT3 gene in childhood acute myelogenous leukemia. *Med Pediatr Oncol* 1999;33 (6):525-9.

[79] Rombouts WJ, Blokland I, Lowenberg B, et al. Biological characteristics and prognosis of adult acute myeloid leukemia with internal tandem duplications in the Flt3 gene. *Leukemia* 2000;14 (4):675-83.

[80] Gilliland DG, Griffin JD. Role of FLT3 in leukemia. *Curr Opin Hematol* 2002;9 (4):274-81.

[81] Horiike S, Yokota S, Nakao M, et al. Tandem duplications of the FLT3 receptor gene are associated with leukemic transformation of myelodysplasia. *Leukemia* 1997;11 (9):1442-6.

[82] Nakao M, Yokota S, Iwai T, et al. Internal tandem duplication of the flt3 gene found in acute myeloid leukemia. *Leukemia* 1996;10 (12):1911-8.

[83] Schnittger S, Schoch C, Dugas M, et al. Analysis of FLT3 length mutations in 1003 patients with acute myeloid leukemia: correlation to cytogenetics, FAB subtype, and prognosis in the AMLCG study and usefulness as a marker for the detection of minimal residual disease. *Blood* 2002;100 (1):59-66.

[84] Lisovsky M, Estrov Z, Zhang X, et al. Flt3 ligand stimulates proliferation and inhibits apoptosis of acute myeloid leukemia cells: regulation of Bcl-2 and Bax. *Blood* 1996;88 (10):3987-97.

[85] Fenski R, Flesch K, Serve S, et al. Constitutive activation of FLT3 in acute myeloid leukaemia and its consequences for growth of 32D cells. *Br J Haematol* 2000;108 (2):322-30.

[86] Kiyoi H, Ohno R, Ueda R, et al. Mechanism of constitutive activation of FLT3 with internal tandem duplication in the juxtamembrane domain. *Oncogene* 2002;21 (16):2555-63.

[87] Mizuki M, Fenski R, Halfter H, et al. Flt3 mutations from patients with acute myeloid leukemia induce transformation of 32D cells mediated by the Ras and STAT5 pathways. *Blood* 2000;96 (12):3907-14.

[88] Iwai T, Yokota S, Nakao M, et al. Internal tandem duplication of the FLT3 gene and clinical evaluation in childhood acute myeloid leukemia. The Children's Cancer and Leukemia Study Group, Japan. *Leukemia* 1999;13 (1):38-43.

[89] Meshinchi S, Woods WG, Stirewalt DL, et al. Prevalence and prognostic significance of Flt3 internal tandem duplication in pediatric acute myeloid leukemia. *Blood* 2001;97 (1):89-94.

[90] Thiede C, Steudel C, Mohr B, et al. Analysis of FLT3-activating mutations in 979 patients with acute myelogenous leukemia: association with FAB subtypes and identification of subgroups with poor prognosis. *Blood* 2002;99 (12):4326-35.

[91] Xu F, Taki T, Yang HW, et al. Tandem duplication of the FLT3 gene is found in acute lymphoblastic leukaemia as well as acute myeloid leukaemia but not in myelodysplastic syndrome or juvenile chronic myelogenous leukaemia in children. *Br J Haematol* 1999;105 (1):155-62.

[92] Van Vlierberghe P, Meijerink JP, Stam RW, et al. Activating FLT3 mutations in CD4+/CD8- pediatric T-cell acute lymphoblastic leukemias. *Blood* 2005;106 (13):4414-5.

[93] Karabacak BH, Erbey F, Bayram I, et al. Fms-like tyrosine kinase 3 mutations in childhood acute leukemias and their association with prognosis. *Asian Pac J Cancer Prev;*11 (4):923-7.

[94] Libura M, Asnafi V, Tu A, et al. FLT3 and MLL intragenic abnormalities in AML reflect a common category of genotoxic stress. *Blood* 2003;102 (6):2198-204.

[95] Armstrong SA, Mabon ME, Silverman LB, et al FLT3 mutations in childhood acute lymphoblastic leukemia. *Blood* 2004;103 (9):3544-6.

[96] Abu-Duhier FM, Goodeve AC, Wilson GA, et al. Identification of novel FLT-3 Asp835 mutations in adult acute myeloid leukaemia. *Br J Haematol* 2001;113 (4):983-8.

[97] Morley GM, Uden M, Gullick WJ, et al. Cell specific transformation by c-fms activating loop mutations is attributable to constitutive receptor degradation. *Oncogene* 1999;18 (20):3076-84.

[98] Yamamoto Y, Kiyoi H, Nakano Y, et al. Activating mutation of D835 within the activation loop of FLT3 in human hematologic malignancies. *Blood* 2001;97 (8):2434-9.

[99] Spiekermann K, Bagrintseva K, Schoch C, et al. A new and recurrent activating length mutation in exon 20 of the FLT3 gene in acute myeloid leukemia. *Blood* 2002;100 (9):3423-5.

[100] Kindler T, Breitenbuecher F, Kasper S, et al. Identification of a novel activating mutation (Y842C) within the activation loop of FLT3 in patients with acute myeloid leukemia (AML). *Blood* 2005;105 (1):335-40.

[101] Jiang J, Paez JG, Lee JC, et al. Identifying and characterizing a novel activating mutation of the FLT3 tyrosine kinase in AML. *Blood* 2004;104 (6):1855-8.

[102] Taketani T, Taki T, Sugita K, et al. FLT3 mutations in the activation loop of tyrosine kinase domain are frequently found in infant ALL with MLL rearrangements and pediatric ALL with hyperdiploidy. *Blood* 2004;103 (3):1085-8.

[103] Wellmann S, Moderegger E, Zelmer A, et al. FLT3 mutations in childhood acute lymphoblastic leukemia at first relapse. *Leukemia* 2005;19 (3):467-8.

[104] Braoudaki M, Karpusas M, Katsibardi K, et al. Frequency of FLT3 mutations in childhood acute lymphoblastic leukemia. *Med Oncol* 2009;26 (4):460-2.

[105] Grabher C, von Boehmer H, Look AT. Notch 1 activation in the molecular pathogenesis of T-cell acute lymphoblastic leukaemia. *Nat Rev Cancer* 2006;6 (5):347-59.

[106] Radtke F, Raj K. The role of Notch in tumorigenesis: oncogene or tumour suppressor? *Nat Rev Cancer* 2003;3 (10):756-67.

[107] Bellavia D, Mecarozzi M, Campese AF, et al. Notch and Ikaros: not only converging players in T cell leukemia. *Cell Cycle* 2007;6 (22):2730-4.

[108] Breit S, Stanulla M, Flohr T, et al. Activating NOTCH1 mutations predict favorable early treatment response and long-term outcome in childhood precursor T-cell lymphoblastic leukemia. *Blood* 2006;108 (4):1151-7.

[109] Chiaramonte R, Basile A, Tassi E, et al. A wide role for NOTCH1 signaling in acute leukemia. *Cancer Lett* 2005;219 (1):113-20.

[110] Sulis ML, Williams O, Palomero T, et al. NOTCH1 extracellular juxtamembrane expansion mutations in T-ALL. *Blood* 2008;112 (3):733-40.

[111] Jundt F, Schwarzer R, Dorken B. Notch signaling in leukemias and lymphomas. *Curr Mol Med* 2008;8 (1):51-9.

[112] Weng AP, Nam Y, Wolfe MS, et al. Growth suppression of pre-T acute lymphoblastic leukemia cells by inhibition of notch signaling. *Mol Cell Biol* 2003;23 (2):655-64.

[113] Reynolds TC, Smith SD, Sklar J. Analysis of DNA surrounding the breakpoints of chromosomal translocations involving the beta T cell receptor gene in human lymphoblastic neoplasms. *Cell* 1987;50 (1):107-17.

[114] Holowiecki J. NOTCH1 pathway: a molecular target in T-cell cancers? *Lancet* 2005;365 (9455):197-9.

[115] Sharma VM, Calvo JA, Draheim KM, et al. Notch1 contributes to mouse T-cell leukemia by directly inducing the expression of c-myc. *Mol Cell Biol* 2006;26 (21):8022-31.

[116] Malecki MJ, Sanchez-Irizarry C, Mitchell JL, et al. Leukemia-associated mutations within the NOTCH1 heterodimerization domain fall into at least two distinct mechanistic classes. *Mol Cell Biol* 2006;26 (12):4642-51.

[117] Ferrando AA. The role of NOTCH1 signaling in T-ALL. *Hematology Am Soc Hematol Educ Program* 2009:353-61.

[118] Aster JC. Deregulated NOTCH signaling in acute T-cell lymphoblastic leukemia/ lymphoma: new insights, questions, and opportunities. *Int J Hematol* 2005;82 (4):295-301.

[119] Espinosa L, Cathelin S, D'Altri T, et al. The Notch/Hes1 pathway sustains NF-kappaB activation through CYLD repression in T cell leukemia. *Cancer Cell;*18 (3):268-81.

[120] Larson Gedman A, Chen Q, Kugel Desmoulin S, et al. The impact of NOTCH1, FBW7 and PTEN mutations on prognosis and downstream signaling in pediatric T-cell acute lymphoblastic leukemia: a report from the Children's Oncology Group. *Leukemia* 2009;23 (8):1417-25.

[121] Screpanti I, Bellavia D, Campese AF, et al. Notch, a unifying target in T-cell acute lymphoblastic leukemia? *Trends Mol Med* 2003;9 (1):30-5.

[122] Pear WS, Aster JC, Scott ML, et al. Exclusive development of T cell neoplasms in mice transplanted with bone marrow expressing activated Notch alleles. *J Exp Med* 1996;183 (5):2283-91.

[123] Pui JC, Allman D, Xu L, et al. Notch1 expression in early lymphopoiesis influences B versus T lineage determination. *Immunity* 1999;11 (3):299-308.

[124] Radtke F, Wilson A, Stark G, et al. Deficient T cell fate specification in mice with an induced inactivation of Notch1. *Immunity* 1999;10 (5):547-58.

[125] Izon DJ, Aster JC, He Y, et al. Deltex1 redirects lymphoid progenitors to the B cell lineage by antagonizing Notch1. *Immunity* 2002;16 (2):231-43.

[126] Rohn JL, Lauring AS, Linenberger ML, et al. Transduction of Notch2 in feline leukemia virus-induced thymic lymphoma. *J Virol* 1996;70 (11):8071-80.

[127] Allman D, Karnell FG, Punt JA, et al. Separation of Notch1 promoted lineage commitment and expansion/transformation in developing T cells. *J Exp Med* 2001;194 (1):99-106.

[128] Bellavia D, Campese AF, Checquolo S, et al. Combined expression of pTalpha and Notch3 in T cell leukemia identifies the requirement of preTCR for leukemogenesis. *Proc Natl Acad Sci U S A* 2002;99 (6):3788-93.

[129] Reizis B, Leder P. Direct induction of T lymphocyte-specific gene expression by the mammalian Notch signaling pathway. *Genes Dev* 2002;16 (3):295-300.

[130] Campese AF, Garbe AI, Zhang F, et al. Notch1-dependent lymphomagenesis is assisted by but does not essentially require pre-TCR signaling. *Blood* 2006;108 (1):305-10.

[131] Bain G, Engel I, Robanus Maandag EC, et al. E2A deficiency leads to abnormalities in alphabeta T-cell development and to rapid development of T-cell lymphomas. *Mol Cell Biol* 1997;17 (8):4782-91.

[132] Busslinger M. Transcriptional control of early B cell development. *Annu Rev Immunol* 2004;22:55-79.

[133] Engel I, Murre C. Disruption of pre-TCR expression accelerates lymphomagenesis in E2A-deficient mice. *Proc Natl Acad Sci U S A* 2002;99 (17):11322-7.

[134] Engel I, Murre C. E2A proteins enforce a proliferation checkpoint in developing thymocytes. *Embo J* 2004;23 (1):202-11.

[135] Huang Z, Nie L, Xu M, et al. Notch-induced E2A degradation requires CHIP and Hsc70 as novel facilitators of ubiquitination. *Mol Cell Biol* 2004;24 (20):8951-62.

[136] Nie L, Xu M, Vladimirova A, et al. Notch-induced E2A ubiquitination and degradation are controlled by MAP kinase activities. *Embo J* 2003;22 (21):5780-92.

[137] Ordentlich P, Lin A, Shen CP, et al. Notch inhibition of E47 supports the existence of a novel signaling pathway. *Mol Cell Biol* 1998;18 (4):2230-9.

[138] Talora C, Campese AF, Bellavia D, et al. Pre-TCR-triggered ERK signalling-dependent downregulation of E2A activity in Notch3-induced T-cell lymphoma. *EMBO Rep* 2003;4 (11):1067-72.

[139] Bash RO, Hall S, Timmons CF, et al. Does activation of the TAL1 gene occur in a majority of patients with T-cell acute lymphoblastic leukemia? A pediatric oncology group study. *Blood* 1995;86 (2):666-76.

[140] Brown L, Cheng JT, Chen Q, et al. Site-specific recombination of the tal-1 gene is a common occurrence in human T cell leukemia. *Embo J* 1990;9 (10):3343-51.

[141] O'Neil J, Shank J, Cusson N, et al. TAL1/SCL induces leukemia by inhibiting the transcriptional activity of E47/HEB. *Cancer Cell* 2004;5 (6):587-96.

[142] Talora C, Cialfi S, Oliviero C, et al. Cross talk among Notch3, pre-TCR, and Tal1 in T-cell development and leukemogenesis. *Blood* 2006;107 (8):3313-20.

[143] Sharma VM, Draheim KM, Kelliher MA. The Notch1/c-Myc pathway in T cell leukemia. *Cell Cycle* 2007;6 (8):927-30.

[144] Weng AP, Millholland JM, Yashiro-Ohtani Y, et al. c-Myc is an important direct target of Notch1 in T-cell acute lymphoblastic leukemia/lymphoma. *Genes Dev* 2006;20 (15):2096-109.

[145] Gutierrez A, Look AT. NOTCH and PI3K-AKT pathways intertwined. *Cancer Cell* 2007;12 (5):411-3.

[146] Beverly LJ, Felsher DW, Capobianco AJ. Suppression of p53 by Notch in lymphomagenesis: implications for initiation and regression. *Cancer Res* 2005;65 (16):7159-68.

[147] Mungamuri SK, Yang X, Thor AD, et al. Survival signaling by Notch1: mammalian target of rapamycin (mTOR)-dependent inhibition of p53. *Cancer Res* 2006;66 (9):4715-24.

[148] Dotto GP. Crosstalk of Notch with p53 and p63 in cancer growth control. *Nat Rev Cancer* 2009;9 (8):587-95.

[149] Chan SM, Weng AP, Tibshirani R, et al. Notch signals positively regulate activity of the mTOR pathway in T-cell acute lymphoblastic leukemia. *Blood* 2007;110 (1):278-86.

[150] Vilimas T, Mascarenhas J, Palomero T, et al. Targeting the NF-kappaB signaling pathway in Notch1-induced T-cell leukemia. *Nat Med* 2007;13 (1):70-7.

[151] Beverly LJ, Capobianco AJ. Perturbation of Ikaros isoform selection by MLV integration is a cooperative event in Notch(IC)-induced T cell leukemogenesis. *Cancer Cell* 2003;3 (6):551-64.

[152] Dohda T, Maljukova A, Liu L, et al. Notch signaling induces SKP2 expression and promotes reduction of p27Kip1 in T-cell acute lymphoblastic leukemia cell lines. *Exp Cell Res* 2007;313 (14):3141-52.

[153] Joshi I, Minter LM, Telfer J, et al. Notch signaling mediates G1/S cell-cycle progression in T cells via cyclin D3 and its dependent kinases. *Blood* 2009;113 (8):1689-98.

[154] Rao SS, O'Neil J, Liberator CD, et al. Inhibition of NOTCH signaling by gamma secretase inhibitor engages the RB pathway and elicits cell cycle exit in T-cell acute lymphoblastic leukemia cells. *Cancer Res* 2009;69 (7):3060-8.

[155] Armstrong F, Brunet de la Grange P, Gerby B, et al. NOTCH is a key regulator of human T-cell acute leukemia initiating cell activity. *Blood* 2009;113 (8):1730-40.

[156] Chiang MY, Xu L, Shestova O, et al. Leukemia-associated NOTCH1 alleles are weak tumor initiators but accelerate K-ras-initiated leukemia. *J Clin Invest* 2008;118 (9):3181-94.

[157] Feldman BJ, Hampton T, Cleary ML. A carboxy-terminal deletion mutant of Notch1 accelerates lymphoid oncogenesis in E2A-PBX1 transgenic mice. *Blood* 2000;96 (5):1906-13.

[158] Girard L, Hanna Z, Beaulieu N, et al. Frequent provirus insertional mutagenesis of Notch1 in thymomas of MMTVD/myc transgenic mice suggests a collaboration of c-myc and Notch1 for oncogenesis. *Genes Dev* 1996;10 (15):1930-44.

[159] Mizuno T, Yamasaki N, Miyazaki K, et al. Overexpression/enhanced kinase activity of BCR/ABL and altered expression of Notch1 induced acute leukemia in p210BCR/ABL transgenic mice. *Oncogene* 2008;27 (24):3465-74.

[160] Mansour MR, Duke V, Foroni L, et al. Notch-1 mutations are secondary events in some patients with T-cell acute lymphoblastic leukemia. *Clin Cancer Res* 2007;13 (23):6964-9.

[161] Gordon WR, Roy M, Vardar-Ulu D, et al. Structure of the Notch1-negative regulatory region: implications for normal activation and pathogenic signaling in T-ALL. *Blood* 2009;113 (18):4381-90.

[162] O'Neil J, Grim J, Strack P, et al. FBW7 mutations in leukemic cells mediate NOTCH pathway activation and resistance to gamma-secretase inhibitors. *J Exp Med* 2007;204 (8):1813-24.

[163] Weng AP, Ferrando AA, Lee W, et al. Activating mutations of NOTCH1 in human T cell acute lymphoblastic leukemia. *Science* 2004;306 (5694):269-71.

[164] Eguchi-Ishimae M, Eguchi M, Kempski H, et al. NOTCH1 mutation can be an early, prenatal genetic event in T-ALL. *Blood* 2008;111 (1):376-8.

[165] Lin YW, Nichols RA, Letterio JJ, et al. Notch1 mutations are important for leukemic transformation in murine models of precursor-T leukemia/lymphoma. *Blood* 2006;107 (6):2540-3.

[166] Asnafi V, Buzyn A, Le Noir S, et al. NOTCH1/FBXW7 mutation identifies a large subgroup with favorable outcome in adult T-cell acute lymphoblastic leukemia (T-ALL): a Group for Research on Adult Acute Lymphoblastic Leukemia (GRAALL) study. *Blood* 2009;113 (17):3918-24.

[167] Park MJ, Taki T, Oda M, et al. FBXW7 and NOTCH1 mutations in childhood T cell acute lymphoblastic leukaemia and T cell non-Hodgkin lymphoma. *Br J Haematol* 2009;145 (2):198-206.

[168] Mansour MR, Sulis ML, Duke V, et al. Prognostic implications of NOTCH1 and FBXW7 mutations in adults with T-cell acute lymphoblastic leukemia treated on the MRC UKALLXII/ECOG E2993 protocol. *J Clin Oncol* 2009;27 (26):4352-6.

[169] Baldus CD, Thibaut J, Goekbuget N, et al Prognostic implications of NOTCH1 and FBXW7 mutations in adult acute T-lymphoblastic leukemia. *Haematologica* 2009;94 (10):1383-90.

[170] Coustan-Smith E, Mullighan CG, Onciu M, et al. Early T-cell precursor leukaemia: a subtype of very high-risk acute lymphoblastic leukaemia. *Lancet Oncol* 2009;10 (2):147-56.

[171] Erbilgin Y, Sayitoglu M, Hatirnaz O, et al. Prognostic significance of NOTCH1 and FBXW7 mutations in pediatric T-ALL. *Dis Markers;*28 (6):353-60.

[172] Masuda S, Kumano K, Suzuki T, et al. Dual antitumor mechanisms of Notch signaling inhibitor in a T-cell acute lymphoblastic leukemia xenograft model. *Cancer Sci* 2009;100 (12):2444-50.

[173] Liu TC, Lin PM, Chang JG, et al. Mutation analysis of PTEN/MMAC1 in acute myeloid leukemia. *Am J Hematol* 2000;63 (4):170-5.

[174] Chow LM, Baker SJ. PTEN function in normal and neoplastic growth. *Cancer Lett* 2006;241 (2):184-96.

[175] Silva A, Yunes JA, Cardoso BA, et al. PTEN posttranslational inactivation and hyperactivation of the PI3K/Akt pathway sustain primary T cell leukemia viability. *J Clin Invest* 2008;118 (11):3762-74.

[176] Gutierrez A, Sanda T, Grebliunaite R, et al. High frequency of PTEN, PI3K, and AKT abnormalities in T-cell acute lymphoblastic leukemia. *Blood* 2009;114 (3):647-50.

[177] Dahia PL, Aguiar RC, Alberta J, et al. PTEN is inversely correlated with the cell survival factor Akt/PKB and is inactivated via multiple mechanismsin haematological malignancies. *Hum Mol Genet* 1999;8 (2):185-93.

[178] Jotta PY, Ganazza MA, Silva A, et al. Negative prognostic impact of PTEN mutation in pediatric T-cell acute lymphoblastic leukemia. *Leukemia;*24 (1):239-42.

[179] Le DT, Shannon KM. Ras processing as a therapeutic target in hematologic malignancies. *Curr Opin Hematol* 2002;9 (4):308-15.

[180] Chung E, Kondo M. Role of Ras/Raf/MEK/ERK signaling in physiological hematopoiesis and leukemia development. *Immunol Res;*49 (1-3):248-68.

[181] Bos JL, Toksoz D, Marshall CJ, et al. Amino-acid substitutions at codon 13 of the N-ras oncogene in human acute myeloid leukaemia. *Nature* 1985;315 (6022):726-30.

[182] Farr CJ, Saiki RK, Erlich HA, et al. Analysis of RAS gene mutations in acute myeloid leukemia by polymerase chain reaction and oligonucleotide probes. *Proc Natl Acad Sci U S A* 1988;85 (5):1629-33.

[183] Needleman SW, Kraus MH, Srivastava SK, et al. High frequency of N-ras activation in acute myelogenous leukemia. *Blood* 1986;67 (3):753-7.

[184] Farr C, Gill R, Katz F, et al. Analysis of ras gene mutations in childhood myeloid leukaemia. *Br J Haematol* 1991;77 (3):323-7.

[185] Guo W, Tang B, Xu S, et al. N-ras mutations in 43 Chinese cases of acute myeloid leukemia. *Chin Med J* (Engl) 1998;111 (4):343-5.

[186] Zhang J, Wang J, Liu Y, et al. Oncogenic Kras-induced leukemogeneis: hematopoietic stem cells as the initial target and lineage-specific progenitors as the potential targets for final leukemic transformation. *Blood* 2009;113 (6):1304-14.

[187] Parikh C, Subrahmanyam R, Ren R. Oncogenic NRAS, KRAS, and HRAS exhibit different leukemogenic potentials in mice. *Cancer Res* 2007;67 (15):7139-46.

[188] Adams JM, Harris AW, Strasser A, et al. Transgenic models of lymphoid neoplasia and development of a pan-hematopoietic vector. *Oncogene* 1999;18 (38):5268-77.

[189] Hawley RG, Fong AZ, Ngan BY, et al. Hematopoietic transforming potential of activated ras in chimeric mice. *Oncogene* 1995;11 (6):1113-23.

[190] Dunbar CE, Crosier PS, Nienhuis AW. Introduction of an activated RAS oncogene into murine bone marrow lymphoid progenitors via retroviral gene transfer results in thymic lymphomas. *Oncogene Res* 1991;6 (1):39-51.

[191] Haupt Y, Harris AW, Adams JM. Retroviral infection accelerates T lymphomagenesis in E mu-N-ras transgenic mice by activating c-myc or N-myc. *Oncogene* 1992;7 (5):981-6.

[192] Braun BS, Tuveson DA, Kong N, et al. Somatic activation of oncogenic Kras in hematopoietic cells initiates a rapidly fatal myeloproliferative disorder. *Proc Natl Acad Sci U S A* 2004;101 (2):597-602.

[193] Chan IT, Kutok JL, Williams IR, et al. Conditional expression of oncogenic K-ras from its endogenous promoter induces a myeloproliferative disease. *J Clin Invest* 2004;113 (4):528-38.

[194] Sabnis AJ, Cheung LS, Dail M, et al. Oncogenic Kras initiates leukemia in hematopoietic stem cells. *PLoS Biol* 2009;7 (3):e59.
[195] von Lintig FC, Huvar I, Law P, et al. Ras activation in normal white blood cells and childhood acute lymphoblastic leukemia. *Clin Cancer Res* 2000;6 (5):1804-10.
[196] Scheele JS, Rhee JM, Boss GR. Determination of absolute amounts of GDP and GTP bound to Ras in mammalian cells: comparison of parental and Ras-overproducing NIH 3T3 fibroblasts. *Proc Natl Acad Sci U S A* 1995;92 (4):1097-100.
[197] Lubbert M, Mirro J, Jr., Miller CW, et al. N-ras gene point mutations in childhood acute lymphocytic leukemia correlate with a poor prognosis. *Blood* 1990;75 (5):1163-9.
[198] Dail M, Li Q, McDaniel A, et al. Mutant Ikzf1, KrasG12D, and Notch1 cooperate in T lineage leukemogenesis and modulate responses to targeted agents. *Proc Natl Acad Sci U S A*;107 (11):5106-11.
[199] Kindler T, Cornejo MG, Scholl C, et al. K-RasG12D-induced T-cell lymphoblastic lymphoma/leukemias harbor Notch1 mutations and are sensitive to gamma-secretase inhibitors. *Blood* 2008;112 (8):3373-82.
[200] Parikh C, Subrahmanyam R, Ren R. Oncogenic NRAS rapidly and efficiently induces CMML- and AML-like diseases in mice. *Blood* 2006;108 (7):2349-57.
[201] Raepple D, von Lintig F, Zemojtel T, et al. Determination of Ras-GTP and Ras-GDP in patients with acute myelogenous leukemia (AML), myeloproliferative syndrome (MPS), juvenile myelomonocytic leukemia (JMML), acute lymphocytic leukemia (ALL), and malignant lymphoma: assessment of mutational and indirect activation. *Ann Hematol* 2009;88 (4):319-24.
[202] Yokota S, Nakao M, Horiike S, et al. Mutational analysis of the N-ras gene in acute lymphoblastic leukemia: a study of 125 Japanese pediatric cases. *Int J Hematol* 1998;67 (4):379-87.
[203] Perentesis JP, Bhatia S, Boyle E, et al. RAS oncogene mutations and outcome of therapy for childhood acute lymphoblastic leukemia. *Leukemia* 2004;18 (4):685-92.
[204] Case M, Matheson E, Minto L, et al. Mutation of genes affecting the RAS pathway is common in childhood acute lymphoblastic leukemia. *Cancer Res* 2008;68 (16):6803-9.
[205] Paulsson K, Horvat A, Strombeck B, et al. Mutations of FLT3, NRAS, KRAS, and PTPN11 are frequent and possibly mutually exclusive in high hyperdiploid childhood acute lymphoblastic leukemia. *Genes Chromosomes Cancer* 2008;47 (1):26-33.
[206] Wiemels JL, Zhang Y, Chang J, et al. RAS mutation is associated with hyperdiploidy and parental characteristics in pediatric acute lymphoblastic leukemia. *Leukemia* 2005;19 (3):415-9.
[207] Wiemels JL, Kang M, Chang JS, et al. Backtracking RAS mutations in high hyperdiploid childhood acute lymphoblastic leukemia. *Blood Cells Mol Dis;*45 (3):186-91.
[208] Coffey MC, Strong JE, Forsyth PA, et al. Reovirus therapy of tumors with activated Ras pathway. *Science* 1998;282 (5392):1332-4.
[209] Gibbs JB, Oliff A, Kohl NE. Farnesyltransferase inhibitors: Ras research yields a potential cancer therapeutic. *Cell* 1994;77 (2):175-8.

[210] Kawamura M, Kikuchi A, Kobayashi S, et al. Mutations of the p53 and ras genes in childhood t(1;19)-acute lymphoblastic leukemia. *Blood* 1995;85 (9):2546-52.

[211] Dosen G, Tenstad E, Nygren MK, et al. Wnt expression and canonical Wnt signaling in human bone marrow B lymphopoiesis. *BMC Immunol* 2006;7:13.

[212] Staal FJ, van Dongen JJ, Langerak AW. Novel insights into the development of T-cell acute lymphoblastic leukemia. *Curr Hematol Malig Rep* 2007;2 (3):176-82.

[213] Weerkamp F, van Dongen JJ, Staal FJ. Notch and Wnt signaling in T-lymphocyte development and acute lymphoblastic leukemia. *Leukemia* 2006;20 (7):1197-205.

[214] Nygren MK, Dosen G, Hystad ME, et al. Wnt3A activates canonical Wnt signalling in acute lymphoblastic leukaemia (ALL) cells and inhibits the proliferation of B-ALL cell lines. *Br J Haematol* 2007;136 (3):400-13.

[215] Doubravska L, Simova S, Cermak L, et al. Wnt-expressing rat embryonic fibroblasts suppress Apo2L/TRAIL-induced apoptosis of human leukemia cells. *Apoptosis* 2008;13 (4):573-87.

[216] Casagrande G, te Kronnie G, Basso G. The effects of siRNA-mediated inhibition of E2A-PBX1 on EB-1 and Wnt16b expression in the 697 pre-B leukemia cell line. *Haematologica* 2006;91 (6):765-71.

[217] Nygren MK, Dosen-Dahl G, Stubberud H, et al. beta-catenin is involved in N-cadherin-dependent adhesion, but not in canonical Wnt signaling in E2A-PBX1-positive B acute lymphoblastic leukemia cells. *Exp Hematol* 2009;37 (2):225-33.

[218] Menssen HD, Siehl JM, Thiel E. Wilms tumor gene (WT1) expression as a panleukemic marker. *Int J Hematol* 2002;76 (2):103-9.

[219] Dey BR, Sukhatme VP, Roberts AB, et al. Repression of the transforming growth factor-beta 1 gene by the Wilms' tumor suppressor WT1 gene product. *Mol Endocrinol* 1994;8 (5):595-602.

[220] Drummond IA, Madden SL, Rohwer-Nutter P, et al. Repression of the insulin-like growth factor II gene by the Wilms tumor suppressor WT1. *Science* 1992;257 (5070):674-8.

[221] Englert C, Hou X, Maheswaran S, et al. WT1 suppresses synthesis of the epidermal growth factor receptor and induces apoptosis. *Embo J* 1995;14 (19):4662-75.

[222] Gashler AL, Bonthron DT, Madden SL, et al. Human platelet-derived growth factor A chain is transcriptionally repressed by the Wilms tumor suppressor WT1. *Proc Natl Acad Sci U S A* 1992;89 (22):10984-8.

[223] Harrington MA, Konicek B, Song A, et al. Inhibition of colony-stimulating factor-1 promoter activity by the product of the Wilms' tumor locus. *J Biol Chem* 1993;268 (28):21271-5.

[224] Hewitt SM, Hamada S, McDonnell TJ, et al. Regulation of the proto-oncogenes bcl-2 and c-myc by the Wilms' tumor suppressor gene WT1. *Cancer Res* 1995;55 (22):5386-9.

[225] Lee TH, Pelletier J. Functional characterization of WT1 binding sites within the human vitamin D receptor gene promoter. *Physiol Genomics* 2001;7 (2):187-200.

[226] Maurer U, Jehan F, Englert C, et al. The Wilms' tumor gene product (WT1) modulates the response to 1,25-dihydroxyvitamin D3 by induction of the vitamin D receptor. *J Biol Chem* 2001;276 (6):3727-32.

[227] Wang ZY, Madden SL, Deuel TF, et al. The Wilms' tumor gene product, WT1, represses transcription of the platelet-derived growth factor A-chain gene. *J Biol Chem* 1992;267 (31):21999-2002.

[228] Werner H, Re GG, Drummond IA, et al. Increased expression of the insulin-like growth factor I receptor gene, IGF1R, in Wilms tumor is correlated with modulation of IGF1R promoter activity by the WT1 Wilms tumor gene product. *Proc Natl Acad Sci U S A* 1993;90 (12):5828-32.

[229] Boublikova L, Kalinova M, Ryan J, et al. Wilms' tumor gene 1 (WT1) expression in childhood acute lymphoblastic leukemia: a wide range of WT1 expression levels, its impact on prognosis and minimal residual disease monitoring. *Leukemia* 2006;20 (2):254-63.

[230] Ellisen LW, Carlesso N, Cheng T, et al. The Wilms tumor suppressor WT1 directs stage-specific quiescence and differentiation of human hematopoietic progenitor cells. *Embo J* 2001;20 (8):1897-909.

[231] Baird PN, Simmons PJ. Expression of the Wilms' tumor gene (WT1) in normal hemopoiesis. *Exp Hematol* 1997;25 (4):312-20.

[232] Menssen HD, Renkl HJ, Rodeck U, et al. Presence of Wilms' tumor gene (wt1) transcripts and the WT1 nuclear protein in the majority of human acute leukemias. *Leukemia* 1995;9 (6):1060-7.

[233] Amin KM, Litzky LA, Smythe WR, et al. Wilms' tumor 1 susceptibility (WT1) gene products are selectively expressed in malignant mesothelioma. *Am J Pathol* 1995;146 (2):344-56.

[234] Bruening W, Gros P, Sato T, et al. Analysis of the 11p13 Wilms' tumor suppressor gene (WT1) in ovarian tumors. *Cancer Invest* 1993;11 (4):393-9.

[235] Campbell CE, Kuriyan NP, Rackley RR, et al. Constitutive expression of the Wilms tumor suppressor gene (WT1) in renal cell carcinoma. *Int J Cancer* 1998;78 (2):182-8.

[236] Ladanyi M, Gerald W. Fusion of the EWS and WT1 genes in the desmoplastic small round cell tumor. *Cancer Res* 1994;54 (11):2837-40.

[237] Langerak AW, Williamson KA, Miyagawa K, et al. Expression of the Wilms' tumor gene WT1 in human malignant mesothelioma cell lines and relationship to platelet-derived growth factor A and insulin-like growth factor 2 expression. *Genes Chromosomes Cancer* 1995;12 (2):87-96.

[238] Loeb DM, Evron E, Patel CB, et al. Wilms' tumor suppressor gene (WT1) is expressed in primary breast tumors despite tumor-specific promoter methylation. *Cancer Res* 2001;61 (3):921-5.

[239] Menssen HD, Bertelmann E, Bartelt S, et al K, Thiel E. Wilms' tumor gene (WT1) expression in lung cancer, colon cancer and glioblastoma cell lines compared to freshly isolated tumor specimens. *J Cancer Res Clin Oncol* 2000;126 (4):226-32.

[240] Oji Y, Ogawa H, Tamaki H, et al. Expression of the Wilms' tumor gene WT1 in solid tumors and its involvement in tumor cell growth. *Jpn J Cancer Res* 1999;90 (2):194-204.

[241] Park S, Schalling M, Bernard A, et al. The Wilms tumour gene WT1 is expressed in *murine mesoderm-derived tissues and mutated in a human mesothelioma.* Nat Genet 1993;4 (4):415-20.

[242] Rodeck U, Bossler A, Kari C, et al. Expression of the wt1 Wilms' tumor gene by normal and malignant human melanocytes. *Int J Cancer* 1994;59 (1):78-82.

[243] Silberstein GB, Van Horn K, Strickland P, et al. Altered expression of the WT1 wilms tumor suppressor gene in human breast cancer. *Proc Natl Acad Sci U S A* 1997;94 (15):8132-7.

[244] Viel A, Giannini F, Capozzi E, et al. Molecular mechanisms possibly affecting WT1 function in human ovarian tumors. *Int J Cancer* 1994;57 (4):515-21.

[245] Walker C, Rutten F, Yuan X, et al. Wilms' tumor suppressor gene expression in rat and human mesothelioma. *Cancer Res* 1994;54 (12):3101-6.

[246] Sugiyama H. WT1 (Wilms' tumor gene 1): biology and cancer immunotherapy. *Jpn J Clin Oncol;*40 (5):377-87.

[247] Kerst G, Bergold N, Gieseke F, et al. WT1 protein expression in childhood acute leukemia. *Am J Hematol* 2008;83 (5):382-6.

[248] Miyagawa K, Hayashi Y, Fukuda T, et al. Mutations of the WT1 gene in childhood nonlymphoid hematological malignancies. *Genes Chromosomes Cancer* 1999;25 (2):176-83.

[249] King-Underwood L, Renshaw J, Pritchard-Jones K. Mutations in the Wilms' tumor gene WT1 in leukemias. *Blood* 1996;87 (6):2171-9.

[250] Heesch S, Goekbuget N, Stroux A, et al. Prognostic implications of mutations and expression of the Wilms tumor 1 (WT1) gene in adult acute T-lymphoblastic leukemia. *Haematologica;*95 (6):942-9.

[251] Tosello V, Mansour MR, Barnes K, et al. WT1 mutations in T-ALL. *Blood* 2009;114 (5):1038-45.

[252] Barragan E, Cervera J, Bolufer P, et al. Prognostic implications of Wilms' tumor gene (WT1) expression in patients with de novo acute myeloid leukemia. *Haematologica* 2004;89 (8):926-33.

[253] Bergmann L, Miething C, Maurer U, et al. High levels of Wilms' tumor gene (wt1) mRNA in acute myeloid leukemias are associated with a worse long-term outcome. *Blood* 1997;90 (3):1217-25.

[254] Chen JS, Coustan-Smith E, Suzuki T, et al. Identification of novel markers for monitoring minimal residual disease in acute lymphoblastic leukemia. *Blood* 2001;97 (7):2115-20.

[255] Garg M, Moore H, Tobal K, et al. Prognostic significance of quantitative analysis of WT1 gene transcripts by competitive reverse transcription polymerase chain reaction in acute leukaemia. *Br J Haematol* 2003;123 (1):49-59.

[256] Kletzel M, Olzewski M, Huang W, et al. Utility of WT1 as a reliable tool for the detection of minimal residual disease in children with leukemia. *Pediatr Dev Pathol* 2002;5 (3):269-75.

[257] Magyarosy E, Varga N, Timar J, et al. Follow-up of minimal residual disease in acute childhood lymphoblastic leukemia by WT1 gene expression in the peripheral blood: the Hungarian experience. *Pediatr Hematol Oncol* 2003;20 (1):65-74.

[258] Schmid D, Heinze G, Linnerth B, et al. Prognostic significance of WT1 gene expression at diagnosis in adult de novo acute myeloid leukemia. *Leukemia* 1997;11 (5):639-43.

[259] Trka J, Kalinova M, Hrusak O, et al. Real-time quantitative PCR detection of WT1 gene expression in children with AML: prognostic significance, correlation with disease status and residual disease detection by flow cytometry. *Leukemia* 2002;16 (7):1381-9.
[260] Gaiger A, Linnerth B, Mann G, et al. Wilms' tumour gene (wt1) expression at diagnosis has no prognostic relevance in childhood acute lymphoblastic leukaemia treated by an intensive chemotherapy protocol. *Eur J Haematol* 1999;63 (2):86-93.
[261] Miwa H, Beran M, Saunders GF. Expression of the Wilms' tumor gene (WT1) in human leukemias. *Leukemia* 1992;6 (5):405-9.
[262] Inoue K, Sugiyama H, Ogawa H, et al. WT1 as a new prognostic factor and a new marker for the detection of minimal residual disease in acute leukemia. *Blood* 1994;84 (9):3071-9.
[263] Inoue K, Ogawa H, Yamagami T, et al. Long-term follow-up of minimal residual disease in leukemia patients by monitoring WT1 (Wilms tumor gene) expression levels. *Blood* 1996;88 (6):2267-78.
[264] Asgarian Omran H, Shabani M, Vossough P, et al. Cross-sectional monitoring of Wilms' tumor gene 1 (WT1) expression in Iranian patients with acute lymphoblastic leukemia at diagnosis, relapse and remission. *Leuk Lymphoma* 2008;49 (2):281-90.
[265] Im HJ, Kong G, Lee H. Expression of Wilms tumor gene (WT1) in children with acute leukemia. *Pediatr Hematol Oncol* 1999;16 (2):109-18.
[266] Kreuzer KA, Saborowski A, Lupberger J, et al. Fluorescent 5'-exonuclease assay for the absolute quantification of Wilms' tumour gene (WT1) mRNA: implications for monitoring human leukaemias. *Br J Haematol* 2001;114 (2):313-8.
[267] Sakatani T, Shimazaki C, Hirai H, et al. Early relapse after high-dose chemotherapy rescued by tumor-free autologous peripheral blood stem cells in acute lymphoblastic leukemia: importance of monitoring for WT1-mRNA quantitatively. *Leuk Lymphoma* 2001;42 (1-2):225-9.
[268] Siehl JM, Thiel E, Leben R, et al. Quantitative real-time RT-PCR detects elevated Wilms tumor gene (WT1) expression in autologous blood stem cell preparations (PBSCs) from acute myeloid leukemia (AML) patients indicating contamination with leukemic blasts. *Bone Marrow Transplant* 2002;29 (5):379-81.
[269] Cilloni D, Gottardi E, De Micheli D, et al. Quantitative assessment of WT1 expression by real time quantitative PCR may be a useful tool for monitoring minimal residual disease in acute leukemia patients. *Leukemia* 2002;16 (10):2115-21.
[270] Busse A, Gokbuget N, Siehl JM, et al. Wilms' tumor gene 1 (WT1) expression in subtypes of acute lymphoblastic leukemia (ALL) of adults and impact on clinical outcome. *Ann Hematol* 2009;88 (12):1199-205.
[271] Ogawa H, Tamaki H, Ikegame K, et al. The usefulness of monitoring WT1 gene transcripts for the prediction and management of relapse following allogeneic stem cell transplantation in acute type leukemia. *Blood* 2003;101 (5):1698-704.

[272] Ostergaard M, Olesen LH, Hasle H, et al. WT1 gene expression: an excellent tool for monitoring minimal residual disease in 70% of acute myeloid leukaemia patients - results from a single-centre study. *Br J Haematol* 2004;125 (5):590-600.

[273] Renneville A, Kaltenbach S, Clappier E, et al. Wilms tumor 1 (WT1) gene mutations in pediatric T-cell malignancies. *Leukemia;*24 (2):476-80.

In: Acute Lymphoblastic Leukemia
Editors: Severo Vecchione and Luigi Tedesco

ISBN: 978-1-61470-872-8
©2012 Nova Science Publishers, Inc.

Chapter II

Mice Deficient for the Slp65 Signaling Protein: A Model for Pre-B Cell Acute Lymphoblastic Leukemia

Van B. T. Ta and Rudi W. Hendriks[*]

Department of Pulmonary Medicine, Erasmus MC Rotterdam, the Netherlands

Abstract

Acute lymphoblastic leukemia (ALL) is characterized by oncogenic transformation of progenitors of the B-cell lineage in the bone marrow. Extensive molecular characterization of genetic abnormalities, in particular chromosomal translocations, have allowed the development of sensitive assays for the identification of underlying molecular defects that are applicable to ALL diagnosis and to monitor response to treatment. The need for further improvement of therapy requires in-depth understanding of the fundamental nature of the disease process and of mechanisms by which lymphoid cells undergo malignant transformation and progression. Research in this area is strongly facilitated by the availability of animal models. Mice deficient for the signaling molecule Slp65 spontaneously develop pre-B cell leukemia. Importantly, deficiency of SLP65 has been reported in a fraction of childhood precursor-B cell ALL cases. Moreover, in precursor-B ALL positive for the BCR-ABL translocation the activity of the BCR-ABL1 kinase fusion protein was linked to expression of the same aberrant SLP65 transcripts. In the B-cell lineage, diversity of the antibody repertoire is generated by recombination of various gene segments at the immunoglobulin (Ig) heavy (H) and light (L) chain loci, which occurs in an ordered manner. Signaling by membrane Ig governs a number of distinct checkpoints in B cell differentiation that shape the antibody repertoire. A central checkpoint is the pre-B cell receptor (pre-BCR), which monitors successful expression of the Ig H chain and signals for proliferation, differentiation and Ig L chain recombination.

---

[*] Correspondence to: Rudi W. Hendriks. Department of Pulmonary Medicine. Room Ee2251a. Erasmus MC Rotterdam. PO Box 2040. NL 3000 CA Rotterdam, The Netherlands. E-mail address: r.hendriks@erasmusmc.nl; Phone: ++31-10-7043700; Fax: ++31-10-7044728.

In pre-B cells cooperative signals initiated from the pre-BCR and the interleukin-7 receptor (IL-7R) govern pre-B cell proliferation. The adapter protein Slp65 and the cytoplasmic tyrosine kinase Btk are key components of signaling pathways downstream of the pre-BCR and cooperate as tumor suppressors. Slp65 is essential for cell cycle exit and developmental progression of large, cycling into small, resting pre-B cells in which Ig L chain recombination is initiated. At this transition, IL-7 responsiveness and expression of the c-myc oncogene is downregulated and the Bcl6 transcriptional repressor is activated, thereby protecting pre-B cells from DNA damage-induced apoptosis during Ig L chain gene recombination. In this review, we discuss recent findings that define the role of Slp65 in pre-B cell differentiation and give insight into molecular mechanisms by which Slp65-deficient pre-B cells undergo oncogenic transformation in the mouse.

Introduction

The development of lymphoid neoplasia is a complex multistep process of genetic alterations and cellular transformations. Lymphoid malignancies are characterized by the frequent occurrence of chromosomal abnormalities, often translocations between proto-oncogenes and Ig or T cell receptor loci [1]. Many of the most known oncogenes, including ABL, Bcl-1 and Bcl-2, were discovered because they are located at translocation breakpoints in leukemia or lymphomas. This has led to the hypothesis that some of these translocations represent the consequence of misregulated V(D)J recombination or Ig heavy chain class switch recombination (CSR) [2]. Alarmingly, and despite success achieved during the last decades in the treatment of these malignancies, their incidence is increasing. The need for further improving therapy requires in-depth understanding of the fundamental nature of the disease process and of the mechanisms by which lymphoid cells undergo malignant transformation and progression. The complexity of the pathogenic mechanism in lymphoid neoplasia is related to the fundamental strategy of the adaptive immune system. The mechanisms of V(D)J recombination, somatic hypermutation and CSR cause genetic instability and impose a constant threat of malignant transformation.

Due to the unique feature of lymphoid cells to somatically rearrange antigen receptor genes, these cells are frequent targets for chromosomal translocations and oncogene activation resulting from recombinase targeting mistakes or incorrect repair of the V(D)J recombination intermediates [3-4]. It was demonstrated in the mouse that chromosomal reinsertion of broken recombination signal sequences (RSS) can target cryptic RSS-like elements via a V(D)J recombination-like mechanism [5]. Moreover, cryptic RSS sequences immediately internal to the deletion breakpoints in the *IKZF1* locus, encoding the transcription factor *IKAROS*, have been identified in human *BCR-ABL1-positive* ALL [6]. Cryptic RSS are estimated to have a density of 1 per 600 bp in the genome and have also been identified in other loci involved in ALL, including *PAX5* and *CDKN2A/B* in humans and *c-Myc* and *Lmo2* in the mouse [7-8]. In addition, recombination activating gene (Rag) proteins, which initiate V(D)J recombination in lymphoid cells, have the ability to rearrange DNA sequences that do not resemble RSS, as reported in follicular lymphoma [9]. Taken together, these findings suggest that gene deletion or translocation arising from aberrant Rag activity contributes to leukemogenesis in human and mouse ALL. In addition, lymphoid development from haematoipoietic stem cells is accompanied by extensive cellular proliferation at specific stages. In the B-cell lineage the pre-B cell receptor (pre-BCR), which monitors successful expression of the Ig H chain, serves as a crucial checkpoint and signals for rapid proliferation and differentiation. We will therefore discuss in this review Slp65-deficient mice as a model system for pre-B cell acute lymphoblastic leukemia, in the context of the normal function of the pre-B cell receptor checkpoint as a crucial proliferation switch in B cell development in the mouse. Slp65 is a signaling protein that is an important transducer of pre-B cell receptor signals (see below) and thereby acts as an important regulator of proliferation.

Malignancies of Pre-B Cells in Human: Acute Lymphoblastic Leukemia

Pre-B cell leukemia is one of the most common forms of childhood malignancy and reflects clonal proliferation of transformed cells as a result of genetic changes. Extensive molecular characterization of these genetic abnormalities, in particular chromosomal translocations, have allowed the development of sensitive assays for the identification of underlying molecular defects, which are applicable to disease diagnosis and to monitor response to treatment. Childhood B-lineage ALL can be divided in different subtypes based on genetic abnormalities. The two main genetic subtypes, *TEL-AML1*-positive and hyperploidy with more than 50 chromosomes, account for 50% of pre-B ALL cases. *BCR-ABL1*-positive ALL, *MLL* and *E2A-PBX1* rearranged ALL each account for less than 5% of pediatric cases of ALL [10]. The *BCR-ABL1* fusion gene is the result of a t(9;22)(q34;q11) translocation and represents the most frequent recurrent genetic aberration leading to ALL in adults [11]. Next to translocations, a large group of pre-B ALL cases has aberrations in loci of various genes, identified by genome-wide hybridization studies [6, 12]. These include transcription factors such as *PAX5* (in ~30% of cases), *IKAROS*, *E2A*, or *EBF1*, cell cycle proteins (*CDKN2A/B, RB*), DNA repair protein *ATM,* the microRNAs Mir-15/16 and the apoptotis regulator *BTG1*. Interestingly, in a small fraction of B-lineage ALL the genes encoding cytokine receptors *CRLF2* (an IL-7R homologue), *IL-7R* and *IL-3R* and the signaling molecules *PTEN* and *SLP65* are affected [6, 12-13]. Loss-of-function mutation of the *IL-7R* gene cause autosomal recessive severe combined immunodeficiency disease, but in B- and T-ALL gain-of-function mutations have been described [6, 12-13]. In pre-B cell leukemias, the mutations were associated with the aberrant expression of CRLF2, and the mutant IL-7R proteins formed a functional receptor with CRLF2 for thymic stromal lymphopoietin (TSLP). Biochemical and functional assays reveal that these activating IL-7R mutations conferred cytokine-independent growth of pre-B cells. In addition, cases have been described in which other mutations affect the same signaling pathway, e.g. in JAK1 or JAK2 [6, 12-13]. Despite impressive progress, there is still a deficiency in our understanding of how consecutive genetic abnormalities ultimately subvert the developmental program of normal precursor-B cells.

Involvement of SLP65 in the Development of B-Lineage ALL in Human

Deficiency of SLP65 has been found in ~50% of childhood precursor-B cell ALL cases [14]. The loss of SLP65 protein was found to be due to defective splicing, leading to premature stop codons. The SLP65 gene contains alternative exons (exons 3a and 3b) located in intron 3 and when these alternative exons are included into the SLP65 mRNA they interrupt the open reading frame of SLP65 and prevent protein expression. Moreover, in precursor-B ALL that where positive for the BCR-ABL translocation the activity of the fusion protein, the BCR-ABL1 kinase, was linked to the expression of the same aberrant SLP65 transcripts [15]. Because other expression profiling studies with a large number of patients reported a low frequency [6, 16], it is not clear whether the loss of SLP65 is a common leukemogenic event. Nevertheless, the reported findings indicate that loss of SLP65 and the accompanying pre-B cell differentiation arrest may be one of the primary causes of precursor-B ALL.

Research in this area is strongly facilitated by the availability of an animal model for this disease: SLP65-deficient mice spontaneously develop pre-B cell leukemia with a similar phenotype as found in humans [17-18]. In contrast, mice deficient for Btk, a kinase that interacts with Slp65, do not develop pre-B cell leukemia. Nevertheless, Btk and Slp65 cooperate as tumor suppressors whereby Btk exerts its tumor suppressor function independently of its kinase activity [19-20]. Combined deficiency of Slp65 and Btk result in a more complete arrest at the pre-B cell stage [19] and a higher incidence of pre-B cell leukemia than compared with single deficient mice [17-18, 21-22], suggesting that the developmental block is one of the tumor-promoting factors. In addition, expression of the pre-BCR is also essential for the development of leukemia, because mice which are Rag-deficient or which cannot express the Ig μ H chain on the surface (e.g. because of deficiency of the pre-BCR component λ5 or due to a disruption of the membrane exon of the Ig μ H chain constant region) are arrested at the pro-B cell stage, but do not develop leukemia [17, 23-24]. Furthermore, Slp65 has a specific function that suppresses malignant transformation because in Btk/Plcγ2 and Irf-4/Irf-8 double-deficient mice with a nearly complete arrest at the large pre-B cell stage no leukemias have been reported [25-26]. We and others have used the Slp65-deficient mouse model to study the basis of pre-B ALL.

B Lymphocyte Development in Mouse Bone Marrow

The earliest committed B cell precursors in the bone marrow are pre-pro-B cells corresponding with Hardy fraction A [27] (Figure 1). These cells have immunoglobulin (Ig) heavy (H) chain alleles which are largely in germline configuration and can be distinguished from other earlier precursors by their ability to differentiate into B cells but not other lymphoid cells. Pre-pro-B cells have low expression of the Rag1 and Rag2 genes [28-30]. B cell development requires a hierarchy involving many transcription factors. In CLP, the helix-loop-helix protein E47, an E2A isoform, induces the expression of early B cell factor 1 (Ebf1) [31-33]. Ebf1 in turn activates expression of the transcription factor Pax5 [34]. The Pax5 gene, encoding the B cell specific activator protein (BSAP) is expressed exclusively in B cells and activates B lineage specific genes and represses B lineage inappropriate genes [35]. Pax5 expression is regulated by the concerted activities of ETS-family transcription factor PU.1 and the interferon regulatory factors IRF-4 and IRF-8 [34, 37]. In addition to E2A, Ebf1 and Pax5, other transcriptional regulators that modulate the developmental progression of B lineage cells have been identified. Prominent among these are Ikaros, Bcl-11 and Foxo1. Ikaros-like proteins recognize binding sites in many lymphocyte-specific genes including TdT, VpreB and λ5 (see below) whereby Ikaros proteins control the expression of λ5 in a developmental specific manner [38-40]. B cell development in Bcl11a-deficient mice is arrested at a stage similar to that described for E2A- or Ebf1-deficient mice and expression of Bcl11a is activated by E2A proteins [41-42].

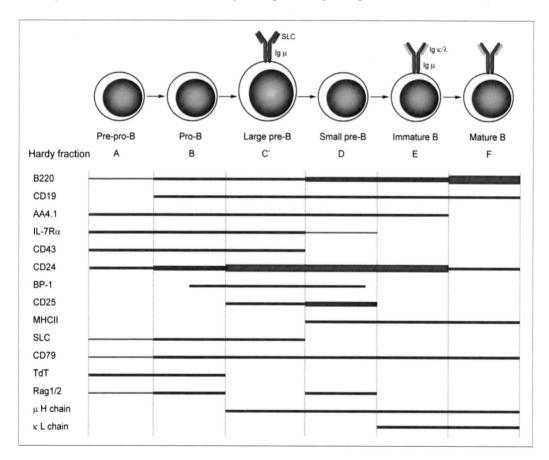

Figure 1. Framework of B cell lineage development based on ordered changes in cell surface molecules. Relative expression levels are indicated by line thickness. AA4.1 is also known as CD93 and PB493; CD24 as HSA (heat stable antigen); CD25 as IL-2R; MHCII, major histocompatibility complex type II; CD79, Igα and Igβ; SLC, surrogate light chain (λ5 and VpreB). TdT and Rag1/2 (recombination activating gene) expression assessed by analysis of mRNA. Figure adapted from ref. [36].

Foxo1-deficient mice show a block at the pro-B cell stage, and Foxo1 directly activates the expression of Rag1 and Rag2 [43]. Collectively, these factors form the transcriptional machinery that promotes commitment to the B cell lineage, suppresses the expression of genes associated with alternative cell fates and coordinates cellular population expansion with developmental progression [36-37].

Ig H Chain Gene Recombination and the Generation of Pre-B Cells

Pro-B cells are distinguished from earlier precursors by a series of cell surface markers [36, 44]. B lineage cells are identified by coexpression of B220, the high molecular weight isoform of Ptprc (CD45), together with leukosialin, CD43 [27]. These early B lineage cells are further subdivided based on expression of CD24, the heat stable antigen (HSA), and BP-1, a zinc-dependent cell surface metallopeptidase (Figure 1). Furthermore, the first step in generating the required antibody diversity is initiated in this stage.

V(D)J recombination is the process which assembles previously scattered variable (V), diversity (D) and joining (J) encoding gene segments to assemble a (pre-) BCR (Figure 2) [44-47]. The reaction is initiated by the lymphoid-specific factors Rag1 and Rag2 [28-29], which recognize RSS that flank all V, D and J gene units and introduce a DNA double strand break (DSB) at the border of the RSS. The resulting DNA DSB is resolved by the DNA repair machinery known as non-homologous end-joining (NHEJ) [48-49]. If these DSB are not properly repaired, they may result in chromosomal translocations and lymphoid malignancies [2-4]. V(D)J recombination is strictly regulated at many different levels. V(D)J recombination is tissue-specific, lineage-specific and developmental stage-specific. Furthermore, V(D)J recombination is temporally ordered and cell cycle regulated, whereby recombination is restricted to the G0-G1 stage of the cell cycle. In large cycling pre-B cells, Rag proteins are transiently downregulated to terminate further Ig H chain gene rearrangement. Moreover, as ongoing recombinase activity during mitosis will interfere with faithful transmission of the genome to daughter cells, Rag2 proteins are degraded during cell division, thus linking V(D)J recombination to the cell cycle [50-52].

The RSS that serve as recognition element for the V(D)J recombinase consist of a conserved heptamer, a spacer of either 12 or 23 nucleotides and a conserved nonamer. Only gene segments flanked by RSS with dissimilar spacer lengths can efficiently rearrange with one another [46, 53]. The NHEJ pathway that resolves V(D)J recombinase-mediated DSB can be schematically divided into three steps (Figure 2): (1) the Ku70/Ku80 heterodimer is recruited to and interacts with the DNA DSB; (2) the DNA-dependent serine/threonine kinase DNA-PKcs and the nuclease Artemis are recruited and activated to modify the DNA ends when needed; and (3) the XRCC-4/DNA-Ligase IV complex together with Cernunnos terminates the reaction by rejoining the broken DNA ends [48, 54]. Imprecise joining of the broken DNA ends contributes considerably to diversity and includes duplication of palindromic sequences (P nucleotides) and deletion or insertion of non-templated nucleotides (N nucleotides) by terminal deoxynucleotidyl transferase (TdT) [55-56]. In eukaryotic cells there are two major pathways of DSB repair, NHEJ and homologous recombination (HR)

[57]. HR repairs DSB using information on the undamaged sister chromatid. NHEJ and HR have overlapping roles in repairing DNA DSBs [58-60].

In the murine Ig H chain locus there are approximately 195 V genes, 13 D genes and 4 J genes dispersed over ~2.5 Mb of DNA on chromosome 12 (Figure 3). Close to half the murine V_H genes belong to the J558 family. The majority of these are located at the 5' end of the V_H cluster, though several are also found interspersed amongst other gene families throughout the locus. The extreme 3' end of the V_H locus comprises the 7183 family [61-62]. Although not all VH genes are functional, random recombination of all V, D and J gene segments and random association of heavy and light chains still produce an enormous diverse repertoire. However, V,D and J genes are not used equally in the pre-immune repertoire, thus limiting the theoretical estimates of combinatorial diversity [63-65].

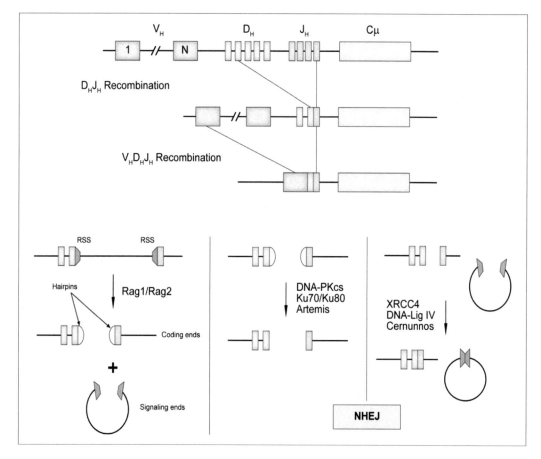

Figure 2. Overview of steps in V(D)J recombination and the involvement of Rag and NHEJ proteins. Schematic representation of the Ig H chain locus and V(D)J recombination process. The V(D)J reaction can be divided into three steps. First, the Rag1/2 complex introduces a DNA DSB at the border between D_H and J_H segments and their respective recombination signal sequences (RSS), creating hairpin-sealed coding ends and blunt signaling ends. Artemis, which is recruited and phosphorylated by the DNA-PKcs/Ku70/Ku80 complex, opens the hairpins through its endonuclease activity. The XRCC4/Cernunnos /DNA-Ligase IV complex finally seals coding and signal joints. NHEJ, non-homologous end-joining. Figure adapted from ref. [47].

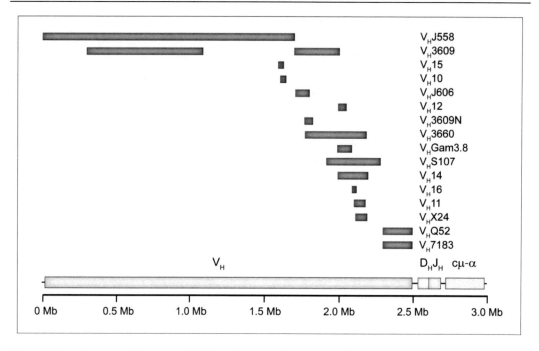

Figure 3. Organization of the mouse Ig H chain locus on chromosome 12.
Schematic map of V_H gene family distribution within the mouse Ig H chain V region according to IMGT (www.imgt.org). The length of boxes indicates the distance spanned by members of the gene families and is not related to the number of genes.

Ig gene recombination occurs in a stepwise fashion and begins with D_H to J_H junction segment rearrangement in pro-B cells [44, 66]. Due to an inexact joining mechanism, the D_H segments can be joined to the J_H in any of the three reading frames (RF). D_H segments are preferentially used in RF1, while RF2 and RF3 are counter selected on the basis of expression of a truncated μ chain protein and stop codons, respectively [67]. After $D_H J_H$ rearrangement, V_H genes become accessible to the V(D)J recombinase and V_H to $D_H J_H$ joining takes place. V_H gene accessibility is dependent on transcriptional regulatory elements and is associated with the onset of germline transcription of V_H genes [68-69]. Furthermore, the Ig H chain locus relocates from the periphery to the center of the nucleus in pro-B cells which facilitates $V_H D_H J_H$ recombination [70] and locus contraction brings the distal V_H gene segments into close proximity with the $D_H J_H$ region [70-72]. Several proteins have been linked to the control of chromatin accessibility of the Ig H chain locus in pro-B cells or with the regulation of the Rag genes, including Pax5, Yy1, Ezh2, FoxP1 and IL-7R signaling via Stat5 [73-77]. Correlating with the activation of the Ig H chain locus are antisense transcripts originating in intergenic regions between V_H gene segments. These transcripts are turned off when the early pro-B cells reach the late pro-B cell stage (Hardy fraction C) [78]. However, the role of these antisense transcripts has not been elucidated yet.

Productive in-frame V(D)J recombination in pro-B cells gives rise to the Ig μ chain, which is expressed by pre-B cells as part of the pre-BCR complex and marks the transition to the pre-B cell stage [24, 79-80].

Pre-B Cells and the Pre-BCR Checkpoint in B Cell Development

The pre-BCR consists of a Ig μ H chain and a surrogate light chain (SLC) associated with the signaling subunits Igα and Igβ. The SLC substitutes the not yet rearranged Ig L chains and is a heterodimer composed of two germline-encoded invariant proteins: λ5, which resembles the constant region of conventional λ light chains and VpreB (**Figure 4**) [80-82]. The pre-BCR is transiently expressed but marks an important checkpoint in B cell development when Ig μ H chains are tested for their ability to associate with the SLC. The primary functions of the pre-BCR are triggering of B cell differentiation, clonal expansion and H chain allelic exclusion. Pre-B cells which express the pre-BCR acquire the capacity to respond to low concentrations of the proliferation factor IL-7 [24, 79-80].

In 1957 Burnet proposed that all B lymphocytes carry unique cell surface receptors for antigen [83]. Each cell expresses on its surface just one kind of antibody and during immunization, antigen selects cells with the corresponding specificity for multiplication and differentiation into antibody-secreting cells. The process which guarantees that each B cell only produces a single antigen receptor is called allelic exclusion [84-85].

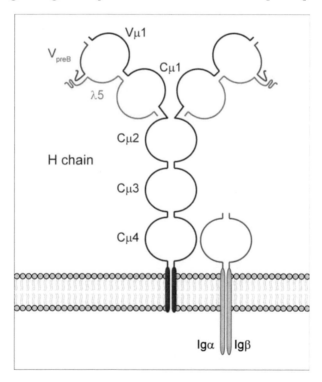

Figure 4. Structure of the pre-BCR.
The pre-BCR complex consists of the heterodimeric Igα/Igβ signal transducer and two covalently associated Ig H chains which are paired with the surrogate light chain, consisting of the invariant proteins λ5 and VpreB. The SLC contains two oppositely charged non-Ig-like tails located at the C-terminus of VpreB and the N-terminus of λ5. The unique tails protrude from the pre-BCR at the position where the CDR3 (complementarity-determining region) of a conventional L chain is located in the BCR.

Allelic exclusion is dependent on correct pre-BCR assembly and pre-BCR signaling [23, 86]. Large-scale contraction of the Ig H chain locus following recombination is instrumental in establishing allelic exclusion. The second allele is repositioned at centromeric heterochromatin at the pre-B cell stage while Ig L recombination takes place [71]. Allelic exclusion of the Ig H chain is initiated in the early embryo when the Ig receptor loci become asynchronously replicating in a stochastic manner with one early and one late allele in each cell [87]. Molecular components including histone modification, nuclear localization and DNA demethylation leads to rearrangement on a single allele and a feedback mechanism that inhibits recombination on the second allele once recombination of the first allele has been successful [84].

Pre-BCR Signaling Pathways

Currently, it still remains controversial as to how pre-BCR mediated signals are initiated. Pre-BCR signaling could be triggered by ligand binding or by cell autonomous aggregation of pre-BCR complexes on the cell surface. The non-Ig-like tail of the SLC component λ5 induces ligand-independent pre-BCR cross-linking and as a result cell-autonomous signaling for pre-B cell expansion [88]. Recently, Jumaa and colleagues [89] have shown that functional pre-BCR formation and autonomous signaling requires the N-linked glycosylation site in the C_H1 domain of Ig μ H chain (N46). However, ligand-mediated cross-linking seems possible since the pre-BCR shapes the V_H repertoire at the transition from pro-B to large pre-B cells [90]. Besides, several groups have identified interactions between the non-Ig tail of λ5 of the pre-BCR to galectin-1 [91-92] and to stromal-cell-associated heparin sulphate [93]. Furthermore, the pre-BCR is a poly-reactive receptor and capable of recognizing multiple (self-)antigens, including DNA, LPS and insulin, via the non-Ig part of λ5 (Kohler 2008). Thus, pre-BCR auto-reactivity may serve to clonally expand those cells that produce a functional μ H chain and ensures that this selection can occur in the absence of foreign antigens. In support of this idea, in SLC-deficient mice mainly autoreactive pre-B cells are selected, resulting in the accumulation of autoreactive antibodies [94]. But also in the presence of SLC, more than half of the antibodies expressed in early B cell compartments of healthy individuals are polyreactive [95].

Activation of pre-BCR signaling involves phosphorylation of immunoreceptor tyrosine based activation motifs (ITAMs) in the cytoplasmic domains of Igα and Igβ by the Src family kinases (Fyn, Lyn and Blk) and the cytosolic protein tyrosine kinase Syk (Figure 5) [79, 96]. This is the first step in the formation of a lipid-raft associated calcium signaling module [97-98]. The binding of Syk to the phosphorylated Igα and Igβ places the active Syk in the right position to allow further phosphorylation of neighboring ITAM sequences. This results in further Syk recruitment and activation [21, 99]. The SH2 domain-containing leukocyte protein of 65 kD, Slp65 (also known as Bash or Blnk) is one of the most prominent targets of Syk kinase activity and is phosphorylated by Syk on several tyrosines. Slp65 and its close relative in T cells (Slp76) are adaptor proteins, which lack intrinsic enzymatic function but regulate the assembly and localization of signaling complexes. They are able to regulate the availability of a substrate to an enzyme and create a scaffold for bridging signaling cascades

[100]. Slp65 is expressed in B cells and myeloid cells and has been mainly reported to function under the (pre-) BCR [79].

Phosphorylated Slp65 provides docking sites for several proteins including the Btk, Grb2, Vav, Nck, and Plcγ2 (Figure 5) [21, 100-101]. Btk is a member of the Tec kinase family, which also includes Tec, Itk, Rlk and Bmx. These molecules have a structure containing a pleckstrin homology domain, followed by a short Tec homology domain, src homology domains and a kinase domain [102-103]. Btk is expressed in B cells, platelets and myeloid cells and activated under a large variety of receptors such as BCR, Fcε, TLR2, TLR4, CD38, CCL5, IL-6R and IL-10R.

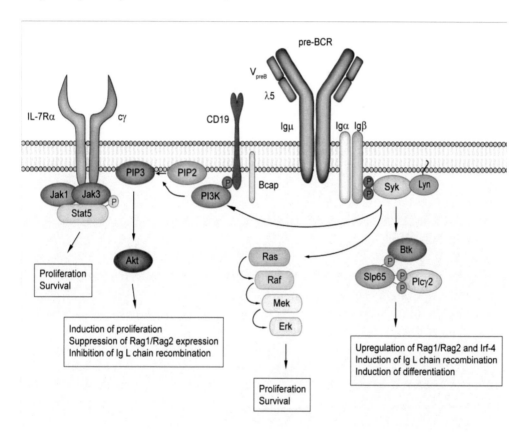

Figure 5. Signaling pathways in pre-B cells: cooperation of IL-7R and pre-BCR signaling. Pre-BCR activation results in activation of Syk, which together with Src family protein kinases, such as Lyn, phosphorylates downstream signaling proteins resulting in pathways involved in proliferation, differentiation and induction of Ig L chain recombination. Activation of Slp65 recruits and activates Btk and Plcγ2 resulting in upregulation of Rag1/Rag2 and Irf-4, induction of Ig L chain recombination and differentiation. An important pathway for proliferation and survival is the activation of the PI3K. Phosphorylation of the co-receptor CD19 and the adaptor protein BCAP (B cell PI3K adaptor) recruit and activate PI3K, resulting in the generation of the second messenger PIP3 (Phosphatidylinositol [3,4,5]-trisphosphate) from PIP2 (Phosphatidylinositol 4,5-bisphosphate). PIP3 recruits Akt, which is the dominant mediator for control of cellular proliferation. Ongoing signaling through the PI3K-Akt pathway induces proliferation, suppresses the Rag1/Rag2 genes and blocks Ig κ gene recombination. Proliferation in pre-B cells is also induced via the pathway involving Erk MAP kinase. In addition to the role of the pre-BCR, signaling via the interleuking-7 receptor (IL-7R) plays a central role in control of survival and proliferation of pre-B cells.

Activation of Plcγ2 by Syk and Btk results in the production of inositol triphosphate (IP3) and diacylglycerol (DAG), both of which are second messengers required for cellular responses [21, 101]. Models of targeted disruption of components of the pre-BCR or downstream signaling proteins have shown the importance of these molecules in pre-BCR signaling [21, 24]. Additionally, active Syk induces phosphorylation and activation of the lipid-modifying kinase phosphoinositide 3 kinase (PI3K), which regulates diverse biological processes, including cell growth, survival, proliferation, migration and metabolism [79, 104].

Regulation of Pre-B Cell Proliferation

Expansion of pre-B cells is severely impaired in mice with targeted disruption of pre-BCR components, including μ H chain, the SLC components λ5 and VpreB, Igα and Igβ and Syk [23, 105-109]. Overexpression or constitutive activation of Syk functions as an oncogene by promoting growth factor independent proliferation of pre-B cells and by inhibiting differentiation [79]. In mice deficient for components of the pre-BCR complex, including Igα, Igβ, SLC or Syk, Ig μ chain positive pre-B cells do not proliferate [24].

In contrast, deficiency of Slp65 or Btk results in an increased proliferative response of pre-B cells to IL-7 in vitro, indicating that Slp65 and Btk are crucially involved in the termination of IL-7 driven proliferation [101]. Slp65 inhibits IL-7R signaling through direct binding to Jak3 in a Btk-independent manner [110] and also by downregulating IL-17R expression [111].

Downstream of the pre-BCR, Syk and the Src family protein tyrosine kinases induce phosphorylation of the co-receptor CD19 and/or the adaptor protein Bcap resulting in the recruitment and activation of PI3K [79, 104]. PI3K activation results in phosphorylation and thereby activation of the serine/threonine kinase Akt, also known as protein kinase B (PKB). Akt inhibits the activities of the forkhead (Foxo) transcription factors (which are mediators of apoptosis and cell-cycle arrest), resulting in cell proliferation and survival [112-113]. Tight regulation of pre-BCR induced signaling is important to avoid abnormal Akt activity, which can result in uncontrolled cellular expansion and malignant transformation. The tumor-suppressor phosphatase with tensin homology (Pten) is the most important negative regulator of the cell survival signaling pathway initiated by PI3K [114].

In addition to the role of the pre-BCR signaling, IL-7R signaling plays a central role in cellular survival, proliferation and maturation. Mice deficient in components of IL-7R signaling have an arrest of B cell development at the pro-B cell stage and impaired V_H to $D_H J_H$ recombination [115]. Expression of the pre-BCR by pro-B cells upregulates IL-7R expression and thereby increases the responsiveness of these cells to IL-7 [101, 115]. Integration of IL-7R signaling and pre-BCR dependent signals to expand the pool of pre-B cells occurs via the D-type cyclin, cyclin D3 [116].

Another downstream signaling cascade involves the mitogen activated protein kinase (MAPK) pathway which functions independently of signaling via Slp65 and Btk [101]. This signaling pathway leads from the Ras GTPase to the extracellular signal regulated kinases (Erk1 and Erk2) [117]. Erk activity has been shown to be important for the pre-BCR to collaborate with IL-7R signaling to drive pre-B cell proliferation [115]. Expression of genes dependent on Erk activation includes genes encoding the proliferation-associated transcription factors c-Myc, c-Fos, Egr-1, Egr-2, Egr-3, Fra-1 and Fra-2 [117-118].

Progression from Large Cycling into Small Resting Pre-B Cells

Upon pre-BCR signaling, cells initially undergo a proliferative burst accompanied by downregulation of SLC components and Rag1/Rag2 protein expression, followed by exit from the cell cycle and transition from large pre-B cells to small pre-B cells. In small resting pre-B cells Ig L chain rearrangement is initiated. Termination of pre-BCR signaling occurs by downregulation of λ5 gene expression and consequently the termination of SLC expression. The pre-BCR activates a negative feedback loop that prevents continuous pre-BCR signaling [79, 119-120].

Pre-BCR signaling leads to activation of Syk, which then phosphorylates Slp65 and thereby regulates pre-B cell differentiation. Slp65 is required for the downregulation of λ5, which terminates SLC expression and the activation of Ig κ L chain recombination by induction of the expression of the transcription factors Aiolos, Irf-4, Foxo3a and Foxo1 [38, 121-122]. At the transition from large cycling into small resting pre-B cells up- and downregulation of specific cell surface markers occurs (Figure 1). Small pre-B cells downregulate expression of sialoglycoprotein CD43, SLC, metallopeptidase BP-1 and IL-7R and upregulate expression of CD2, CD25, MHCII [36, 101]. Slp65 or Btk-deficient cells fail to efficiently modulate the expression of these developmentally regulated markers, including CD43, c-kit, SLC, IL-7R and BP-1. When we analyzed the kinetics of pre-B cell differentiation *in vivo* using 5-bromo-2-deoxyuridine (BrdU) incorporation, Btk-deficient cells manifested a specific ~3 hour developmental delay within the small pre-B cell compartment, when compared with wild-type cells. Therefore, Btk and Slp65 are critical for the efficient transit through the small pre-B cell compartment, thereby regulating cell surface phenotype changes during the developmental progression of cytoplasmic Ig μ H chain expressing pre-B cells into immature IgM[+] B cells. Moreover, Btk- and Slp65-deficient pre-B cells have a specific defect in Ig L chain recombination [101].

Transcription factors that are important for Ig κ rearrangement are E2A, Pax5, Irf-8 and Spi-B [122-124]. Germline transcription of the Ig L chain loci is associated with the regulation of accessibility of the Ig loci to the VDJ recombinase, because germline transcription precedes VDJ recombination of the Ig L chain [125]. There are two type of light chains, Ig κ and Ig λ, which are expressed at a ratio of approximately 20:1 in mice [123]. Ig κ genes are activated and undergo recombination before Ig λ, which contributes to the preferential usage of the Ig κ L chain in mature B cells [123, 126].

In the absence of Btk mainly Ig λ L chain germline transcription and recombination is impaired, whereas in Btk/SLP-65 double-deficient pre-B cells, both κ and λ L chain germline transcripts are severely reduced [101].

Beyond the Pre-B Cell Stage: Immature and Mature B Cells

After successful rearrangement of the Ig H and L chain locus, the immature B cells are the first B lineage cells to express surface BCR, they display surface IgM but little or no IgD. Expression of the BCR is a second key checkpoint in B cell development for monitoring the production of a functional Ig L chain and to eliminate autoreactive BCR. The receptor consists of randomly selected Ig H and L chains and has an unpredictable specificity that includes the ability to bind self. Indeed, it has been found that about 50% of BCR are autoreactive in humans and mice [95, 127-128]. Induction of B cell tolerance can occur by clonal deletion, cell inactivation (anergy) or receptor editing. Receptor editing is the process that alters antigen receptors by allowing secondary rearrangements of mainly the Ig L chain. This process is the dominant tolerance mechanism for developing B cells [128-130]. When autoreactive B cells encounter self-antigen that induces signaling through the BCR, developmental progression is blocked and secondary V(D)J recombination can take place. Immature B cells differ from mature B cells in that they are particularly susceptible to BCR-induced apoptosis. Thus the BCR is an essential regulator of immature B cell development.

Immature B cells that emigrate from the bone marrow (BM) to the periphery are referred to as transitional B cells. Transitional B cells can be distinguished from mature B cells by a series of cell surface markers. Transitional B cells are short-lived and only 10-30% of these cells enter the long-lived mature peripheral B cell compartment. Transitional B cells are unable to proliferate and are unable to generate an immune response upon BCR cross-linking [36, 131]. The transitional cells that lack autoreactivity enter the pool of mature recirculating B cells in the spleen. These cells are termed follicular B cells because of their localization to the B cell follicle region [132]. This is the final maturation stage of developing BM B cells (Figure 6).

Marginal zone (MZ) B cells are a second population of mature splenic B lymphocytes which are specifically located in the marginal zone of the spleen [134]. MZ B cells are pre-selected to express a BCR repertoire that is biased and they respond rapidly to antigenic challenge.

Another B cell subset is the B-1 B cells, which are found in the peritoneal and pleural cavities, spleen and gut. B-1 cells persist largely by self-renewal. In contrast to follicular and MZ B cells, B-1 cells are primarily generated from progenitors in the fetal liver and neonatal BM and can be divided into the $CD5^+$ B-1a and $CD5^-$ B-1 B cells. The most distinctive feature of B-1a cells is the production of 'natural antibodies', autoantibodies with specificities that include glycoproteins, phosphorylcholine, phosphatidylcholine but which are not pathogenic (Figure 6). The choice of differentiation into any of the three subsets is dependent on BCR signaling [36]. However, recently in our lab it was found that constitutive active Btk expression did not change follicular, marginal zone, or B-1 B cell fate choice, but resulted in selective expansion and survival of B-1 cells. Therefore, constitutive Btk activation and consequently active BCR signaling results in defective B cell tolerance [135].

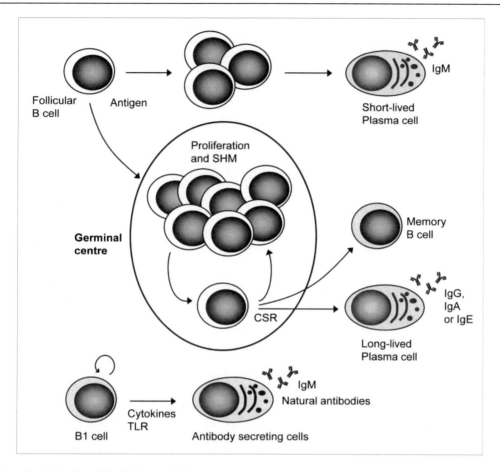

Figure 6. Activation of B cells in germinal centers.
Productive interaction of follicular B cells with antigen results in proliferation and differentiation. The primary response generates pre-germinal center plasma cells that are short-lived and usually secrete IgM. Some activated follicular B cells form a germinal center. Antigen-activated lymphoblasts that enter a germinal center are subjected to multiple rounds of SHM and antigen selection. Cells that express high-affinity antigen receptors are selected for survival with subsequent differentiation to memory B cells or post-germinal center plasma cells. Post-germinal center plasma cells that undergo Ig H chain CSR typically home to the bone marrow where they reside and become long-lived [133]. Upon activation of a distinct population of B cells, B-1 cells, by cytokine and/or TLR activation antibody secreting cells are formed which secrete natural IgM antibodies, which often recognize bacterial antigens. SHM, somatic hypermutation; CSR, class switch recombination.

The Germinal Center Reaction

After being stimulated with antigen, mature B cells undergo two additional processes of antigen receptor diversification. Class switch recombination (CSR) and somatic hypermutation (SHM) occur mainly in specialized structures in secondary lymphoid organs called germinal centers (Figure 6). CSR and SHM are initiated by activation-induced cytidine deaminase (Aicda/Aid) (Figure 7) [137-138]. Aid is a single-stranded DNA deaminase that targets cytidine residues and thereby creates uracil-guanine mismatches in DNA that can be processed by many different pathways to produce mutations or DSB [139-141].

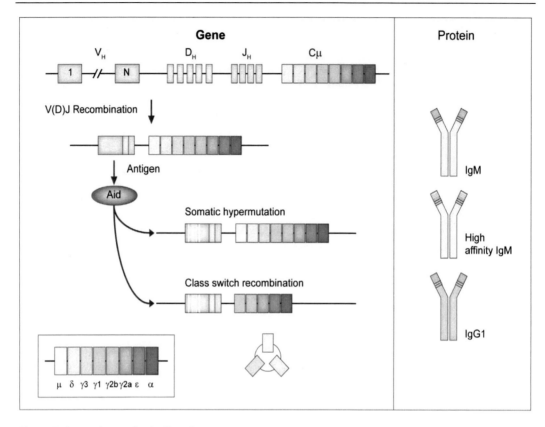

Figure 7. Generating antibody diversity.
Antibodies are encoded by immunoglobulin genes; these include V, D and J regions and C regions. In pro-B cells an immunoglobulin gene includes the full range of V,D, J and C regions. V(D)J recombination generates an antibody (IgM) with a variable region that recognizes a particular antigen. When the B cell encounters antigen, two other processes — both catalysed by the Aid protein — are triggered. Somatic hypermutation generates mutations (thin white lines) in the variable regions, potentially generating an IgM with higher affinity for its antigen. Class switch recombination results in the excision of some of the constant regions, generating antibodies with distinct effector functions (IgG1 is shown here). Figure adapted from ref. [136].

SHM introduces point mutations in the V_H regions of Ig H and L chains. B cells expressing high affinity Ig are selected by limited amounts of antigen, resulting in affinity maturation. CSR is a recombination reaction that does not affect the antigen binding specificity of an antibody but exchanges the constant region of the Ig H chain and thereby producing antibodies with distinct effector functions.

During CSR the Ig H chain isotype switches from IgM to IgG, IgA or IgE. Aid expression is normally restricted to germinal center B cells but when expressed in non-germinal center cells, Aid can induce mutation in various highly transcribed genes and thereby acts as a genome-wide mutator [142-144]. Furthermore, Aid can initiate chromosomal translocations between c-Myc and the Ig H locus [145]. Thus, all three processes responsible for diversification of the antigen receptor genes, V(D)J recombination, SHM and CSR, can initiate the formation of oncogenic translocations [1, 138].

Mechanism of Malignant Transformation of Slp65-Deficient Pre-B Cells

Several lines of evidence have indicated a role for unregulated Rag activity in Slp65-deficient pre-B cell leukemia. First, Rag proteins are expressed in strongly proliferating Slp65-deficient pre-B cells [17-18]. Second, Slp65-deficient pre-B cell leukemias mostly co-express Ig H chain, SLC and Ig L chain [19]. Third, in human pre-B cell leukemia SLP65 deficiency correlates with RAG expression and ongoing V_H gene rearrangement activity [146]. However, we found by inactivation of Rag that the V(D)J recombinase is not essential for malignant transformation of Slp65-deficient pre-B cells [147]. Nevertheless, we cannot formally exclude that V(D)J recombination somehow contributes to malignant transformation, as the incidence of leukemias in our model of Btk/Slp65-double deficient mice with the autoreactive 3-83µδ transgene was low (~11%) and therefore did not allow an accurate and reliable comparison of tumor frequencies in Rag1-deficient, DNA-PK-deficient and V(D)J recombination-competent mice [147, 148]. Although we have shown that V(D)J recombination-mediated defects are not essential for leukemogenesis in Slp65-deficient pre-B cells, they may still contribute to malignant transformation.

Similar to Slp65-deficient mice Eµ-*myc* transgenic mice, which express c-Myc under the control of the IgH intronic enhancer, develop rapid-onset pre-B cell malignancies [149]. The c-Myc proto-oncogene is a broadly expressed transcription factor that is implicated in various cellular processes – cell growth, loss of differentiation and apoptosis. Elevated or deregulated Myc expression has been found in a wide range of human cancers, and is often associated with aggressive, poorly differentiated tumors. Such cancers include breast, colon, cervical, small-cell lung carcinomas, osteosarcomas, gliobastomas, melanomas and myeloid leukemias [150]. In Burkitt's lymphoma c-MYC is oncogenically activated as a result of a translocation between chromosome 8 and the Ig H chain locus or the Ig κ or λ L chain locus [151-152]. Interestingly, the incidence of lymphomas in Eµ-*myc* mice is greatly reduced by the introduction of a human IgH transgene [153]. In addition, loss of Btk or PLC-γ2 synergizes with deregulation of c-Myc during lymphoma formation in Eµ-*myc* mice [154-155]. The presence of the Eµ-*myc* transgene substantially increased the proliferative potential of B cell progenitors in response to IL-7 [154-155]. Activation of c-Myc is required for progression of quiescent cells into the S phase of the cell cycle, but c-Myc can also induce the p53 protein, which protects against oncogenic transformation of proliferating cells [156]. c-Myc activates the p19^{Arf} tumor suppressor that interferes with the E3 ubiquitin protein ligase Mdm2 and thereby stabilizes and activates p53, resulting in cell-cycle arrest or apoptosis. In Myc-induced lymphomagenesis the p19^{Arf}–Mdm2–p53 circuitry is often disrupted, indicating that c-Myc activation strongly selects for spontaneous inactivation of this pathway [157].

Recent findings show that Slp65 downregulates IL-7 mediated proliferation and survival through direct inhibition of Jak3 [110]. The IL-7R pathway promotes cellular survival, proliferation and maturation, involving induction of the proto-oncogene c-Myc [158]. B cell development can be partially restored in Jak3-deficient mice when they are bred to mice co-expressing a rearranged Ig H chain transgene and a c-Myc transgene [159]. Loss of Btk synergizes with deregulation of the c-Myc oncogene during lymphoma formation [154]. We found that disruption of the p19^{Arf}–Mdm2–p53 tumor suppressor pathway plays an important role in malignant transformation of Slp65-deficient pre-B cells [148]. Our findings reveal striking parallels in pre-B cell tumor formation between Slp65-deficient and Eµ-*myc* Tg mice. First, in both models the expression of a pre-rearranged Ig H chain transgene in early B cell differentiation reduces oncogenic transformation [148, 153]. Second, malignant transformation of both Slp65-deficient and Eµ-*myc* Tg pre-B cells involves disruption of the p19^{Arf}–Mdm2–p53 tumor suppressor pathway [148, 157]. Third, somatic hypermutation-associated, Aid-induced DNA damage is not required for tumor development in either of the two models [148, 160]. The finding that Slp65-deficient pre-B cell tumors display disruptions of the p19^{Arf}–Mdm2–p53 pathway implies that oncogenic transformation of Slp65-deficient pre-B cells does not exclusively result from sustained IL-7R signaling and endocrine IL-7 production. Slp65 regulates the activity of the forkhead-box transcription factors Foxo3a and Foxo1, which do not only promote Ig L chain recombination, but also suppress Myc-driven lymphomagenesis via direct p19^{Arf} activation [79, 161]. These parallels suggest that oncogenic Myc activation contributes to malignant transformation of Slp65-deficient pre-B cells. In addition, disruption of the p19^{Arf}–Mdm2–p53 tumor suppressor pathway also plays an essential role in the pre-B cell transformation process mediated by Abelson murine leukemia virus [162].

There are also differences between the Slp65-deficient and Eµ-*myc* Tg tumor models. Many Eµ-*myc* lymphomas sustained either p53 or p19^{Arf} loss of function and elevation of Mdm2 levels. Almost all Slp65-deficient or Btk/Slp65-double deficient leukemias expressed substantial levels of p19^{Arf}, suggesting inactivation of the p53 response, as p53 is a negative regulator of p19^{Arf}. Arf is highly expressed in many human tumors that contain p53 and in up to 40% of Burkitts lymphomas [163]. P19^{Arf} has also p53-independent functions, e.g it promotes the progression of lymphomas by mediating autophagy, a process of lysosome-mediated self-digestion that occurs during periods of nutrient deprivation [164-165]. Autophagy plays a complex role in the initiation and progression of tumors. It appears that autophagy suppresses tumor initiation, but promotes the survival of established tumors [166]. Silencing of p19^{Arf} inhibits the progression of Myc-driven lymphoma cells containing mutant or no p53 [165]. Thus, Slp65-deficient leukemias may retain p19^{Arf} to promote survival under metabolic stress. Autophagy inhibitors chloroquine and 3-methyladenine are effective anti-tumor drugs for Burkitts lymphoma and chronic myeloid leukemia [167-169]. Chloroquine-induced cell death was dependent on p53 but not on the modulators Atm or Arf [167]. Therefore, it would be interesting to test the effect of small molecule inhibitors of autophagy on the survival of Slp65-deficient tumors and to administer Chloroquine to Slp65/Btk-double deficient mice and follow the mice for tumor-free suvival.

It is tempting to speculate that transformation of Slp65-deficient pre-B cells is dependent on early oncogenic events that induce constitutive Jak3-Stat5 signaling at the pro-B cell stage. Furthermore, signaling via the IL-7R represses Bcl6 and its negative regulation of p19^{Arf} [170]. Therefore, Slp65-deficient pre-B cells which have acquired constitutive IL-7R signaling will be cleared via the p19^{Arf}–Mdm2–p53 pathway which protects against malignant transformation. The dramatic increase in tumor incidence when both Slp65 and p53 are lacking supports this notion [148]. However, after initiation of malignant transformation, expression of p19^{ARF} protects the cells against metabolic stress. Thus, p53 mediated apoptosis is an important mechanism in preventing transformation of Slp65 deficient pre-B cells.

This leads us to propose the following mechanism for malignant transformation of Slp65-deficient pre-B cells (Figure 8). The absence of Slp65 results in sustained expression of the pre-BCR and the IL-7R in large cycling pre-B cells. Since IL-7R signaling induces c-Myc this results in constitutively high levels of c-Myc. At this stage, Foxo transcription factors that normally suppress c-Myc-driven lymphomagenesis via direct activation of $p19^{Arf}$ are not properly activated because of the absence of Slp65. Furthermore, IL-7R signaling and aberrant pre-BCR signaling represses Bcl6 and thereby induces $p19^{Arf}$ expression. Subsequently, Slp65-deficient pre-B cells acquiring sporadic alterations in the $p19^{Arf}$–Mdm2–p53 are selected to become malignant. Furthermore, expression of $p19^{Arf}$ in Slp65-deficient leukemias possibly promotes survival under metabolic stress. Malignant transformation of Slp65-deficient pre-B cells thus is not a one hit model, but a complex multi-step process that requires different acquired mutations.

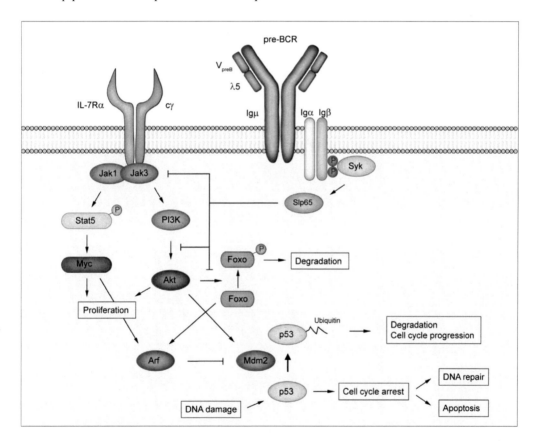

Figure 8. Model for tumor suppression in pre-B cells.
Signaling via Slp65 inhibits IL-7R signaling and induces activation of Foxo. Acativation of Arf occurs via Foxo proteins as well as through sustained and increased signaling induced by overexpressed Myc. Once expressed, the Arf protein interferes with the activity of Mdm2, leading to p53 stabilization and the triggering of a complex p53-dependent transcriptional program. The activation of p53 classically occurs in response to many other cellular stresses that produce DNA damage. Target genes induced by p53 can generate different biological outcomes depending on the tissue type and convergence of different activating signals. Arf induction primarily triggers cell-cycle arrest.

The role for Btk in suppression of malignant transformation remains unclear. It is conceivable that the increased frequency of malignant transformation in Slp65/Btk-double deficient mice reflects the increased pool size of proliferating pre-B cells. Mice that are double deficient for Btk/Plc-γ2 and Irf-4/Irf-8, however, are arrested at the large pre-B cell stage. Most of these mutant pre-B cells express pre-BCR on their cell surface, but so far the development of pre-B cell leukemia has not been reported [25-26]. Therefore, a complete block at the large pre-B cell stage is not sufficient to initiate malignant transformation. The absence of Btk might alter the proliferative capacity of Slp65-deficient pre-B cells. However, Btk does not cooperate with Slp65 in the suppression of the Jak3-Stat5 signaling pathway. Instead, Btk seems to play a role in the accumulation of $p27^{Kip1}$ and to induce cell cycle arrest [110]. A third possibility would be that Btk influences the malignant transformation of pre-B cells by c-Abl. C-Abl is a Src family non-receptor protein tyrosine kinase [171]. Alteration of the c-Abl structure and function as a consequence of chromosomal translocation (Bcr-Abl) results in fusion protein.

This translocation accounts for the majority of cases of human chronic myeloid leukemia and a part of the human ALL cases [172-173]. In human pre-B ALL Btk contributes to multiple aspects of the BCR-ABL1-driven survival signaling [174]. Our current model is that Slp65 and Btk act on different levels and thereby synergistically increase the incidence of leukemias.

Future Directions

In the past few years, our understanding of the function of the adaptor protein Slp65 in pre-B cell proliferation and differentiation has increased and consequently our understanding of the role of Slp65 in preventing malignant transformation. Still intriguing questions remain to be answered.

Pre-BCR signaling is different from BCR signaling in that BCR signaling is induced by antigen binding. The non-Ig-like tail of the SLC component λ5 induces ligand-independent pre-BCR cross-linking and as a result cell-autonomous signaling, which is essential for pre-B cell expansion [88]. The importance of a ligand for the pre-BCR is not clear; it is possible that a ligand exists on stromal cells, on other pre-B cells or on the membrane of the same cell. High-level pre-BCR expression on Slp65-deficient leukemic cells is thought to contribute to their strong proliferative capacity and therefore the specificities of the pre-BCR of malignant pre-B cells should be investigated. Furthermore, Slp65-deficient pre-B cells have high levels of IL-7R and pre-BCR, both of which provide proliferative signals. It is therefore conceivable that cell division in these cells may be accompanied by genomic instability, ultimately leading to oncogenic transformation. To investigate the involvement of genomic instability in proliferating large pre-B cells, we have performed comparative genomic hybridization analyses of pre-B cell tumor samples from Slp65-deficient mice. Our first results indeed point to the presence in these tumors of gene duplications and deletions, which may help us to identify oncogenes or tumor suppressors involved malignant transformation of Slp65-deficient pre-B cells. Finally, cancer may not only be caused by alterations in oncogenes or tumor suppressor genes, but also by defective expression of microRNA genes. MicroRNA genes can regulate many cellular processes and aberrant microRNA expression has been associated with the development and progression of tumors [175-177]. Examples include miR-15a and miR-16-1, which are deleted or downregulated in cases of chronic lymphocytic leukemia [178]. Importantly, regions of the genome that are consistently involved in chromosomal rearrangements in cancer but that lack oncogenes or tumor suppressor genes appear to harbor microRNA genes [177]. Therefore, it would be interesting to investigate microRNAs that are suppressed in Slp65-deficient leukemias.

Acknowledgment

These studies were partly supported by the Netherlands Organization for Scientific Research (NWO/Mozaiek) and the Dutch Cancer Society (KWF/NKB).

References

[1] Kuppers R, Dalla-Favera R. 2001. Mechanisms of chromosomal translocations in B cell lymphomas. *Oncogene* 20: 5580-94.

[2] Schlissel MS, Kaffer CR, Curry JD. 2006. Leukemia and lymphoma: a cost of doing business for adaptive immunity. *Genes Dev* 20: 1539-44.

[3] Roth DB. 2003. Restraining the V(D)J recombinase. *Nat Rev Immunol* 3: 656-66.

[4] Marculescu R, Vanura K, Montpellier B, Roulland S, Le T, Navarro JM, Jager U, McBlane F, Nadel B. 2006. Recombinase, chromosomal translocations and lymphoid neoplasia: targeting mistakes and repair failures. *DNA Repair (Amst)* 5: 1246-58.

[5] Curry JD, Schulz D, Guidos CJ, Danska JS, Nutter L, Nussenzweig A, Schlissel MS. 2007. Chromosomal reinsertion of broken RSS ends during T cell development. *J Exp Med* 204: 2293-303.

[6] Mullighan CG, Goorha S, Radtke I, Miller CB, Coustan-Smith E, Dalton JD, Girtman K, Mathew S, Ma J, Pounds SB, Su X, Pui CH, Relling MV, Evans WE, Shurtleff SA, Downing JR. 2007. Genome-wide analysis of genetic alterations in acute lymphoblastic leukaemia. *Nature* 446: 758-64.

[7] Mullighan CG, Downing JR. 2009. Genome-wide profiling of genetic alterations in acute lymphoblastic leukemia: recent insights and future directions. *Leukemia* 23: 1209-18.

[8] Merelli I, Guffanti A, Fabbri M, Cocito A, Furia L, Grazini U, Bonnal RJ, Milanesi L, McBlane F. RSSsite: a reference database and prediction tool for the identification of cryptic Recombination Signal Sequences in human and murine genomes. *Nucleic Acids Res* 38 Suppl: W262-7.

[9] Raghavan SC, Swanson PC, Wu X, Hsieh CL, Lieber MR. 2004. A non-B-DNA structure at the Bcl-2 major breakpoint region is cleaved by the RAG complex. *Nature* 428: 88-93.

[10] Meijerink JP, den Boer ML, Pieters R. 2009. New genetic abnormalities and treatment response in acute lymphoblastic leukemia. *Semin Hematol* 46: 16-23.

[11] Rowley JD. 1973. Letter: A new consistent chromosomal abnormality in chronic myelogenous leukaemia identified by quinacrine fluorescence and Giemsa staining. *Nature* 243: 290-3.

[12] Kuiper RP, Schoenmakers EF, van Reijmersdal SV, Hehir-Kwa JY, van Kessel AG, van Leeuwen FN, Hoogerbrugge PM. 2007. High-resolution genomic profiling of childhood ALL reveals novel recurrent genetic lesions affecting pathways involved in lymphocyte differentiation and cell cycle progression. *Leukemia* 21: 1258-66.

[13] Shochat C, Tal N, Bandapalli OR, Palmi C, Ganmore I, Te Kronnie G, Cario G, Cazzaniga G, Kulozik AE, Stanulla M, Schrappe M, Biondi A, Basso G, Bercovich D, Muckenthaler MU, Izraeli S. 2011. Gain-of-function mutations in interleukin-7 receptor-{alpha} (IL7R) in childhood acute lymphoblastic leukemias. *J Exp Med (in press)*.

[14] Jumaa H, Bossaller L, Portugal K, Storch B, Lotz M, Flemming A, Schrappe M, Postila V, Riikonen P, Pelkonen J, Niemeyer CM, Reth M. 2003. Deficiency of the adaptor SLP-65 in pre-B-cell acute lymphoblastic leukaemia. *Nature* 423: 452-6.

[15] Klein F, Feldhahn N, Harder L, Wang H, Wartenberg M, Hofmann WK, Wernet P, Siebert R, Muschen M. 2004. The BCR-ABL1 kinase bypasses selection for the expression of a pre-B cell receptor in pre-B acute lymphoblastic leukemia cells. *J Exp Med* 199: 673-85.

[16] Imai C, Ross ME, Reid G, Coustan-Smith E, Schultz KR, Pui CH, Downing JR, Campana D. 2004. Expression of the adaptor protein BLNK/SLP-65 in childhood acute lymphoblastic leukemia. *Leukemia* 18: 922-5.

[17] Flemming A, Brummer T, Reth M, Jumaa H. 2003. The adaptor protein SLP-65 acts as a tumor suppressor that limits pre-B cell expansion. *Nat Immunol* 4: 38-43.

[18] Hayashi K, Yamamoto M, Nojima T, Goitsuka R, Kitamura D. 2003. Distinct signaling requirements for Dmu selection, IgH allelic exclusion, pre-B cell transition, and tumor suppression in B cell progenitors. *Immunity* 18: 825-36.

[19] Kersseboom R, Middendorp S, Dingjan GM, Dahlenborg K, Reth M, Jumaa H, Hendriks RW. 2003. Bruton's tyrosine kinase cooperates with the B cell linker protein SLP-65 as a tumor suppressor in Pre-B cells. *J Exp Med* 198: 91-8.

[20] Middendorp S, Zijlstra AJ, Kersseboom R, Dingjan GM, Jumaa H, Hendriks RW. 2005. Tumor suppressor function of Bruton tyrosine kinase is independent of its catalytic activity. *Blood* 105: 259-65.

[21] Jumaa H, Hendriks RW, Reth M. 2005. B cell signaling and tumorigenesis. *Annu Rev Immunol* 23: 415-45.

[22] Khan WN, Alt FW, Gerstein RM, Malynn BA, Larsson I, Rathbun G, Davidson L, Muller S, Kantor AB, Herzenberg LA, et al. 1995. Defective B cell development and function in Btk-deficient mice. *Immunity* 3: 283-99.

[23] Kitamura D, Rajewsky K. 1992. Targeted disruption of mu chain membrane exon causes loss of heavy-chain allelic exclusion. *Nature* 356: 154-6.

[24] Hendriks RW, Middendorp S. 2004. The pre-BCR checkpoint as a cell-autonomous proliferation switch. *Trends Immunol* 25: 249-56.

[25] Xu S, Lee KG, Huo J, Kurosaki T, Lam KP. 2007. Combined deficiencies in Bruton tyrosine kinase and phospholipase Cgamma2 arrest B-cell development at a pre-BCR+ stage. *Blood* 109: 3377-84.

[26] Lu R, Medina KL, Lancki DW, Singh H. 2003. IRF-4,8 orchestrate the pre-B-to-B transition in lymphocyte development. *Genes Dev* 17: 1703-8.

[27] Hardy RR, Carmack CE, Shinton SA, Kemp JD, Hayakawa K. 1991. Resolution and characterization of pro-B and pre-pro-B cell stages in normal mouse bone marrow. *J Exp Med* 173: 1213-25.

[28] Schatz DG, Oettinger MA, Baltimore D. 1989. The V(D)J recombination activating gene, RAG-1. *Cell* 59: 1035-48.

[29] Oettinger MA, Schatz DG, Gorka C, Baltimore D. 1990. RAG-1 and RAG-2, adjacent genes that synergistically activate V(D)J recombination. *Science* 248: 1517-23.

[30] Igarashi H, Gregory SC, Yokota T, Sakaguchi N, Kincade PW. 2002. Transcription from the RAG1 locus marks the earliest lymphocyte progenitors in bone marrow. *Immunity* 17: 117-30.

[31] Kee BL, Murre C. 1998. Induction of early B cell factor (EBF) and multiple B lineage genes by the basic helix-loop-helix transcription factor E12. *J Exp Med* 188: 699-713.

[32] Ikawa T, Kawamoto H, Wright LY, Murre C. 2004. Long-term cultured E2A-deficient hematopoietic progenitor cells are pluripotent. *Immunity* 20: 349-60.

[33] Beck K, Peak MM, Ota T, Nemazee D, Murre C. 2009. Distinct roles for E12 and E47 in B cell specification and the sequential rearrangement of immunoglobulin light chain loci. *J Exp Med* 206: 2271-84.

[34] Decker T, Pasca di Magliano M, McManus S, Sun Q, Bonifer C, Tagoh H, Busslinger M. 2009. Stepwise activation of enhancer and promoter regions of the B cell commitment gene Pax5 in early lymphopoiesis. *Immunity* 30: 508-20.

[35] Cobaleda C, Schebesta A, Delogu A, Busslinger M. 2007. Pax5: the guardian of B cell identity and function. *Nat Immunol* 8: 463-70.

[36] Hardy RR, Kincade PW, Dorshkind K. 2007. The protean nature of cells in the B lymphocyte lineage. *Immunity* 26: 703-14.

[37] Nutt SL, Kee BL. 2007. The transcriptional regulation of B cell lineage commitment. *Immunity* 26: 715-25.

[38] Thompson EC, Cobb BS, Sabbattini P, Meixlsperger S, Parelho V, Liberg D, Taylor B, Dillon N, Georgopoulos K, Jumaa H, Smale ST, Fisher AG, Merkenschlager M. 2007. Ikaros DNA-binding proteins as integral components of B cell developmental-stage-specific regulatory circuits. *Immunity* 26: 335-44.

[39] Georgopoulos K. 2002. Haematopoietic cell-fate decisions, chromatin regulation and ikaros. *Nat Rev Immunol* 2: 162-74.

[40] Reynaud D, Demarco IA, Reddy KL, Schjerven H, Bertolino E, Chen Z, Smale ST, Winandy S, Singh H. 2008. Regulation of B cell fate commitment and immunoglobulin heavy-chain gene rearrangements by Ikaros. *Nat Immunol* 9: 927-36.

[41] Liu P, Keller JR, Ortiz M, Tessarollo L, Rachel RA, Nakamura T, Jenkins NA, Copeland NG. 2003. Bcl11a is essential for normal lymphoid development. *Nat Immunol* 4: 525-32.

[42] Ikawa T, Kawamoto H, Goldrath AW, Murre C. 2006. E proteins and Notch signaling cooperate to promote T cell lineage specification and commitment. *J Exp Med* 203: 1329-42.
[43] Amin RH, Schlissel MS. 2008. Foxo1 directly regulates the transcription of recombination-activating genes during B cell development. *Nat Immunol* 9: 613-22.
[44] Meffre E, Casellas R, Nussenzweig MC. 2000. Antibody regulation of B cell development. *Nat Immunol* 1: 379-85.
[45] Schlissel MS. 2003. Regulating antigen-receptor gene assembly. *Nat Rev Immunol* 3: 890-9.
[46] Jung D, Giallourakis C, Mostoslavsky R, Alt FW. 2006. Mechanism and control of V(D)J recombination at the immunoglobulin heavy chain locus. *Annu Rev Immunol* 24: 541-70.
[47] Soulas-Sprauel P, Rivera-Munoz P, Malivert L, Le Guyader G, Abramowski V, Revy P, de Villartay JP. 2007. V(D)J and immunoglobulin class switch recombinations: a paradigm to study the regulation of DNA end-joining. *Oncogene* 26: 7780-91.
[48] Weterings E, Chen DJ. 2008. The endless tale of non-homologous end-joining. *Cell Res* 18: 114-24.
[49] Bassing CH, Alt FW. 2004. The cellular response to general and programmed DNA double strand breaks. *DNA Repair (Amst)* 3: 781-96.
[50] Lee J, Desiderio S. 1999. Cyclin A/CDK2 regulates V(D)J recombination by coordinating RAG-2 accumulation and DNA repair. *Immunity* 11: 771-81.
[51] Liu Y, Zhang L, Desiderio S. 2009. Temporal and spatial regulation of V(D)J recombination: interactions of extrinsic factors with the RAG complex. *Adv Exp Med Biol* 650: 157-65.
[52] Matthews AG, Oettinger MA. 2009. RAG: a recombinase diversified. *Nat Immunol* 10: 817-21.
[53] Schatz DG. 2004. V(D)J recombination. *Immunol Rev* 200: 5-11.
[54] van Gent DC, van der Burg M. 2007. Non-homologous end-joining, a sticky affair. *Oncogene* 26: 7731-40.
[55] Komori T, Okada A, Stewart V, Alt FW. 1993. Lack of N regions in antigen receptor variable region genes of TdT-deficient lymphocytes. *Science* 261: 1171-5.
[56] Gilfillan S, Benoist C, Mathis D. 1995. Mice lacking terminal deoxynucleotidyl transferase: adult mice with a fetal antigen receptor repertoire. *Immunol Rev* 148: 201-19.
[57] Agarwal S, Tafel AA, Kanaar R. 2006. DNA double-strand break repair and chromosome translocations. *DNA Repair (Amst)* 5: 1075-81.
[58] Essers J, van Steeg H, de Wit J, Swagemakers SM, Vermeij M, Hoeijmakers JH, Kanaar R. 2000. Homologous and non-homologous recombination differentially affect DNA damage repair in mice. *Embo J* 19: 1703-10.
[59] Mills KD, Ferguson DO, Essers J, Eckersdorff M, Kanaar R, Alt FW. 2004. Rad54 and DNA Ligase IV cooperate to maintain mammalian chromatid stability. *Genes Dev* 18: 1283-92.
[60] Couedel C, Mills KD, Barchi M, Shen L, Olshen A, Johnson RD, Nussenzweig A, Essers J, Kanaar R, Li GC, Alt FW, Jasin M. 2004. Collaboration of homologous

recombination and nonhomologous end-joining factors for the survival and integrity of mice and cells. *Genes Dev* 18: 1293-304.

[61] Chevillard C, Ozaki J, Herring CD, Riblet R. 2002. A three-megabase yeast artificial chromosome contig spanning the C57BL mouse Igh locus. *J Immunol* 168: 5659-66.

[62] Johnston CM, Wood AL, Bolland DJ, Corcoran AE. 2006. Complete sequence assembly and characterization of the C57BL/6 mouse Ig heavy chain V region. *J Immunol* 176: 4221-34.

[63] Feeney AJ, Goebel P, Espinoza CR. 2004. Many levels of control of V gene rearrangement frequency. *Immunol Rev* 200: 44-56.

[64] Schroeder HW, Jr., Hillson JL, Perlmutter RM. 1987. Early restriction of the human antibody repertoire. *Science* 238: 791-3.

[65] Malynn BA, Yancopoulos GD, Barth JE, Bona CA, Alt FW. 1990. Biased expression of JH-proximal VH genes occurs in the newly generated repertoire of neonatal and adult mice. *J Exp Med* 171: 843-59.

[66] Chowdhury D, Sen R. 2004. Regulation of immunoglobulin heavy-chain gene rearrangements. *Immunol Rev* 200: 182-96.

[67] Gu H, Kitamura D, Rajewsky K. 1991. B cell development regulated by gene rearrangement: arrest of maturation by membrane-bound D mu protein and selection of DH element reading frames. *Cell* 65: 47-54.

[68] Yancopoulos GD, Alt FW. 1985. Developmentally controlled and tissue-specific expression of unrearranged VH gene segments. *Cell* 40: 271-81.

[69] Alt FW, Blackwell TK, Yancopoulos GD. 1987. Development of the primary antibody repertoire. *Science* 238: 1079-87.

[70] Kosak ST, Skok JA, Medina KL, Riblet R, Le Beau MM, Fisher AG, Singh H. 2002. Subnuclear compartmentalization of immunoglobulin loci during lymphocyte development. *Science* 296: 158-62.

[71] Roldan E, Fuxa M, Chong W, Martinez D, Novatchkova M, Busslinger M, Skok JA. 2005. Locus 'decontraction' and centromeric recruitment contribute to allelic exclusion of the immunoglobulin heavy-chain gene. *Nat Immunol* 6: 31-41.

[72] Sayegh CE, Jhunjhunwala S, Riblet R, Murre C. 2005. Visualization of looping involving the immunoglobulin heavy-chain locus in developing B cells. *Genes Dev* 19: 322-7.

[73] Fuxa M, Skok J, Souabni A, Salvagiotto G, Roldan E, Busslinger M. 2004. Pax5 induces V-to-DJ rearrangements and locus contraction of the immunoglobulin heavy-chain gene. *Genes Dev* 18: 411-22.

[74] Corcoran AE, Riddell A, Krooshoop D, Venkitaraman AR. 1998. Impaired immunoglobulin gene rearrangement in mice lacking the IL-7 receptor. *Nature* 391: 904-7.

[75] Hu H, Wang B, Borde M, Nardone J, Maika S, Allred L, Tucker PW, Rao A. 2006. Foxp1 is an essential transcriptional regulator of B cell development. *Nat Immunol* 7: 819-26.

[76] Liu H, Schmidt-Supprian M, Shi Y, Hobeika E, Barteneva N, Jumaa H, Pelanda R, Reth M, Skok J, Rajewsky K. 2007. Yin Yang 1 is a critical regulator of B-cell development. *Genes Dev* 21: 1179-89.

[77] Su IH, Basavaraj A, Krutchinsky AN, Hobert O, Ullrich A, Chait BT, Tarakhovsky A. 2003. Ezh2 controls B cell development through histone H3 methylation and Igh rearrangement. *Nat Immunol* 4: 124-31.

[78] Bolland DJ, Wood AL, Johnston CM, Bunting SF, Morgan G, Chakalova L, Fraser PJ, Corcoran AE. 2004. Antisense intergenic transcription in V(D)J recombination. *Nat Immunol* 5: 630-7.

[79] Herzog S, Reth M, Jumaa H. 2009. Regulation of B-cell proliferation and differentiation by pre-B-cell receptor signalling. *Nat Rev Immunol* 9: 195-205.

[80] Melchers F. 2005. The pre-B-cell receptor: selector of fitting immunoglobulin heavy chains for the B-cell repertoire. *Nat Rev Immunol* 5: 578-84.

[81] Kudo A, Melchers F. 1987. A second gene, VpreB in the lambda 5 locus of the mouse, which appears to be selectively expressed in pre-B lymphocytes. *Embo J* 6: 2267-72.

[82] Sakaguchi N, Melchers F. 1986. Lambda 5, a new light-chain-related locus selectively expressed in pre-B lymphocytes. *Nature* 324: 579-82.

[83] Burnet FM. 1957. A modification of Jerne's theory of antibody production using the concept of clonal selection. *Aust. J. Sci.* 20: 67-9.

[84] Cedar H, Bergman Y. 2008. Choreography of Ig allelic exclusion. *Curr Opin Immunol* 20: 308-17.

[85] Vettermann C, Schlissel MS. 2010. Allelic exclusion of immunoglobulin genes: models and mechanisms. *Immunol Rev* 237: 22-42.

[86] Papavasiliou F, Misulovin Z, Suh H, Nussenzweig MC. 1995. The role of Ig beta in precursor B cell transition and allelic exclusion. *Science* 268: 408-11.

[87] Mostoslavsky R, Singh N, Tenzen T, Goldmit M, Gabay C, Elizur S, Qi P, Reubinoff BE, Chess A, Cedar H, Bergman Y. 2001. Asynchronous replication and allelic exclusion in the immune system. *Nature* 414: 221-5.

[88] Ohnishi K, Melchers F. 2003. The nonimmunoglobulin portion of lambda5 mediates cell-autonomous pre-B cell receptor signaling. *Nat Immunol* 4: 849-56.

[89] Ubelhart R, Bach MP, Eschbach C, Wossning T, Reth M, Jumaa H. 2010. N-linked glycosylation selectively regulates autonomous precursor BCR function. *Nat Immunol* 11: 759-65.

[90] ten Boekel E, Melchers F, Rolink AG. 1997. Changes in the V(H) gene repertoire of developing precursor B lymphocytes in mouse bone marrow mediated by the pre-B cell receptor. *Immunity* 7: 357-68.

[91] Gauthier L, Rossi B, Roux F, Termine E, Schiff C. 2002. Galectin-1 is a stromal cell ligand of the pre-B cell receptor (BCR) implicated in synapse formation between pre-B and stromal cells and in pre-BCR triggering. *Proc Natl Acad Sci U S A* 99: 13014-9.

[92] Mourcin F, Breton C, Tellier J, Narang P, Chasson L, Jorquera A, Coles M, Schiff C, Mancini SJ. 2011. Galectin-1 expressing stromal cells constitute a specific niche for pre-BII cell development in mouse bone marrow. *Blood*.

[93] Bradl H, Wittmann J, Milius D, Vettermann C, Jack HM. 2003. Interaction of murine precursor B cell receptor with stroma cells is controlled by the unique tail of lambda 5 and stroma cell-associated heparan sulfate. *J Immunol* 171: 2338-48.

[94] Keenan RA, De Riva A, Corleis B, Hepburn L, Licence S, Winkler TH, Martensson IL. 2008. Censoring of autoreactive B cell development by the pre-B cell receptor. *Science* 321: 696-9.

[95] Wardemann H, Yurasov S, Schaefer A, Young JW, Meffre E, Nussenzweig MC. 2003. Predominant autoantibody production by early human B cell precursors. *Science* 301: 1374-7.

[96] Sanchez M, Misulovin Z, Burkhardt AL, Mahajan S, Costa T, Franke R, Bolen JB, Nussenzweig M. 1993. Signal transduction by immunoglobulin is mediated through Ig alpha and Ig beta. *J Exp Med* 178: 1049-55.

[97] Gupta N, DeFranco AL. 2007. Lipid rafts and B cell signaling. *Semin Cell Dev Biol* 18: 616-26.

[98] Lingwood D, Simons K. 2010. Lipid rafts as a membrane-organizing principle. *Science* 327: 46-50.

[99] Kurosaki T, Johnson SA, Pao L, Sada K, Yamamura H, Cambier JC. 1995. Role of the Syk autophosphorylation site and SH2 domains in B cell antigen receptor signaling. *J Exp Med* 182: 1815-23.

[100] Koretzky GA, Abtahian F, Silverman MA. 2006. SLP76 and SLP65: complex regulation of signalling in lymphocytes and beyond. *Nat Rev Immunol* 6: 67-78.

[101] Hendriks RW, Kersseboom R. 2006. Involvement of SLP-65 and Btk in tumor suppression and malignant transformation of pre-B cells. *Semin Immunol* 18: 67-76.

[102] Lewis CM, Broussard C, Czar MJ, Schwartzberg PL. 2001. Tec kinases: modulators of lymphocyte signaling and development. *Curr Opin Immunol* 13: 317-25.

[103] Kurosaki T, Hikida M. 2009. Tyrosine kinases and their substrates in B lymphocytes. *Immunol Rev* 228: 132-48.

[104] Deane JA, Fruman DA. 2004. Phosphoinositide 3-kinase: diverse roles in immune cell activation. *Annu Rev Immunol* 22: 563-98.

[105] Shimizu T, Mundt C, Licence S, Melchers F, Martensson IL. 2002. VpreB1/VpreB2/lambda 5 triple-deficient mice show impaired B cell development but functional allelic exclusion of the IgH locus. *J Immunol* 168: 6286-93.

[106] Gong S, Nussenzweig MC. 1996. Regulation of an early developmental checkpoint in the B cell pathway by Ig beta. *Science* 272: 411-4.

[107] Pelanda R, Braun U, Hobeika E, Nussenzweig MC, Reth M. 2002. B cell progenitors are arrested in maturation but have intact VDJ recombination in the absence of Ig-alpha and Ig-beta. *J Immunol* 169: 865-72.

[108] Cheng AM, Rowley B, Pao W, Hayday A, Bolen JB, Pawson T. 1995. Syk tyrosine kinase required for mouse viability and B-cell development. *Nature* 378: 303-6.

[109] Turner M, Mee PJ, Costello PS, Williams O, Price AA, Duddy LP, Furlong MT, Geahlen RL, Tybulewicz VL. 1995. Perinatal lethality and blocked B-cell development in mice lacking the tyrosine kinase Syk. *Nature* 378: 298-302.

[110] Nakayama J, Yamamoto M, Hayashi K, Satoh H, Bundo K, Kubo M, Goitsuka R, Farrar MA, Kitamura D. 2009. BLNK suppresses pre-B-cell leukemogenesis through inhibition of JAK3. *Blood* 113: 1483-92.

[111] Schebesta M, Pfeffer PL, Busslinger M. 2002. Control of pre-BCR signaling by Pax5-dependent activation of the BLNK gene. *Immunity* 17: 473-85.

[112] Brunet A, Bonni A, Zigmond MJ, Lin MZ, Juo P, Hu LS, Anderson MJ, Arden KC, Blenis J, Greenberg ME. 1999. Akt promotes cell survival by phosphorylating and inhibiting a Forkhead transcription factor. *Cell* 96: 857-68.
[113] Coffer PJ, Burgering BM. 2004. Forkhead-box transcription factors and their role in the immune system. *Nat Rev Immunol* 4: 889-99.
[114] Cully M, You H, Levine AJ, Mak TW. 2006. Beyond PTEN mutations: the PI3K pathway as an integrator of multiple inputs during tumorigenesis. *Nat Rev Cancer* 6: 184-92.
[115] Milne CD, Paige CJ. 2006. IL-7: a key regulator of B lymphopoiesis. *Semin Immunol* 18: 20-30.
[116] Cooper AB, Sawai CM, Sicinska E, Powers SE, Sicinski P, Clark MR, Aifantis I. 2006. A unique function for cyclin D3 in early B cell development. *Nat Immunol* 7: 489-97.
[117] Gold MR. 2008. B cell development: important work for ERK. *Immunity* 28: 488-90.
[118] Yasuda T, Sanjo H, Pages G, Kawano Y, Karasuyama H, Pouyssegur J, Ogata M, Kurosaki T. 2008. Erk kinases link pre-B cell receptor signaling to transcriptional events required for early B cell expansion. *Immunity* 28: 499-508.
[119] Parker MJ, Licence S, Erlandsson L, Galler GR, Chakalova L, Osborne CS, Morgan G, Fraser P, Jumaa H, Winkler TH, Skok J, Martensson IL. 2005. The pre-B-cell receptor induces silencing of VpreB and lambda5 transcription. *Embo J* 24: 3895-905.
[120] van Loo PF, Dingjan GM, Maas A, Hendriks RW. 2007. Surrogate-light-chain silencing is not critical for the limitation of pre-B cell expansion but is for the termination of constitutive signaling. *Immunity* 27: 468-80.
[121] Herzog S, Hug E, Meixlsperger S, Paik JH, DePinho RA, Reth M, Jumaa H. 2008. SLP-65 regulates immunoglobulin light chain gene recombination through the PI(3)K-PKB-Foxo pathway. *Nat Immunol* 9: 623-31.
[122] Johnson K, Hashimshony T, Sawai CM, Pongubala JM, Skok JA, Aifantis I, Singh H. 2008. Regulation of immunoglobulin light-chain recombination by the transcription factor IRF-4 and the attenuation of interleukin-7 signaling. *Immunity* 28: 335-45.
[123] Geier JK, Schlissel MS. 2006. Pre-BCR signals and the control of Ig gene rearrangements. *Semin Immunol* 18: 31-9.
[124] Muljo SA, Schlissel MS. 2003. A small molecule Abl kinase inhibitor induces differentiation of Abelson virus-transformed pre-B cell lines. *Nat Immunol* 4: 31-7.
[125] Reth M, Petrac E, Wiese P, Lobel L, Alt FW. 1987. Activation of V kappa gene rearrangement in pre-B cells follows the expression of membrane-bound immunoglobulin heavy chains. *Embo J* 6: 3299-305.
[126] Schlissel MS. 2004. Regulation of activation and recombination of the murine Igkappa locus. *Immunol Rev* 200: 215-23.
[127] Merrell KT, Benschop RJ, Gauld SB, Aviszus K, Decote-Ricardo D, Wysocki LJ, Cambier JC. 2006. Identification of anergic B cells within a wild-type repertoire. *Immunity* 25: 953-62.
[128] Shlomchik MJ. 2008. Sites and stages of autoreactive B cell activation and regulation. *Immunity* 28: 18-28.

[129] Nemazee D. 2006. Receptor editing in lymphocyte development and central tolerance. *Nat Rev Immunol* 6: 728-40.
[130] Halverson R, Torres RM, Pelanda R. 2004. Receptor editing is the main mechanism of B cell tolerance toward membrane antigens. *Nat Immunol* 5: 645-50.
[131] Chung JB, Silverman M, Monroe JG. 2003. Transitional B cells: step by step towards immune competence. *Trends Immunol* 24: 343-9.
[132] Rolink AG, Andersson J, Melchers F. 2004. Molecular mechanisms guiding late stages of B-cell development. *Immunol Rev* 197: 41-50.
[133] Benner R, Hijmans W, Haaijman JJ. 1981. The bone marrow: the major source of serum immunoglobulins, but still a neglected site of antibody formation. *Clin Exp Immunol* 46: 1-8.
[134] Martin F, Kearney JF. 2000. B-cell subsets and the mature preimmune repertoire. Marginal zone and B1 B cells as part of a "natural immune memory". *Immunol Rev* 175: 70-9.
[135] Kersseboom R, Kil L, Flierman R, van der Zee M, Dingjan GM, Middendorp S, Maas A, Hendriks RW. 2010. Constitutive activation of Bruton's tyrosine kinase induces the formation of autoreactive IgM plasma cells. *Eur J Immunol* 40: 2643-54.
[136] Ramiro AR, Nussenzweig MC. 2004. Immunology: aid for AID. *Nature* 430: 980-1.
[137] Honjo T, Nagaoka H, Shinkura R, Muramatsu M. 2005. AID to overcome the limitations of genomic information. *Nat Immunol* 6: 655-61.
[138] Jankovic M, Nussenzweig A, Nussenzweig MC. 2007. Antigen receptor diversification and chromosome translocations. *Nat Immunol* 8: 801-8.
[139] Chaudhuri J, Tian M, Khuong C, Chua K, Pinaud E, Alt FW. 2003. Transcription-targeted DNA deamination by the AID antibody diversification enzyme. *Nature* 422: 726-30.
[140] Dickerson SK, Market E, Besmer E, Papavasiliou FN. 2003. AID mediates hypermutation by deaminating single stranded DNA. *J Exp Med* 197: 1291-6.
[141] Ramiro AR, Stavropoulos P, Jankovic M, Nussenzweig MC. 2003. Transcription enhances AID-mediated cytidine deamination by exposing single-stranded DNA on the nontemplate strand. *Nat Immunol* 4: 452-6.
[142] Wang CL, Harper RA, Wabl M. 2004. Genome-wide somatic hypermutation. *Proc Natl Acad Sci U S A* 101: 7352-6.
[143] Liu M, Duke JL, Richter DJ, Vinuesa CG, Goodnow CC, Kleinstein SH, Schatz DG. 2008. Two levels of protection for the B cell genome during somatic hypermutation. *Nature* 451: 841-5.
[144] Pasqualucci L, Neumeister P, Goossens T, Nanjangud G, Chaganti RS, Kuppers R, Dalla-Favera R. 2001. Hypermutation of multiple proto-oncogenes in B-cell diffuse large-cell lymphomas. *Nature* 412: 341-6.
[145] Ramiro AR, Jankovic M, Eisenreich T, Difilippantonio S, Chen-Kiang S, Muramatsu M, Honjo T, Nussenzweig A, Nussenzweig MC. 2004. AID is required for c-myc/IgH chromosome translocations in vivo. *Cell* 118: 431-8.
[146] Sprangers M, Feldhahn N, Liedtke S, Jumaa H, Siebert R, Muschen M. 2006. SLP65 deficiency results in perpetual V(D)J recombinase activity in pre-B-lymphoblastic leukemia and B-cell lymphoma cells. *Oncogene*.

[147] Ta VB, de Haan AB, de Bruijn MJ, Dingjan GM, Hendriks RW. 2011. Pre-B-cell leukemias in Btk/Slp65-deficient mice arise independently of ongoing V(D)J recombination activity. *Leukemia* 25: 48-56.

[148] Ta VB, de Bruijn MJ, ter Brugge PJ, van Hamburg JP, Diepstraten HJ, van Loo PF, Kersseboom R, Hendriks RW. 2010. Malignant transformation of Slp65-deficient pre-B cells involves disruption of the Arf-Mdm2-p53 tumor suppressor pathway. *Blood* 115: 1385-93.

[149] Adams JM, Harris AW, Pinkert CA, Corcoran LM, Alexander WS, Cory S, Palmiter RD, Brinster RL. 1985. The c-myc oncogene driven by immunoglobulin enhancers induces lymphoid malignancy in transgenic mice. *Nature* 318: 533-8.

[150] Pelengaris S, Khan M, Evan G. 2002. c-MYC: more than just a matter of life and death. *Nat Rev Cancer* 2: 764-76.

[151] Neri A, Barriga F, Knowles DM, Magrath IT, Dalla-Favera R. 1988. Different regions of the immunoglobulin heavy-chain locus are involved in chromosomal translocations in distinct pathogenetic forms of Burkitt lymphoma. *Proc Natl Acad Sci U S A* 85: 2748-52.

[152] Dave SS, Fu K, Wright GW, Lam LT, Kluin P, Boerma EJ, Greiner TC, Weisenburger DD, Rosenwald A, Ott G, Muller-Hermelink HK, Gascoyne RD, Delabie J, Rimsza LM, Braziel RM, Grogan TM, Campo E, Jaffe ES, Dave BJ, Sanger W, Bast M, Vose JM, Armitage JO, Connors JM, Smeland EB, Kvaloy S, Holte H, Fisher RI, Miller TP, Montserrat E, Wilson WH, Bahl M, Zhao H, Yang L, Powell J, Simon R, Chan WC, Staudt LM. 2006. Molecular diagnosis of Burkitt's lymphoma. *N Engl J Med* 354: 2431-42.

[153] Nussenzweig MC, Schmidt EV, Shaw AC, Sinn E, Campos-Torres J, Mathey-Prevot B, Pattengale PK, Leder P. 1988. A human immunoglobulin gene reduces the incidence of lymphomas in c-Myc-bearing transgenic mice. *Nature* 336: 446-50.

[154] Habib T, Park H, Tsang M, de Alboran IM, Nicks A, Wilson L, Knoepfler PS, Andrews S, Rawlings DJ, Eisenman RN, Iritani BM. 2007. Myc stimulates B lymphocyte differentiation and amplifies calcium signaling. *J Cell Biol* 179: 717-31.

[155] Wen R, Chen Y, Bai L, Fu G, Schuman J, Dai X, Zeng H, Yang C, Stephan RP, Cleveland JL, Wang D. 2006. Essential role of phospholipase C gamma 2 in early B-cell development and Myc-mediated lymphomagenesis. *Mol Cell Biol* 26: 9364-76.

[156] Sherr CJ. 1998. Tumor surveillance via the ARF-p53 pathway. *Genes Dev* 12: 2984-91.

[157] Eischen CM, Weber JD, Roussel MF, Sherr CJ, Cleveland JL. 1999. Disruption of the ARF-Mdm2-p53 tumor suppressor pathway in Myc-induced lymphomagenesis. *Genes Dev* 13: 2658-69.

[158] Morrow MA, Lee G, Gillis S, Yancopoulos GD, Alt FW. 1992. Interleukin-7 induces N-myc and c-myc expression in normal precursor B lymphocytes. *Genes Dev* 6: 61-70.

[159] Dillon SR, Schlissel MS. 2002. Partial restoration of B cell development in Jak-3(-/-) mice achieved by co-expression of IgH and E(mu)-myc transgenes. *Int Immunol* 14: 893-904.

[160] Nepal RM, Zaheen A, Basit W, Li L, Berger SA, Martin A. 2008. AID and RAG1 do not contribute to lymphomagenesis in Emu c-myc transgenic mice. *Oncogene* 27: 4752-6.

[161] Bouchard C, Lee S, Paulus-Hock V, Loddenkemper C, Eilers M, Schmitt CA. 2007. FoxO transcription factors suppress Myc-driven lymphomagenesis via direct activation of Arf. *Genes Dev* 21: 2775-87.

[162] Radfar A, Unnikrishnan I, Lee HW, DePinho RA, Rosenberg N. 1998. p19(Arf) induces p53-dependent apoptosis during abelson virus-mediated pre-B cell transformation. *Proc Natl Acad Sci U S A* 95: 13194-9.

[163] Basso K, Margolin AA, Stolovitzky G, Klein U, Dalla-Favera R, Califano A. 2005. Reverse engineering of regulatory networks in human B cells. *Nat Genet* 37: 382-90.

[164] Sherr CJ. 2006. Divorcing ARF and p53: an unsettled case. *Nat Rev Cancer* 6: 663-73.

[165] Humbey O, Pimkina J, Zilfou JT, Jarnik M, Dominguez-Brauer C, Burgess DJ, Eischen CM, Murphy ME. 2008. The ARF tumor suppressor can promote the progression of some tumors. *Cancer Res* 68: 9608-13.

[166] Balaburski GM, Hontz RD, Murphy ME. 2010. p53 and ARF: unexpected players in autophagy. *Trends Cell Biol* 20: 363-9.

[167] Maclean KH, Dorsey FC, Cleveland JL, Kastan MB. 2008. Targeting lysosomal degradation induces p53-dependent cell death and prevents cancer in mouse models of lymphomagenesis. *J Clin Invest* 118: 79-88.

[168] Amaravadi RK, Yu D, Lum JJ, Bui T, Christophorou MA, Evan GI, Thomas-Tikhonenko A, Thompson CB. 2007. Autophagy inhibition enhances therapy-induced apoptosis in a Myc-induced model of lymphoma. *J Clin Invest* 117: 326-36.

[169] Carew JS, Nawrocki ST, Kahue CN, Zhang H, Yang C, Chung L, Houghton JA, Huang P, Giles FJ, Cleveland JL. 2007. Targeting autophagy augments the anticancer activity of the histone deacetylase inhibitor SAHA to overcome Bcr-Abl-mediated drug resistance. *Blood* 110: 313-22.

[170] Duy C, Yu JJ, Nahar R, Swaminathan S, Kweon SM, Polo JM, Valls E, Klemm L, Shojaee S, Cerchietti L, Schuh W, Jack HM, Hurtz C, Ramezani-Rad P, Herzog S, Jumaa H, Koeffler HP, de Alboran IM, Melnick AM, Ye BH, Muschen M. 2010. BCL6 is critical for the development of a diverse primary B cell repertoire. *J Exp Med* 207: 1209-21.

[171] Pendergast AM. 2002. The Abl family kinases: mechanisms of regulation and signaling. *Adv Cancer Res* 85: 51-100.

[172] Heisterkamp N, Stephenson JR, Groffen J, Hansen PF, de Klein A, Bartram CR, Grosveld G. 1983. Localization of the c-abl oncogene adjacent to a translocation break point in chronic myelocytic leukaemia. *Nature* 306: 239-42.

[173] Wong S, Witte ON. 2004. The BCR-ABL story: bench to bedside and back. *Annu Rev Immunol* 22: 247-306.

[174] Feldhahn N, Klein F, Mooster JL, Hadweh P, Sprangers M, Wartenberg M, Bekhite MM, Hofmann WK, Herzog S, Jumaa H, Rowley JD, Muschen M. 2005. Mimicry of a constitutively active pre-B cell receptor in acute lymphoblastic leukemia cells. *J Exp Med* 201: 1837-52.

[175] Iorio MV, Croce CM. 2009. MicroRNAs in cancer: small molecules with a huge impact. *J Clin Oncol* 27: 5848-56.
[176] Croce CM. 2009. Causes and consequences of microRNA dysregulation in cancer. *Nat Rev Genet* 10: 704-14.
[177] Croce CM. 2008. Oncogenes and cancer. *N Engl J Med* 358: 502-11.
[178] Calin GA, Dumitru CD, Shimizu M, Bichi R, Zupo S, Noch E, Aldler H, Rattan S, Keating M, Rai K, Rassenti L, Kipps T, Negrini M, Bullrich F, Croce CM. 2002. Frequent deletions and down-regulation of micro- RNA genes miR15 and miR16 at 13q14 in chronic lymphocytic leukemia. *Proc Natl Acad Sci U S A* 99: 15524-9.

In: Acute Lymphoblastic Leukemia
Editors: Severo Vecchione and Luigi Tedesco

ISBN: 978-1-61470-872-8
©2012 Nova Science Publishers, Inc.

Chapter III

Childhood Acute Lymphoblastic Leukemia

*Adriana Zámečníkova**

Kuwait Cancer Control Center, Department of Hematology,
Laboratory of Cancer Genetics, Kuwait

Abstract

Acute lymphoblastic leukemia (ALL) is a malignant disorder of the bone marrow in which a lymphoid precursor cell becomes genetically altered resulting in dysregulated proliferation and clonal expansion of neoplastic cells. It is the most common malignancy in children, representing nearly one third of all pediatric cancers. The disease has a bimodal distribution; there is an early incidence peak at 2 to 5 years of age, where they represent about 80% of the childhood leukemias and with a second incidence peak at around 50 years old. Although there are some identified factors associated with increased risk of developing the disease, the etiology of acute lymphoblastic leukemia remains largely unknown. A small percentage of cases are associated with inherited genetic abnormalities, with the best characterized being Down's syndrome and congenital immunodeficiencies. In addition to genetics, parental and environmental factors have been suggested to contribute to susceptibility, supported by the observation that the type and frequency of childhood ALL vary by geographic region and ethnicity. Improvement in molecular biology research as well as better cytogenetic techniques revealed that childhood acute lymphoblastic leukemia is a highly heterogeneous disease, comprising many entities. A number of genetic subtypes has been and continue to be discovered in pediatric ALL and it has been repeatedly shown that recurrent genetic abnormalities are present in the majority of successfully karyotyped patients with ALL. In addition, several new cryptic abnormalities have been discovered recently using genome-wide surveys, leading to identification of previously unrecognized diversity among individual patients.

---

* Correspodence to : Zámečníkova Adriana, Kuwait Cancer Control Center, Department of Hematology, Laboratory of Cancer Genetics, P.O.Box 42262, Shuwaikh -70653, Kuwait. E-mail: annaadria@yahoo.com; Tel: 00965 4821363; Fax: 00965 481007.

More importantly, recurrent chromosomal abnormalities observed in leukemia cells have shown correlations between specific genomic alterations and clinical-biological features of patients with diagnostic and prognostic significance. The recognition of these anomalies has contributed greatly to our understanding of disease pathogenesis, leading to the concept of risk-adapted treatment strategies and intensive therapy approaches for patients. Due to the exponential growth in our understanding, the treatment ofchildhood acute lymphoblastic leukemia is a success story in modern oncology with the potential to change the medicine fundamentally. This review provides insight into clinical and biological characteristics of ALL in children, as well as highlights some of the recently described prognostic markers that might serve as new and potential therapeutic targets for future drug development.

Introduction

Acute lymphoblastic leukemia (ALL) is a malignant disorder of the bone marrow in which a lymphoid precursor cell becomes genetically altered resulting in dysregulated proliferation, survival and accumulation of neoplastic cells. It is the most common malignancy of childhood, representing nearly one third of all pediatric cancers [1-4]. The disease has a bimodal distribution; there is an early incidence peak at 2 to 5 years of age, decreasing in incidence with increasing age before a second incidence peak at around 50 years old. The incidence of ALL among children ages 2 to 3 years is approximately 10-fold higher than that for children who are 19 years old. Approximately 2% to 5% of ALL occurs in infants (children less than 1 year old) [5-6].

Childhood ALL has unique clinical, epidemiological and biological features. It is the most common leukemia in children representing about 75-80% of childhood leukemias while it accounts for only 20% of adult acute leukemia [3, 4]. It is slightly more common in males than females and this difference is greatest among pubertal children. The male preponderance is particularly evident in children with T-cell ALL. For unexplained reasons, the incidence of ALL is substantially higher for white than for black children and in advanced (not developing) countries. In addition, there appear to be geographic and racial differences in the frequency and age distribution of pediatric malignancy. For example, in North Africa and the Middle East, non-Hodgkin's lymphoma is the most common childhood malignancy and ALL is relatively rare [7-10].

Etiology of Childhood Acute Lymphoblastic Leukemia

Although pediatric ALL is the most common cancer in childhood, its etiology remains largely unknown. Confirmed responsibility of certain factors explains less than 10% of disease incidence, leaving 90% of cases with an unknown etiology. While the cause in most cases is not known, certain clinical and epidemiologic associations have been suggested and there are some identified factors associated with an increased risk of developing ALL (Figure 1) [2, 11].

Etiology of childhood acute lymphoblastic leukemia

Prenatal origin	Inherited predisposition	Enviromental
Errors in normal DNA processing Mothers recently infected with influenza, varicella, or other viruses Parental exposures to chemicals and solvents Prenatal exposures to genotoxic agents Maternal age	Family history of cancer Constitutional chromosomal anomalies Fanconi anemia Neurofibromatosis Shwachman syndrome Congenital immunodeficiency Inherited variation of specific genes	Exposure to ionizing radiation Exposure to herbicides and pesticides, electromagnetic fields Maternal use of alcohol, contraceptives, cigarettes Exposures to genotoxic chemicals and solvents Chemical contamination of ground water

Figure 1. Etiology of childhood acute lymphoblastic leukemia.

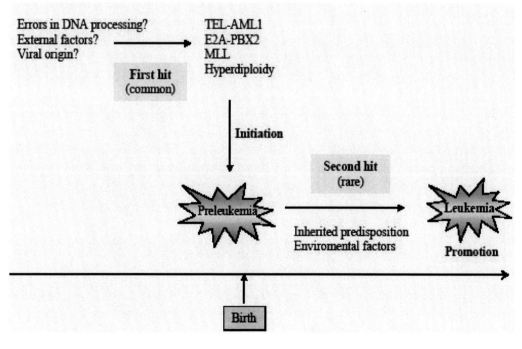

Figure 2. Natural course of childhood leukaemia.

Prenatal Origin

Recent reports have suggested that development of childhood acute lymphoblastic leukaemia often occurs *in utero* during fetal development. Evidence in support of this comes from genetic studies of identical infant twins with concordant leukemia showing concordance with identical, clonal fusion gene sequences in both twins. Similarly, it has been demonstrated that pediatric ALL patients with specific chromosomal abnormalities had blood cells carrying the abnormalities at the time of birth. By retrospective analysing blood samples obtained at birth it was demonstrated, that that foetal initiation is a common phenomenon in childhood ALL [12].

However, there is compelling evidence that such an event is insufficient and that the development of leukaemia requires at least one additional genetic event after birth besides the initial translocation ("two hit" model). This is consistent with the hypothesis that childhood acute lymphoblastic leukaemia develops as a multiple step process involving both foetal initiation and postnatal promotion (Figure 2) [2, 11-12].

Inherited Predisposition

Hereditary factors are presumed to have a role in the predisposition of pediatric acute leukemias, including ALL. This is suggested by several findings, such as association of childhood ALL with family history of haematological neoplasm, association between inherited, predisposing genetic syndromes and childhood ALL as well as with inherited variations of some specific genes. It is likely, that the development of leukemia in these cases is not likely to be caused by a single factor but rather by interaction of inherited genetic predisposition and exposure to certain factor(s) [2, 11].

Several constitutional genetic syndromes have been associated with childhood leukemia, with the best characterized being Down's syndrome. Children with Down syndrome and an extra chromosome 21 are at a 10- to 15-fold increased risk of developing acute leukemia, including both acute lymphoblastic leukemia and acute myeloid leukemia (AML) with a cumulative risk for developing leukemia of approximately 2.1% by age 5 years and 2.7% by age 30 years [2,13]. Approximately two thirds of the cases of acute leukemia in children with Down syndrome are ALL. Increased risk of developing ALL is also associated with certain genetic conditions, including neurofibromatosis, Shwachman syndrome and congenital immunodeficiencies (ie, Wiskott-Aldrich syndrome, X-linked agammaglobulinemia, severe combined immunodeficiency, Bloom syndrome and ataxia-telangiectasia). In addition, some genetic bone marrow failure syndromes, such as Fanconi anaemia, which is a rare autosomal recessive disorder, have inherited genetic predisposition for developing leukemia. Some of these diseases, like ataxia telangiectasia, Bloom syndrome and the Li Fraumeni syndrome, are associated with abnormalities in DNA repair mechanisms indicating that damage to DNA and improper repair initiates or promotes childhood leukaemia. Finally, risk of infant leukaemia has been associated with genetic polymorphisms of NQ01 (NAD(P)H:quinone oxidoreductase) and MTHFR (methylenetetrahydrofolate reductase), as well as HLA class II alleles [14-16].

Environmental Factors

Many external factors have been investigated as potential risk factors for developing childhood ALL, however only few risk factors have been firmly established. Some known environmental risk factors presumed to play a role in developing acute leukemia include exposure to ionizing radiation and certain toxic chemicals (such as benzene). Some studies have shown an increased risk of leukemia in children exposed to diagnostic ionizing radiation in utero; however this experience contrasts with observations of survivors of the atomic bomb, as there was no increase in the incidence of leukemia in children exposed to radiation in utero [2, 3]. Radiography of a mother's abdomen during pregnancy may increase a child's risk of ALL and the evidence of such association was confirmed in studies of animals. Chemotherapy, particularly with alkylating agents can facilitate the development of acute leukemia. Other apparent associations include maternal use of alcohol, tobacco and contraceptives, parental occupational exposures to chemicals, exposure to herbicides and pesticides and chemical contamination of ground water with contaminants such as trihalomethanes, chloroform, zinc, cadmium, and arsenic [2]. A number of reports suggested an increased risk of ALL among children who are not firstborn, children being born to a mother over 35 years of age or to one who previously had spontaneous abortions and among those whose mothers took antibiotics during their pregnancies while breastfeeding has been found to be protective [2,11].

A Critical Role for Infection?

There has been intense interest in the possible role played by bacterial or viral infections in the pathogenesis of leukemia. Few associations have been firmly established, including the link of the Epstein-Barr virus (EBV) to cases of endemic Burkitt's lymphoma and the L3 subtype of ALL, and the association of the human T cell leukaemia/lymphoma virus type I with adult T-cell leukemia/lymphoma [2, 11].

Some reports have suggested an increased risk for ALL in children born to mothers recently infected with various viruses such as influenza and varicella. However; no direct link has been established between prenatal viral exposure and the development of leukemia in children. Similarly, no direct association between childhood viral infections and leukemic risk has been confirmed and the role of viral exposure in the development of childhood acute lymphoblastic leukaemia remains uncertain. Recent epidemiological studies indirectly support the theory that early protection from viral infection may play a role in the development of some subtypes of leukaemia; further supported by the observations that children with more contacts with other infants had a lower risk of developing childhood leukaemia than others [2,17].

Classification of Acute Lymphoblastic Leukemia

Historically, acute lymhoblastic leukemia was classified using the French-American-British (FAB) criteria as having L1 morphology, L2 morphology, or L3 morphology. The widely used French-American-British classification is now considered to not be relevant and is replaced by the new WHO classification system which includes former FAB classifications ALL-L1 and L2, while FAB L3 is now considered Burkitt's leukemia/lymphoma [18]. The division of acute lymphoblastic leukaemia to subtypes is based on morphology of the leukaemic cells, immunophenotyping and cytogenetics (MIC classification: Morphology, Immunophenotype, Cytogenetics). In immunophenotyping, the cell type of the leukaemic blasts is identified with monoclonal antibodies, which allows the recognition of the lineage involved in the malignant process, and the degree of maturation of the malignant cell [18-19].

Broadly, ALL cases can be classified as either B- or T-lineage; however both often express aberrant myeloid or lymphoid associated antigens. B-cell lineage ALL defined by the expression of CD19, HLA-DR, CD10 (cALLa), and other B-cell associated antigens is the most common subtype of childhood leukaemia, accounting for 80-85% of childhood ALL cases. Approximately 80% of B-precursor ALL express the cALLa, CD10 antigen [20-22. Depending on the stage of B-cell maturation B-cell precursor cases can be further subclassified as:

- Early precursor-B cell ALL (no surface or cytoplasmic immunoglobulin)
- Precursor-B cell ALL (blasts express immunoglobulins in the cytoplasm)
- B-cell ALL (presence of surface immunoglobulin).

Approximately three quarters of patients with B-precursor ALL have the early pre-B phenotype. Early pre-B phenotype comprises most of infant ALL. B-cell leukemia, which accounts for only about 3% of ALL cases is a rare case of childhood ALL. B-cell ALL is a systemic manifestation of Burkitt's leukaemia/lymphoma and Burkitt's-like non-Hodgkin's lymphoma in which the leukaemic clone represents a more developed B cell with immunoglobulins on cell surface (L3 in the French-American-British system) [19-20].

T-cell ALL is identified by the expression of T-cell–associated surface antigens CD2, CD7, CD5, or CD3. Approximately 15% of children with newly diagnosed ALL have the T-cell phenotype associated with specific clinical features such as male sex, older age, leukocytosis, and mediastinal mass [22-23].

The recent WHO International panel on ALL recommends the use of the following classification [18, 19]:

- Acute lymphoblastic leukemia/lymphoma (former FAB L1/L2)
- Burkitt's leukemia/lymphoma (former FAB L3)
- Biphenotypic acute leukemia (Table 1).

Table 1. Classification of acute lymphoblastic leukemia

Classification of acute lymphoblastic leukemia
Acute lymphoblastic leukemia/lymphoma (Former FAB L1/L2)
Precursor B acute lymphoblastic leukemia/lymphoma
Cytogenetic subtypes:
t(12;21)(p12,q22) TEL/AML-1
t(1;19)(q23;p13) PBX/E2A
t(9;22)(q34;q11) ABL/BCR
t(V,11)(V;q23); V/MLL rearranged
Hyperdiploid >50
Hypodiploid
Precursor T acute lymphoblastic leukemia/lymphoma
Burkitt's leukemia/lymphoma (Former FAB L3)
Biphenotypic acute leukemia

Table 2. Common chromosomal rearrangements in childhood B-ALL

Common chromosomal rearrangements in childhood B-ALL					
Rearrangement	Genes Involved	Protein	Function of Protein	Phenotype
t(12;21)(p13;q22)	*TEL-AML1*	Runt/transactivating domain	Transcription regulation	Pre-B
t(9;12)(q34;p13)	*ABL-TEL*	HLH protein tyrosine kinase		
t(1;19)(q23;p13)	*E2A-PBX1*	Fusion proteins	Transcription factor	Pre-B
t(17;19)(q22;p13)	*E2A-HLF*			
t(9;22)(q34;q11)	*BCR-ABL1*	p190 p210 p230	Tyrosine kinase	B- or T
t(2;8)(p12;q24)	*IGK-C-MYC*	Basic HLH protein	Transcription factor	B
t(8;14)(q24;q32)	*C-MYC-IGH*			
t(8;22)(q24;q11)	*C-MYC-IGL*			
i(9q)	?	?	?	Pre-B
del(9q)(p21-22)	*MTS1/MTS2*	p16^{INK4A}/p15^{INK4B}	Cyclin-dependent kinase inhibitors	B- or T
t/dic(9;12)	?	?	?	Early-pre-B or pre-B
t(4;11)(q21;q23)	*AF4-MLL*	Fusion proteins	Transcriptional regulation	Early-pre-B T-lineage biphenotypic
t(11;19)(q23;p13)	*MLL-ENL*			
t(V ;11)	*MLL-V*			
i(17q)	?	?	?	Pre-B
del(6q)	?	?	?	B- or T

Genetic Aberrations in Childhood Acute Lymphoblastic Leukemia

Due to the rapid progress in the field of molecular biology and improvements in molecular techniques, the diagnosis and treatment of ALL is rapidly changing and improving. Increased application of new techniques has led to the identification of many cytogenetic or submicroscopic molecular anomalies, and at present recurring genomic abnormalities can be identified in about 80 % of pediatric ALL patients [1, 2, 24].

A number of genetic subtypes with distinct clinical and prognostic features have been and continue to be discovered in pediatric ALL [24-26]. These nonrandom rearrangements can be classified as one of two types: numerical or structural. Numerical aberrations include changes in the number of individual chromosomes such as chromosomal gains or losses and changes in the number of sets of chromosomes (polyploidy) resulting in hyperdiploidy or hypodiploidy, respectively. Structural changes include a wide variety of rearrangements including translocations, inversions, isochromosomes, deletions as well as submicroscopic molecular anomalies (Figure 3). Although the frequency and types of genetic alterations differ between pediatric and adult ALL subtypes, the general mechanism(s) leading to malignant transformation are similar. They include activation of protooncogenes, dysregulation of gene expression; deletion or functional inactivation of tumor-suppressor genes along with gene mutations and numerical changes (Table 2) [4; 24].

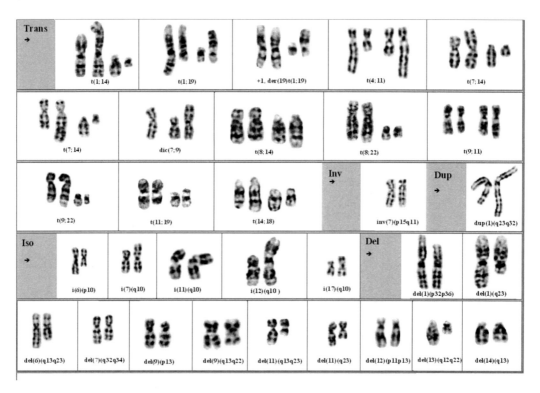

Figure 3. The most common structural rearrangements found in pediatric B- ALL.

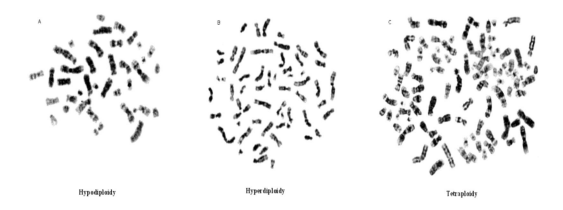

Figure 4. Ploidy groups in ALL. (A) Hypodiploidy, (B) Hyperdiploidy (C), Tetraploidy.

Numerical Chromosome Abnormalities

Altered chromosome numbers either alone or in combination with structural changes, are frequently found in childhood ALL [24, 27]. These include low hyperdiploidy (modal number 47 to 50), high hyperdiploidy (>50 chromosomes), hypodiploidy with less than 45 chromosomes as well as gain or loss of a single chromosome (Figure 4).

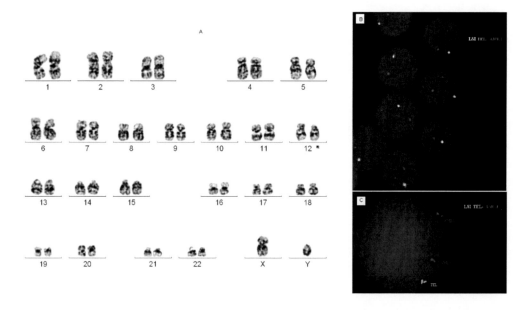

Figure 5. (A) Karyotype of a child with ALL, cryptic t(12;21) and deletion of the short arm of chromosome 12 in (B). Fluorescence in situ hybridization with Dual Color *TEL-AML1* translocation probe showing the fusion *TEL-AML1* signal from the same patient. One of the green signals (*TEL*) is missing as a result of 12p deletion. (C) Interphase nucleus showing 2 orange (*AML1*) and one green signal (*TEL*) in a patient without *TEL-AML1* fusion but with deletion of *TEL* from 12p13.

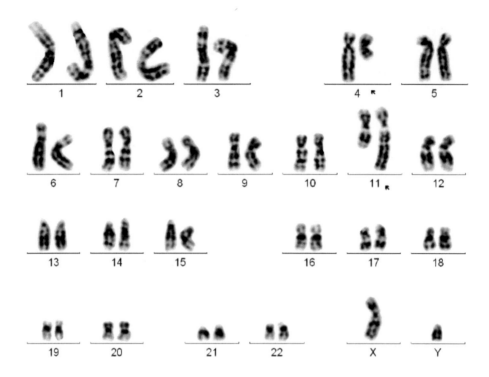

Figure 6. Metaphase cell with chromosome translocation t (4;11)(q21;q23).

High hyperdiploidy (51-67 chromosomes) is the most common chromosomal abnormality in childhood acute lymphoblastic leukemia peaking at 3-5 years, and occurring in approximately 30% of all cases [24, 28]. High hyperploid karyotypes are characterized by the presence of non-random trisomies or tetrasomies of certain chromosomes. While every chromosome may be involved; certain karyotypes seem to prevail. Although high hyperdiploid clones are rarely identical, gains in chromosomes X, 4, 5, 6, 8, 10, 14, 17, 18, as well as 21 appear to be the most frequent and are dominant in the group with >50 chromosomes [4, 28]. Almost all cases with >50 are of precursor B-cell type, and generally occur in children with favorable prognostic factors (age 1-10 years, low WBC count at presentation and FAB L1 or L2 morphology).

Hyperdiploidy in children is associated with favorable prognosis, particularly high hyperploidy with chromosomal numbers of >50. Combination of trisomies of trisomies of chromosomes 4, 10 and 17 in children with hyperdiploid ALL is associated with an extremely favorable prognosis. Moreover, the presence of triple trisomy of +4,+10,+17 at diagnosis appear to have a protective effect against relapse. The good prognosis is thought to be related to leukaemic cell higher sensitivity to a number of anti-leukaemic drugs. In addition, hyperdiploid leukemia cells are particularly susceptible to undergoing apoptosis, which may account for the favorable outcome commonly observed for these cases [28-31].

However, outcome of children with hyperdiploid ALL is heterogeneous and depends on age, sex, WBC counts and other factors. In addition, in a substantial number of patients, hyperdiploidy is associated with additional chromosome rearrangements, duplication 1q, deletion of 6q, i(7q) and i(17q) being the most common [24, 28, 32]. The presence of 1q and

6q rearrangements have no known prognostic impact, whereas the presence of i(17q) is associated with a poor prognosis. The occurrence of non-random structural rearrangements, found in about 40% to 70% of cases indicates that in the substantial number of cases, hyperdiploidy is probably a secondary event and that numerical aberrations emerged during the progression of leukaemia [29, 31]. Moreover, as the quality of hyperdiploid metaphases is frequently substandard, it is possible that structural chromosome aberrations may be overlooked in a significant number of patients.

ALL with Hypodiploidy

Hypodiploidy, characterized by a specific pattern of chromosome losses, occurs rarely in pediatric ALL. In most series of pediatric patients, hypodiploid chromosome numbers were found in 2%-7% of children with ALL. Hypodiploid lines have fewer than 45 chromosomes per cell and may be divided into three groups: near-haploid (23-29 chromosomes), low hypodiploid (chromosome number 30-40, and high hypodiploid with chromosome number 41-44. Near-haploid cases almost always have only numerical changes, and appear to be restricted to children of young age [27]. Structural chromosomal rearrangements are more frequent in the low hypodiploid group and are associated with and an older age at diagnosis (median age 15 years). Patients with high hypodiploid karyotypes show frequent structural aberrations, mainly translocations and complex karyotypes [32, 33]. Interestingly, many ALL patients with hypodiploidy also have a second leukemic line with hyperdiploid population and frequently show retention of two copies of the same chromosomes as are involved in the hyperdiploid karyotypes.

Hypodiploid karyotype in pediatric ALL is usually associated with a precursor B-cell type, less frequently T-cell type and predominantly FAB L2 morphology. Patients with hypodiploid karyotype are at high risk for treatment failure with a short median survival and poor prognosis. Survival analysis showed a significant trend for progressively worse outcome with a decreasing chromosome number, and the worst outcome of children with 24 to 28 chromosomes (Table 3) [32, 33].

Table 3. Characterization of ploidy groups

Characterization of ploidy groups				
Genetic subgroup	Phenotype	Clinical features	Frequency	Prognosis
High-hyperdiploid	B-precursor	Age 2-10 years, low white blood cell count, no aggressive features	20%-30%	Excellent
Hypodiploid	B-precursor T-cell	No aggressive features	7%–8%	Poor
Near-tetraploid	B-precursor T-cell	Older age, no aggressive features	1%-2%	Poor

Table 4. Characteristics and Clinical Outcomes in genetic subgroups in childhood ALL

Genetic subgroup	Phenotype	Clinical features at presentation	Frequency	Prognosis
High-hyperploidy	B-precursor	Age 2-10 years, low LDH, low WBC count, no aggressive features	20%-30%	Excellent
Hypodiploidy	B-precursor, T-cell	No aggressive features	7%–8%	Unfavorable
t(12;21)	B-precursor CD10+, HLA-DR+	Age 2 to 9 years, low WBC count, no aggressive features	20%-30%	Excellent
11q23/ MLL t(4;11)(q21;q23)	Early pre-B, B-precursor, bilineage ALL, T-ALL, CD19+,CD10-,CD15+, CD65+, NG2+, expression of myeloid markers	Older age, high WBC and blast counts, organomegaly, CNS involvement	8% 2%	Poor, particularly in infants
t(1;19) der(19)t(1;19)	B-precursor CD19+,CD10+,CD22+, CD34-	High WBC, non-white race, absence of hyperdiploidy	5%-6%% 25% in pre-B ALL	
t(8;14)(q24;q32)/ C-MYC	Mature B cell, FAB L3 (Burkitt's leukemia) CD10, CD19, CD20, CD22, CD79a, bright sIgH	Older age, high WBC and blast counts at presentation, organomegaly, CNS disease, extramedullary masses	1–3% 85–90% in B-cell ALL	70%- 80% are cured
t(9;22)(q34;q11)	B-precursor, T-cell CD10+, expression of myeloid markers	Older age, high WBC and blast counts at presentation, organomegaly, CNS disease	3% to 5%	Poor 20–30% are cured

LDH, lactate dehydrogenase; WBC, white blood cell count; CNS, central nervous system.

Chromosomal Translocations

A number of recurrent chromosomal translocations have been recognized as primary pathogenetic changes in childhood ALL. Molecular cloning of these rearrangements has led to the discovery of many genes including protooncogenes, genes that act as transcription-regulating factors and genes that are involved in the regulation of DNA repair and apoptosis. Most of the cloned chromosome rearrangements lead to the formation of fusion genes resulting in aberrant expression of genes encoding active kinases and transcription factors. Another mechanism of chromosomal translocation is the juxtaposition of transcription factor genes to the neighborhood of active promoter or enhancer elements of transcriptionally active T-cell receptor (TCR) or immunoglobulin (IG) genes, leading to their overexpression [3,4,24]. Most of these rearrangements are balanced translocations that are closely associated with certain clinical and biological features in childhood ALL. These include genetic alterations in B-precursor ALL such as t(12;21), t(9;22), t(1;19), a variety of **MLL** gene rearrangements and the chromosomal translocation t(8;14) found almost exclusively in mature B-cell ALL (Table 4). Other specific rearrangements include TCR rearrangements closely correlated with T-lineage leukemias (Table 5).

Table 5. Rearrangements closely correlated with T-lineage leukemias

Genetic lesions in pediatric T-ALL				
Abnormality	Genes involved	Protein domain	Frequency (%)	Molecular findings/Comments
TCR GENETIC LESIONS				
t(1;14)(p32;q11)/ t(1;7)(p32;q34)	TAL1-TRD TAL1-TRB	Transcription factor Transcription factor	<3 <1	TAL1 expression 60%
t(1;7)(p34;q34)	LCK-TRB	Signal transduction	<1	
t(1;7)(p32;q35)	TAL1-TRB	Transcription factor	<1	
t(7;9)(q34;q32)	TAL2-TRB	Transcription factor	<1	
t(7;9)(q34;q34)	NOTCH1-TRB	Transcription factor	2	
t(7;9)(q34;p34)	TAN1-TRB	Signal transduction	<1	
t(7;10)(q35;q24)	RHOM2-TRB	Transcription factor	<1	
t(7;10)(q34;q24)/ t(10;14)(q24;q11)	HOX11-TRB HOX11-TRA/D	Transcription factor Transcription factor	<7 <1	HOX11 expression 30%, favorable ?
t(7;11)(q34;p13)	LMO2-TRB	Transcription factor	<1	LMO2 expression 30%
t(7;11)(q35;p13)	RHOM2-TRB	Transcription factor	<1	
inv(7)(p15q34), t(7;7)	HOXA cluster-TRB	Transcription factor	5	CD2-, CD4+
t(7;19)(q34;p13)	LYL1-TRB	Transcription factor	<1	CD34+, poor prognosis

Table 5. (Continued)

\multicolumn{5}{c	}{Genetic lesions in pediatric T-ALL}
Abnormality	Genes involved	Protein domain	Frequency (%)	Molecular findings/Comments
t(8;14)(q24;q11)	MYC-TRA	Transcription factor	<1	aggressive course
t(11;14)(p15;q11)	LMO1-TRD	Transcription factor	<1	LMO1 expression 45%
t(11;14)(p13;q11)	LMO2-TRA/D	Transcription factor	10	LMO2 expression 45%
t(11;14)(p15;q11)	RHMO1-TRD	Transcription factor	<1	
t(11;14)(p13;q11)	RHMO2-TRD	Transcription factor	5-7	
t(14;14)(q11;q32.1)	TCL1-TRD	Transcription factor	<1	
t(14;21)(q11;q22)	BHLH1-TRA	Transcription factor	<1	
Fusion genes				
1p32 deletion (cryptic)	*SIL-TAL1*	Transcription factor	9–30	*TAL1* expression 40%
t(10;11)(p12;q14)	*CALM-AF10*	Transcription factor	4-10	often cryptic
t(11;19)(q23;p13)	*MLL-ENL*	Transcription factor	3-10	Early pre-B, T-cell
t(5;14)(q35;q32) (cryptic)	*HOX11L2-BCL11B*	Transcription factor	20	
t(9;9)(q34;q34) (episomal or hsr)	*NUP214-ABL1*	Tyrosine kinase	6	
t(9;14)(q34;q32) (cryptic)	*EML1-ABL1*	Tyrosine kinase	<1	
t(9;12)(q34;p13)	*ETV6-ABL1*	Tyrosine kinase	<1	
t(9;22)(q34;q11)	*BCR-ABL1*	Tyrosine kinase	1	Poor prognosis
Cryptic deletions/ amplifications				
INK4/ARF/9p21 INK4B/ CDKN2B	MTS1/ MTS2	CDK inhibitors	9 -12	by FISH 60%-80% 20%
del (6q)	*MYB?*	?	15	by FISH 15%-32%
9q34amplification	*NUP214-ABL1*	tyrosine kinase	3 to 6	33% by array-CGH aggressive disease?
del(11)(p12p13)	*LMO2?*	?	<1	4% by array-CGH

t(12;21)/ TEL-AML1 *(ETV6- RUNX1)*

The cryptic t(12;21)(p12;q22) is the most frequent chromosomal abnormality in paediatric cancer, observed in up to 30% of children with B-lineage ALL, while it is rare or absent in adults and in infants (3% of adults) [34, 35]. It was long considered a rarity, as it was detected in less than 0.05% of patients analyzed with conventional cytogenetics. Because the t(12;21) is difficult to detect, molecular techniques and FISH is applied to detect this cryptic rearrangement (Figure 5).

The t(12;21) rearrangement results in the fusion of the *TEL* (translocation-ets-leukaemia; *ETV6*) gene on chromosome 12 to the *AML1* ((acute myeloid leukaemia-1; *RUNX1, CBFA2*) gene on chromosome 21. The *TEL* gene encodes a sequence-specific transcriptional repressor containing a HLH domain and a ETS-DNA binding domain, which belongs to ETS family of transcription factors. The *AML1* gene, on the other hand, encodes a transcription factor with a DNA-binding domain related to *Drosophila Runt* protein and a variety of transcripts giving rise to different proteins [34]. Both, *AML1* and *TEL* are one of the most frequently rearranged genes in leukaemias, observed in a variety of different myeloid and lymphoid malignancies. In the ALL associated *TEL-AML1* hybrid gene formed by t(12;21), the 5' region of the *TEL* gene is fused in-frame to almost the entire *AML1* (*RUNX1*) locus. In the resulting chimeric protein, the helix-loop-helix (HLH) domain of *TEL* joins to the DNA-binding and transactivation domains of *AML1*. The TEL-AML1 protein is a transcriptional repressor, which dominantly blocks the AML1-dependent transactivation, therefore the fusion alters the normal function of AML. In addition, the TEL-AML fusion protein is able to form heterodimers with the normal TEL protein, suggesting hybrid protein may alter the normal function of TEL [34-35].

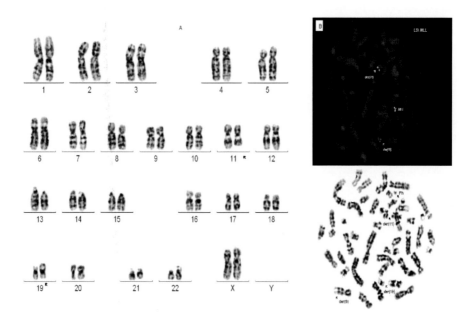

Figure 7. (A) Karyotype showing the chromosomal translocation t(11;19)(q23;p13). (B) Fluorescence in situ hybridization with Dual Color Break-Apart MLL probe showing the split signal of MLL as a result of t(11;19) (red signal on chromosome 19).

There is a persuasive evidence for in utero origin of several leukemia translocations including *TEL-AML1* and it was suggested that *TEL-AML1* arises prenatally as an early or initiating event in most cases. However, this translocation has been detected in approximately 1% of newborns, which is 100x the leukaemia rate in children. This suggests that additional or secondary and complementary genetic events are required to the development or progression of leukaemia [36]. Interestingly, most cases of ALL with *TEL-AML1* fusions have deletion of the nonrearranged or normal *TEL* allele. The nontranslocated allele of *TEL* is deleted in about 75% of the patients with t(12;21) and seems to be a secondary event in the *TEL-AML1*-positive ALL, raising the possibility is that the loss of *TEL* itself may be second genetic 'hit' [37].

Children with the t(12;21) translocation are generally 2 to 9 years of age showing favourable prognostic features at diagnosis. Most of cases are associated with B-precursor ALL with expression of CD10+, HLA-DR+ and with frequent coexpression of myeloid markers CD13 and CD33. Patients with the *TEL-AML1* fusion have an excellent outcome due to good response to chemotherapy with almost 100% remissions. Moreover, children with *TEL AML1* fusion seem to have a better outcome after relapse than other patients [35, 38].

Abnormalities Involving 11q23/MLL

Chromosomal rearrangements of the 'mixed lineage leukemia' or myeloid/lymphoid leukemia (*MLL, ALL-1, HRX, Htrx-1*) gene located at 11q23 are among the most frequent chromosomal rearrangements in a variety of hematopoietic malignancies [39, 40]. About 70% of *MLL* rearrangements are detected by conventional cytogenetics. In the remaining cases the abnormality is detected by molecular techniques and/or fluorescence in situ hybridization studies (FISH).

The *MLL* gene contains 36 exons, and encodes a 3969 amino acid protein which functions as a positive regulator of *HOX* gene expression and has an important role in normal hematopoietic growth and differentiation. To date, over 70 chromosome partners of *MLL* have been described. In most of these rearrangements the translocation breakpoints occur within an 8.3 kb breakpoint cluster region (BCR) resulting in the in-frame joining of the *MLL* gene with a partner gene [39,40].

Abnormalities of 11q23 occur in approximately 8% of childhood ALL cases. *MLL* rearrangements are particularly common in two groups of patients — in infants where they represent about 60% to 80% of acute leukemias, and in those who had previous therapy with topoisomerase II inhibitors. They are frequently associated with young age, female sex, high white blood cell (WBC) count, and they are more likely than other children with ALL to have organomegaly and central nervous system (CNS) disease [40]. It is found mainly in B-cell precursor ALL, positive for TdT, HLA-DR, and CD19 but not CD10. Leukemic cells with 11q23 abnormalities frequently coexpress myeloid antigens, such as CD13, CD15, or CD33 and there is a strong association between 11q23 abnormalities and the expression of CD65+, and the human homolog of the rat chondroitin sulfate proteoglycan NG2 [4, 24, 40].

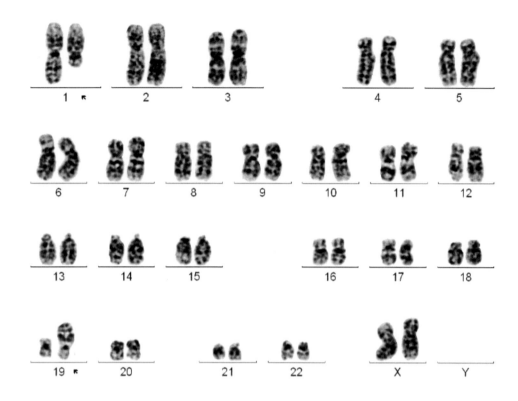

Figure 8. Karyotype from the bone marrow cell showing the balanced t(1;19).

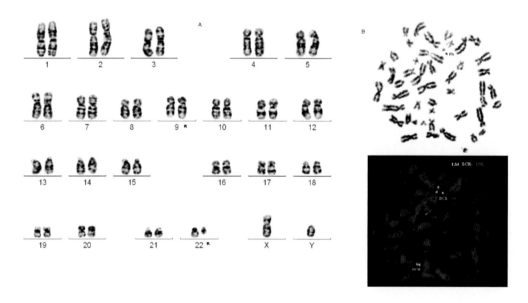

Figure 9. (A) Karyotype of a patient showing the Philadelphia chromosome translocation t(9;22)(q34;q11). (B) Fluorescence in situ hybridization with Dual color *BCR-ABL1* probe showing the fusion signal on Philadelphia chromosome.

The most common translocation involving 11q23 is translocation t(4;11)(q21;q23), generating the fusion gene *MLL-AF4* and representing about one-third of all 11q23 cases (Figure 6). It is mainly found in B-cell precursor ALL, with L1 or L2 morphology. The presence of a t(4;11) translocation is associated with unfavorable presenting features such as young age, high white blood cell count and organomaly. The t(4;11) is the most common translocation in infant patients with ALL where it is associated with a worse prognosis among children with ALL [24, 40, 41].

The t(11;19)(q23;p13.3) translocations fusing *MLL* to *AF9* is a less frequent rearrangement, found in approximately 1% of children with ALL, and occurs in both B-precursor and T-cell ALL (Figure 7). While the outcome for infants with t(11;19) is poor, the prognosis appears to be relatively favorable for children with the T-cell phenotype [41].

Recently, microarray analyses have shown that *MLL*+ acute leukemias have specific gene expression signatures and that *MLL*-positive leukemic cells resemble very immature progenitor cells. In fact, a proposal by the World Health Organization considers 11q23+/*MLL*+ as a separate entity [19, 42, 43].

t(1;19)(q23;p13) and Pre-B-ALL

The t(1;19)(q23;p13), is one of the most common recurring translocations in childhood ALL, representing 5%-6% of all cases. A strong association exists between t(1;19) and pre-B-ALL, especially in children, where it occurs in 25% to 30% of patients. The characteristic immunophenotyping profile is a positive expression of CD10, CD19, CD22+ and cytoplasmic immunoglobulin with a complete absence of CD34. It is also seen in 1% of children with early pre-B-cell ALL and occasionally with a transitional pre-B phenotype [4, 24, 44].

The translocation t(1;19)(q23;p13) involves fusion of the N-terminal transactivation domain of TCF3 (E2A) gene on chromosome 19 to the C-terminal DNA-binding homeodomain of *PBX1* gene on chromosome 1. The product of the hybrid gene is a TCF3 (E2A)/PBX1 fusion protein, which acts as a transcription factor. The rearrangement may occur in two principal forms and it can be observed as either a balanced translocation or as an unbalanced translocation der(19)t(1;19) resulting in trisomy for 1q23 1qter (Figure 8). The unbalanced form appears to be more common than the balanced t(1;19) rearrangement (75% vs 25%). Most cases with pre-B-ALL and with a balanced t(1;19) are pseudodiploid, and hyperdiploidy is only occasionally seen in these group of patients.

Clinical characteristics of pre-B-ALL with t(1;19) include presentation with high WBC counts and high LDH levels whether the translocation is balanced or derivative(24, 44). TCF3/PBX1 genotype was initially associated with inferior outcome compared with patients lacking this translocation. Intensified chemotherapy improved outcome of patients with the t(1;19). At present, patients with the t(1;19) receiving contemporary therapy have a favorable overall outcome; however the t(1;19) appear to be an independent risk factor for isolated CNS relapse [45, 46].

Philadelphia-chromosome Positive ALL

The chromosomal translocation t(9;22)(q34;q11), forming the Philadelphia chromosome is observed in 3% to 5% of children with ALL (Figure 9). While the t(9;22)(q34;q11) occurs rarely in children, it is observed in up to 20% to 30% of adults with ALL, making it the most common chromosomal abnormality in the latter group [4]. The result of the t(9;22) translocation is a hybrid *BCR-ABL1* gene that is transcribed into a chimeric *BCR-ABL1* mRNA. The chimerical BCR-ABL oncoprotein has altered tyrosine kinase activity leading to uncontrolled cell proliferation, reduced apoptosis and impaired cell adhesion [4, 24].

Clinically, Philadelphia-positive ALL in children is associated with older age (children older than 10 years). Patients have frequently increased leukocyte and blast counts. Lymphadenopathy and splenomegaly as well as CNS disease is more common in children with Ph-positive ALL than in children without Ph. Almost all cases of Ph^+ ALL have a B-precursor phenotype and other immunophenotypes are rare. This subgroup is associated with increased expression of CD10 and frequent co-expression of myeloid markers (present in 40% to 65% of Ph^+ ALL cases). Pre-B and T cell phenotypes are seen in 5–10% of patients with Ph-positive ALL [24, 47].

Children with Ph-positive ALL have a dismal prognosis even with innovative and intensified strategies. With intensive chemotherapy alone, only 20–30% of children with Ph+ ALL are cured. Therefore, allogeneic BMT is generally considered for this subgroup of patients, particularly when the disease it is associated with either a high WBC count or slow early response to initial therapy. However, BCR-ABL-targeted strategies have demonstrated promising efficacy in Ph+ ALL in recent studies. While tyrosine kinase inhibitors (TKIs) appear to have limited activity against Ph+ ALL as a single agent, their combination with chemotherapy showed promising results. Recent studies of combination of imatinib with a standard chemotherapy regimen have shown 88% 3-year event-free survival for Ph+ patients, suggesting that administration of a targeted agent in conjunction with chemotherapy regimen may be the initial treatment of choice for Ph+ ALL in children [48, 49].

B Cell ALL and t(8;14)(q24;q32) and its Variants

The chromosomal translocation t(8;14)(q24;q32) fusing the C-*MYC* gene located at 8q24 with the immunoglobulin heavy chain gene (*IGH*) at band 14q32 constitute about 1–3% of all pediatric ALL cases (Figure 10). Less frequently, the C-*MYC* gene is involved in variant translocations fusing the C-*MYC* gene with one of the IG genes located on chromosomes 2p12 (IG kappa) or 22q11 (IG lambda). Among them, the frequency of the most common translocation t(8;14)(q24;q32) is about 85% and the frequency of variant translocations t(2;8)(p12;q24) and t(8;22)(q24;q11) is estimated to be approximately 15% and 5%, respectively [4, 24, 50].

All of these translocations affect the site of the C-*MYC* proto-oncogene at band 8q24 resulting in a juxtaposition of C-*MYC* to the neighborhood of active enhancer elements of an immunoglobulin gene. *MYC* is transcription factor that acts in the nucleus and is known to play a central role in the regulation of cell division and cell death. As a result of the rearrangement, the gene encoding the MYC transcription factor is exposed to the enhancer elements of an immunoglobulin gene causing overexpression of *MYC* leading to deregulation of multiple cell processes [50, 51].

The chromosomal translocation t(8;14)(q24;q32) is a highly specific and recurrent rearrangement in mature B-cell malignancies accounting for less than 5% of all cases of ALL in children [50]. *C-MYC* gene rearrangement found in these cases is identical to the karyotypic and molecular findings for Burkitt leukaemia/lymphoma, which may present clinically as *de novo* acute lymphoblastic leukaemia. In fact, WHO classifies Burkitt's lymphoma with bone marrow or peripheral blood involvement and ALL-L3 as the same disease [19]. Almost all patients with ALL and *C-MYC* gene rearrangement have typical L3 morphology and the t(8;14)(q24;q32) or its variants can be detected in 85–90% of B cell ALL of L3 morphology.

Children in the leukemic phase often present at older age with high WBC and blast counts, hepatosplenomegaly, extramedullary masses and frequent and early CNS involvement. Cells usually express the B-cell-specific surface markers CD10, CD19, CD20, CD22, together with bright expression of surface immunoglobulin. Cases with L3 morphology and *C-MYC* translocation was reported to be associated with rapidly progressive clinical course due to an unusually high rate of turnover of malignant cells. At present its treatment is completely different than for other forms of childhood ALL, including more intensive chemotherapy than standard ALL and CNS prophylaxis. While with intensive chemotherapy protocols, applied for Burkitt's lymphomas, a majority of these patients are cured, the prognosis remains to be dismissal in a substantial number of cases, particularly in older children with abdominal tumors and CNS disease [50, 51].

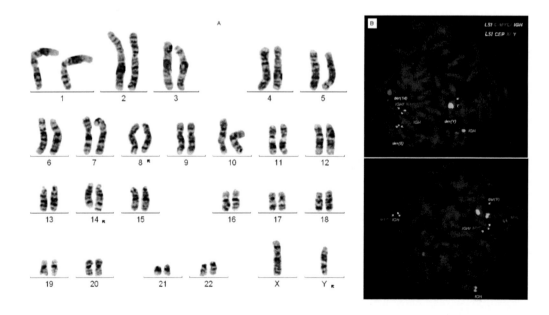

Figure 10. (A) Karyotype of the patient showing the chromosomal translocation t(8;14)(q22;q32) and der(Y)t(1;Y) rearrangements. (B) Fluorescence in situ hybridization with Dual color dual fusion *MYC-IGH* probe showing the fusion signal on der(14) and der(8) chromosomes.

Tumor Suppressor Genes and Allelic Losses

Tumor suppressor genes are essential for normal cell development and their products normally provide negative control of cell proliferation and prevent oncogenesis. Their activity may be neutralized by different mechanisms including deletions of variable amounts of chromosome material, hypermethylation of the promoter region or point mutation. Deletion or functional inactivation of tumor-suppressor genes is an infrequent phenomenon in pediatric leukemias and only few tumor suppressor genes have been reported to contribute to malignant transformation in childhood ALL [1, 3, 24].

One such frequent mutation is a deletion in the short arm of 12p, secondary to the TEL-AML1 translocation (Figure 5). Partial deletions of the nonrearranged or normal *TEL* allele from chromosome 12p are by now well characterized and it was suggested that del(12p) occurs postnatally as a secondary aberration to translocation [36, 37]. Del(6q) involving 6q21 is found in about 4% to 6% of childhood B-cell acute lymphoblastic leukemia patients after conventional cytogenetic analysis, in 30% after FISH analysis, in 5 to 25% of cases in loss of heterozygosity studies. The frequency in B-cell ALL is somewhat less than in childhood T-cell acute lymphoblastic leukemia where del(6q) is one of the most frequent chromosomal anomalies occurring in 10-20% of cases. Del(6q) is often part of complex karyotypes, often associated with numerical changes in B-cell ALL and 14q11 or del(9p) abnormalities in T-cell phenotype [24, 52]. Monosomy 7 or chromosome 7 deletions are relatively infrequent in childhood ALL. . Monosomy 7 and deletions of 7p are associated with unfavarable prognosis in children with ALL, while deletions of 7q are not associated with an dismal prognosis [53]. Isochromosomes are relatively unusual in pediatric ALL and they include i(6p), i(7q), i(9q), and i(17q). They occur in about 1-4% of call cases of lymphoblastic leukemia, mostly associated with a precursor B-cell immunophenotype [1, 3, 24].

Deletions in Cell Cycle Checkpoint Genes/ Abnormalities of the Short Arm of Chromosome 9

Another important class of tumor suppressor genes is cyclin-dependent kinase (CDK) inhibitors that encode for proteins that inhibit the cyclin-dependent kinases. Specific deletions involving the short arm of chromosome 9 are among the most frequent cytogenetic aberratios. Different mechanisms of such deletions have been described including 9p deletions, interstitial deletions, unbalanced translocations, or loss of the entire chromosome. All of these cases involve missing of segment 9p21-pter where two known tumor suppressor genes are located, namely $p16^{INK4A}$ and the structurally homologous gene, $p15^{INK4B}$. Both of the genes encode for proteins that inhibit the cyclin-dependent kinases and negatively regulate the cell cycle by inhibiting CDK phosphorylation of Rb protein. The main mechanism for $p16^{INK4A}$ inactivation is biallelic deletions, with frequent codeletions of $p15^{INK4B}$ which is located centromeric to $p16^{INK4A}$. [1, 3, 24].

Inactivation of $p16^{INK4A}$ and $p15^{INK4B}$ genes by deletion and/or gene methylation is among the most consistent genetic defects found in childhood ALL found in about of 7% to 10%

cases. An association with high-risk clinical features such as older age, high WBC and blasts counts, lymphadenopathy splenomegaly bulky disease and T-cell immunophenotype has been reported by some but not all studies [3, 24].

Another mechanism of loss of part of the short arms of chromosomes 9 and 12 is the formation of a dicentric chromosome t/dic(9;12)(p11-12)(p11-13). This unbalanced translocation result in hypodiploidy with loss of chromosomes 9 and or 12. The deletion of can occur in various parts of 9p11, where the translocation can fall anywhere in a 300-kb segment. There is a strong association with dic(9;12) and pre-B/early-pre-B-cell ALL phenotype, positivity for CD10 and male gender in children. dic(9;12) is an infrequent chromosomal rearrangement in childhood ALL, found in about 1% of children with ALL.. As a sole abnormality it has been reported to have a very low relapse rate and an excellent prognosis [54].

Acute Lymphoblastic Leukemia in Infancy

Infant or congenital leukemias are defined by a diagnosis within the first year or the first two years of life, account for about 5% of all leukemic cases in childhood. Acute lymphoblastic leukemia in infancy is uncommon, comprising 2% to 5% of cases of childhood ALL. ALL in infancy is a biologically distinctive disorder with characteristic epidemiological and clinical features [55, 56]. Most of infant ALL cases are characterized by unfavorable features such as hyperleukocytosis at presentation, hepatosplenomegaly, and central nervous system (CNS) disease. ALL in infants is also associated with an immature immunophenotype and frequent coexpression of lymphoid and myeloid antigens such as CD13, CD15, or CD33 [56].

Cytogenetic analyses in infants have revealed, that karyotypic anomalies detected in infants have an unique pattern and it has been repeatedly shown, that the type and frequency of chromosomal aberrations detected in infant leukamias are clearly different from those in older children and adults. According to these studies, most infants with ALL have an abnormality of 11q23 and/or molecular genetic rearrangement of the *MLL* gene [57, 58]. In general, infants with *MLL* gene rearrangements tend to be younger than 6 months and have higher white blood cell counts, than infants without *MLL* gene rearrangements, both of which are considered to be poor prognostic indicators. The blast cells most commonly are positive for TdT, HLA-DR, CD19 and CDw65, while there is a significant association of *MLL-AF4* rearrangement with a lack of CD10 (cALLa antigen) expression [55-57]. While the incidence of MLL gene rearrangements among children with ALL who are older than 1 year, ranges from 4% to 7%, the frequency of 11q23 abnormalities among infants with ALL is about 60% to 80%. On the other hand, the most common chromosomal translocations seen in older children with ALL are under represented in infant series. Similarly, high hyperdiploidy, a well known numeric anomaly in childhood ALL is only occasionally seen in infancy [56-58].

Most infants with an 11q23 breakpoint have a t(4;11)(q21;q23) occurring in about 40% of infants with ALL [57]. The next most common abnormality is t(11;19)(q23;p13) involving the ENL gene on 19p13.3. The t(11;19) occurs in approximately 1% of infant ALL cases and occurs in both B-precursor and T-cell ALL. In addition, a large number of *MLL* gene partners, apart from the AF4 gene of the t(4;11), have been described in infant ALL [56-58].

As rearrangements of the *MLL* gene known to be often related to genotoxic exposure these findings provide further supportive evidence that MLL rearrangements in infant leukemia may be the result of an environmental factor. In addition, there is strong epidemiological and molecular evidence that MLL gene rearrangements in infant leukemias occur in utero, probably in response to natural or synthetic genotoxic compounds substances (e.g. infection, topoisomerase II inhibitors, pesticides and carcinogens). Furthermore, the foetal origin of infant leukemia has been established by demonstration that children diagnosed with leukaemia at age 5 months to 2 yrs already had MLL-AF4 fusion gene in their neonatal blood spots (Guthrie cards) [5, 11]. Moreover, genetic studies of identical twins with concordant leukemia demonstrated that the concordance of both of identical twins having leukaemia with MLL-AF4 fusion gene seems to be almost 100%. These findings indicate that leukaemia to be foetal in origin in most if not all cases of infant leukaemia, particularly with fusions of *MLL* gene [2, 11, 12].

Despite current attempts to improve the outcome of ALL in infants, children younger than 1 years of age continue to have a poor therapeutic outcome. Adverse prognostic factors include the presence of an **MLL** gene rearrangement, age less than 6 months, high presenting leukocyte counts, CD10 negativity and slow early response to therapy. Most of infants with ALL experience very low event-free survival, indicating that this group of children needs innovative treatment approaches. These may include current clinical trials testing cytarabine-intensive regimens and targeted therapies, such as FLT3-inhibitors to improve the outcome of MLL-rearranged ALL in infants [59].

Genetic Changes Associated with T-ALL

T-cell acute lymphoblastic leukemia (T-ALL) is a malignant disease resulting from the accumulation of genetic alterations of T lymphoid precursor cells. It comprises about 15% of childhood AL, predominantly affecting boys of older age. T-ALL is a heterogeneous disease with distinct clinical and biological features that are different from those associated with B-lineage ALL. Patients are often presenting with high WBC counts, lymphadenophaty and extramedullary disease [60, 61]. Blasts show T-cell immunophenotype that corresponds to the common thymocyte stage and less frequently to prothymocyte stage of differentiation. Immunophenotyping is positive for TdT and variably positive for CD2, CD3, CD4, CD5, CD7, and CD8. Less frequently, immunophenotype reveal prothymocyte stage of differentiation (CD4, CD8-).

Cytogenetic and molecular genetic studies revealed that the types and frequencies of genetic abnormalities detected in pediatric T-ALL are clearly different from those observed in B-lineage ALL. Hyperdiploidy found in about 25% of B-lineage childhood ALL is uncommon in T-ALL and, when present, is not associated with any survival advantage [60]. Tetraploidy is seen in approximately 5% of cases, while single chromosomal losses and trisomies are rare in T-ALL [61]. Chromosomal translocations are less commonly found than in B precursor ALL cases and about 50% to 70% of patients have a normal karyotype [60,

61]. In approximately 25–50% of children recurrent genetic rearrangements are identified. A variety of genetic rearrangements occur in pediatric T-cell acute lymphoblastic leukemia; however many of these translocations occur with a low frequency. These include chromosomal translocations leading to aberrant expression of transcription factors and constitutively activated tyrosine kinases, mutation or methylation of promoters of genes involved in T-cell development as well as chromosomal deletions leading to the loss of tumor suppressor genes. In addition, a substantial number of cases have cryptic abnormalities, as shown by fluorescent in situ hybridization (FISH) or other molecular methods [60-63].

Translocations Involving T Cell Receptors Genes

A variety of chromosomal translocations have been identified by conventional karyotyping involving specific chromosome breakpoints known to harbor genes implicated in T-cell development. In about one-third of childhood T-ALL patients rearrangements of T cell receptors genes (TCR) have been detected. Breakpoints involving T-cell receptor gene clusters are recurrent on 14q11.2 (*TRA@* or *TRD@*) and 7q34 (*TRB@*). The *TRG@* locus at 7p14-15 appear to be restricted to ataxia telangiectasia patients with T-cell ALL (Figure 11). As a result of rearrangement, the strong promoter and enhancer elements of the *TCR* genes are juxtaposed to transcription factor genes leading to T-cell malignancies [61, 62].

T-cell ALL with rearrangements of T cell receptors genes represents a heterogeneous subgroup of ALL in which a variety of partner genes have been identified (Figure 11). These include chromosomal abnormalities affecting 7q34 such as t(1;7)(p32;q34) disrupting *TAL1(TCL5/SCL)*, t(1;7)(p34;q34) activating *LCK*, t(7;9)(q34;q34.3) affecting *NOTCH1*, t(7;19)(q34;p13.2) involving *LYL1* and inv(7)(p15.3;q34)/t(7;7)(p15.3;q34) leading to transcriptional activation of *HOXA* genes [64-66].

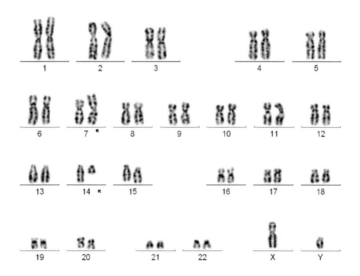

Figure 11. Translocation t(7;14) in an ataxia telangiectasia patients with T-cell ALL.

Childhood Acute Lymphoblastic Leukemia

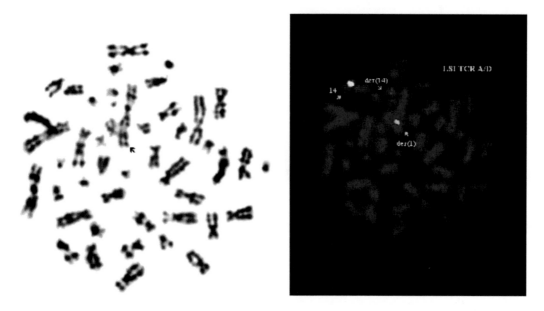

Figure 12. Rearrangement of TCR A/D as a result of t(1;14) in T-ALL.

Table 6. Prognostic factors in childhood ALL

Targeted therapies in childhood ALL		
Mechanism	Agent	Comment
BCR-ABL1 tyrosine kinase inhibition	Imatinib. Dasatinib Nilotinib	Ph+
FLT3 receptor tyrosine kinase inhibition	Lestaurtanib Midostaurin	MLL+, high hyperdiploid
mTOR kinase inhibitors	Rapamycin, Temsirolimus	relapsed ALL
aurora kinase inhibitors	MLN8237	relapsed ALL
multi-kinase inhibitors	Sorafenib	relapsed ALL
proteasome inhibitors	Bortezomib	relapsed ALL
histone deacetylase inhibitors	vorinostat (SAHA)	relapsed ALL
DNA methyltransferase inhibitors	Decitabine	relapsed ALL
CD Marker Antibodies	Rituximab, Epratuzimab, Alemtuzumab	relapsed ALL

Others: conjugated CD marker antibodies, BCL2 antagonists, farnesyltransferase inhibitors, TAM tyrosine kinase inhibitors, gamma secretase inhibitors (T-cell ALL, NOTCH mutations), JAK tyrosine kinase inhibition (Down syndrome and Latino/Hispanic patients).

Chromosome 14 alterations associated with *TRA@/TRD@* rearrangements are among the most common observed by conventional cytogenetics in T-ALL, found up to 20% of all T-ALL cases [61]. One example is t(1;14)(p32;q11.2) and its variant t(1;7)(p32;q34) associated with organomegaly and high WBC count (Figure 12). The two chromosome anomalies share identical features and in both cases the result of the rearrangement is disruption of *TAL1* and its ectopic expression. Another frequent translocation is t(11;14)(p13;q11.2) and its variant t(7;11)(q35;p13) observed in up to 10% of children with T-ALL. As a result of these translocations, fusion with *TRA@/TRD@* or *TRB@* constitutively activates the *LMO2* gene.

Truncation of the promoter/control region of *LMO2* leads to its dysregulation, especially in T-cells. In addition, in as many as 30% of T-ALL cases, high levels of LMO2 expression have been detected without visible chromosomal rearrangement [63, 64].

Non TCR Genetic Lesions in T-ALL

Non-TCR genetic lesions include a variety of chromosomal translocations leading to gene fusions, as well as chromosomal deletions leading to the loss of tumor suppressor genes. Moreover, T-cell oncogenes such as *TAL1 (SCL), NOTCH1, LYL1, LMO2, TLX1(HOX11)* and *TLX3 (HOX11L2)* are typically overexpressed, without evidence of any visible chromosomal rearrangement. Among then, activating mutations of *NOTCH1* have been found in 56% of all molecular subtypes of T-ALL [61, 64-66].

In addition, a number of cytogenetically cryptic anomalies, such as microdeletions, cryptic interstitial deletions, duplications and amplifications have been revealed by FISH and other molecular studies studies. Among these, submicroscopic deletions are very frequent. One example is a submicroscopic interstitial deletion of *TAL1 (SCL, TCLS)* located at 1p32 generating the *SIL-TAL1* fusion gene found in 9–30% of childhood T-ALL. Furthermore, a high number of patients with T-ALL cases (about 60%) have submicroscopic deletions of *TAL1* (1p32) as shown by fluorescent in situ hybridization or molecular methods. Similarly, FISH and other molecular methods have shown that homozygous deletions of *CDKN2A (INK4A)* resulting in loss of G1 control of cell cycle occur in 60% to 80% of children with T-ALL. Similarly, homozygous deletions of *CDKN2B (INK4B)* at locus 9p21 are observed in as many as 20% of children with T-ALL [61]. A recurrent cryptic translocation t(5;14)(q35.1;q32.2) resulting in the activation of the *TLX3 (HOX11L2)* homeobox gene at 5q35.1 has been observed in approximately 20% of pediatric patients with T-ALL. Terminal and interstitial deletions of variable size of the long arm of chromosome 6 are known structural aberrations in pediatric ALL, representing about 15% of T-ALL cases [61, 62]. Furthermore, a variety of cryptic abnormalities such as duplications of 9q34 region, 9q34 amplification of *ABL1*, duplication of 6q23 region and submicroscopic deletions at del(11)(p12p13) involving *LMO2* ware identified in a number of pediatric T-ALL cases by the array comparative genome hybridization (array-CGH) method [65-67].

Future Directions

The recognition of cytogenetic and molecular genetic abnormalities in childhood ALL has contributed greatly to our understanding of the pathogenesis and prognosis of the disease. Advances in our understanding have led to new treatment strategies including the use of risk-adapted treatment protocols in which therapy is tailored according to risk groups (Table 6). With improvements in diagnosis and treatment, the outcome for children with acute lymphoblastic leukemia has improved dramatically. At present, the treatment of ALL in children is a success story in pediatric oncology resulting in complete remission (CR) rates of 97% to 99% and in 5-year event-free survival rates of 75% to 86% [24].

Table 7. Potential targets for novel therapies in pediatric ALL

Targeted therapies in childhood ALL		
Mechanism	Agent	Comment
BCR-ABL1 tyrosine kinase inhibition	Imatinib. Dasatinib Nilotinib	Ph+
FLT3 receptor tyrosine kinase inhibition	Lestaurtanib Midostaurin	MLL+, high hyperdiploid
mTOR kinase inhibitors	Rapamycin, Temsirolimus	relapsed ALL
aurora kinase inhibitors	MLN8237	relapsed ALL
multi-kinase inhibitors	Sorafenib	relapsed ALL
proteasome inhibitors	Bortezomib	relapsed ALL
histone deacetylase inhibitors	vorinostat (SAHA)	relapsed ALL
DNA methyltransferase inhibitors	Decitabine	relapsed ALL
CD Marker Antibodies	Rituximab, Epratuzimab, Alemtuzumab	relapsed ALL

Others: conjugated CD marker antibodies, BCL2 antagonists, farnesyltransferase inhibitors, TAM tyrosine kinase inhibitors, gamma secretase inhibitors (T-cell ALL, NOTCH mutations), JAK tyrosine kinase inhibition (Down syndrome and Latino/Hispanic patients).

Despite this success, a significant number of children either relapse or fail to ever achieve a complete remission [68-71]. Moreover, differences in treatment response and outcome may still be observed in the groups of patients with the same genetic subtypes or within the same risk classification group. Furthermore, about 25% of children with ALL still lack defined genetic hallmarks indicating in these groups of children cryptic molecular genetic events impact disease biology and therapeutic response [68].

To identify genetic lesions undetected by conventional methods, researchers have developed new promising applications of large-scale genomic technologies. Recent genome-wide association studies have identified several genetic lesions associated with childhood ALL with diagnostic and prognostic significance. These include genetic alterations targeting transcriptional regulators, genetic alterations affecting genes involved in cell cycle regulation and genes encoding proteins regulating intracellular signaling, altered expression of apoptosis genes, chromosome deletions amplifications, as well as inherited genetic variations in susceptibility to ALL. Activating *RAS* pathway mutations including *KRAS2, NRAS, FLT3, BRAF* and *PTPN11* genes are particularly frequent in high hyperdiploid (>50 chromosomes). Mutations in the RAS signaling pathway may be observed in about one third of the cases, raising the possibility of targeted therapeutic interventions in high hyperdiploid pediatric ALLs [72-74]. Mutation of genes encoding tyrosine kinases is uncommon in pediatric *BCR-ABL1*-negative ALL. Alteration of specific genes in this pathway include deletion of *IKZF1* (encoding the lymphoid transcription factor IKAROS) and activating mutations in the Janus kinases *JAK1 JAK2* and *JAK3* [75]. Pediatric *BCR-ABL1*-negative ALL patients characterized by deletion of *IKZF1* and *JAK*-mutations showed gene expression signatures similar to *BCR-ABL1*-positive ALL. Genetic alterations in this group of patient are associated with high-risk ALL, suggesting that tyrosine kinase signaling pathway may be a potential target for novel therapies (Table 7) [68, 76]. Genome-wide association studies are beginning to be applied successfully to the study of childhood leukemia, broadly segregating patients defined by traditional measures. Because of the diverse nature of the disease, future goals include further characterization of the leukemic cells that can be used for improved diagnosis and risk classification in pediatric ALL. In addition, molecular characterization of the leukemic cells with combination of cytogenetic techniques may lead to better understanding of the disease pathogenesis and delineation of new therapeutic targets which may change the medicine fundamentally [77].

References

[1] Carroll WL, Bhojwani D, Min DJ, et al. Pediatric Acute Lymphoblastic Leukemia. *Hematology* 2003;1:102-131.
[2] Greaves, M. Childhood leukaemia. *British Med J,* 2002;324:283-287.
[3] Pui CH, Relling MV, Downing JR. Acute lymphoblastic leukemia. *N Engl J Med* 2004;350:1535-1548.
[4] Faderl S, Kantarjian HM, Talpaz M, et al. Clinical Significance of Cytogenetic Abnormalities in Adult Acute Lymphoblastic Leukemia. *Blood* 1998; 91:3995-4019.
[5] Forestier E; Schmiegelow K. The Incidence Peaks of the Childhood Acute Leukemias Reflect Specific Cytogenetic Aberrations. *J Ped Hematol/Oncol* 2006;28:486-495.
[6] Erik F, Kjeld S. The Incidence Peaks of the Childhood Acute Leukemias Reflect Specific Cytogenetic Aberrations. J Pediatric Hematol Oncology 2006;28:486-495.
[7] Carroll WL. Racial and Ethnic Factors in Outcomes of Children With Acute Lymphoblastic Leukemia. *JAMA* 2004;291:2541-2541.
[8] Matasar MJ, Ritchie EK, Consedine N, et al. Incidence rates of the major leukemia subtypes among U.S. Hispanics, Blacks, and non-Hispanic Whites. 2006; *Leukemia Lymphoma* 47:2365-2370.
[9] Bhatia S, Sather HN, Heerema NA, et al. Racial and ethnic differences in survival of children with acute lymphoblastic leukemia. *Blood* 2002;100:1957-1964.
[10] Aldrich MC, Zhang L, Wiemels JL, et al. Cytogenetics of Hispanic and White Children with Acute Lymphoblastic Leukemia in California. *Cancer Epidem Biomarkers Prevention* 2006;15:578-581.
[11] Dickinson HO. The causes of childhood leukemia. *British Med J* 2005;330:1279-1280.
[12] Hjalgrim LL, Madsen HO, Melbye M, Jørgensen P, Christiansen M, Andersen MT, Pallisgaard N, Hokland P, Clausen N, Ryder LP, Schmiegelow K, Hjalgrim H. Presence of clone-specific markers at birth in children with acute lymphoblastic leukaemia. *British J Cancer* 2002;87:994–999.
[13] Whitlock JA. Down syndrome and acute lymphoblastic leukaemia. *Br J Haematol* 2006;135:595-602.
[14] Wiemels JL, Pagnamenta A, Taylor GM, Eden OB, Alexander FE, Greaves MF, et al. A lack of a functional NAD(P)H:quinone oxidoreductase allele is selectively associated with pediatric leukemias that have MLL fusions. C*ancer Res* 1999; 59:4095–4099.

[15] Taylor GM, Dearden S, Payne N, Ayres M, Gokhale DA, Birch JM, et al. Evidence that an HLA-DQA1-DQB1 haplotype influences susceptibility to childhood common acute lymphoblastic leukaemia in males provides further support for an infection-related aetiology. *Br J Cancer* 1998;78:561–565.

[16] Wiemels JL, Smith RN, Taylor GM, Eden OB, Alexander FE, Greaves MF, et al. Methylenetetrahydrofolate reductase (MTHFR) polymorphisms and risk of molecularly defined subtypes of childhood acute leukemia. Proc Natl Acad Sci USA 2001; 98:4004–4009.

[17] McNally RJQ, Eden TOB. An infectious aetiology for childhood leukaemia: a review of the evidence. *Br J Haematology* 2004;127:243-63.

[18] Harris NL, Jaffe ES, Diebold J, Flandrin G, Muller-Hermelink HK, Vardiman J, Lister TA, Bloomfield CD. World Health Organization Classification of Neoplastic Diseases of the Hematopoietic and Lymphoid Tissues: Report of the Clinical Advisory Committee Meeting. *J Clin Oncol* 1997;17:3835-3849.

[19] Harris NL, Jaffe ES, Diebold J, Flandrin G, Muller-Hermelink HK, Vardiman J, Lister TA, Bloomfield CD. The World Health Organization classification of hematological malignancies report of the Clinical Advisory Committee Meeting, Airlie House, Virginia, November 1997. *Mod Pathol* 2000;13:193-207.

[20] Campana D, Behm FG. Immunophenotyping of leukemia. *J Immunol Methods* 2000 21;243:59-75.

[21] Jeha S, Behm F, Pei D, Sandlund JT, Ribeiro RC, Razzouk BI, Rubnitz JE, Hijiya N, Howard SC, Cheng C, Pui CH. Prognostic significance of CD20 expression in childhood B-cell precursor acute lymphoblastic leukemia. Blood. 2006;108:3302-3304.

[22] Suggs JL, Cruse JM, Lewis RE. Aberrant myeloid marker expression in precursor B-cell and T-cell leukemias. *Exp Mol Pathol* 2007;83:471-473.

[23] Lewis RE, Cruse JM, Sanders CM, Webb RN, Tillman BF, Beason KL, Lam J, Koehler J. The immunophenotype of pre-TALL/LBL revisited. *Exp Mol Pathol* 2006;81:162-5.

[24] Pui CH, Robison LL, Look AT. Acute lymphoblastic leukaemia. *Lancet* 2008; 371:1030-1043.

[25] Schneider NR, Carroll AJ, Shuster JJ, et al. Jeanette Pullen, Michael P. Link, Michael J. Borowitz, Bruce M. Camitta, Julie A. Katz, and Michael D. Amylon. New recurring cytogenetic abnormalities and association of blast cell karyotypes with prognosis in childhood T-cell acute lymphoblastic leukemia: a Pediatric Oncology Group report of 343 cases. *Blood.* 2000; 96:2543-2549.

[26] Forestier E, Johansson B, Gustafsson G, Borgström G, Kerndrup G, Johannsson J, Heim S. Prognostic impact of karyotypic findings in childhood acute lymphoblastic leukaemia: a Nordic series comparing two treatment periods. For the Nordic Society of Paediatric Haematology and Oncology (NOPHO) Leukaemia Cytogenetic Study Group. *Br J Haematol* 2000;110:147-53.

[27] Harrison CJ, Moorman AV, Broadfield ZJ, Cheung KL, Harris RL, Reza Jalali G, Robinson HM, Barber KE, Richards SM, Mitchell CD, Eden TO, Hann IM, Hill FG, Kinsey SE, Gibson BE, Lilleyman J, Vora A, Goldstone AH, Franklin IM, Durrant J, Martineau M; Childhood and Adult Leukaemia Working Parties. Three distinct

subgroups of hypodiploidy in acute lymphoblastic leukaemia. *Br J Haematol* 2004;125:552-559.

[28] Paulsson K, Johansson B. High hyperdiploid childhood acute lymphoblastic leukemia. *Genes Chromosomes Cancer.* 2009;48:637-660.

[29] Paulsson K, Panagopoulos I, Knuutila S, Jee KJ, Garwicz S, Fioretos T, Mitelman F, Johansson B. Formation of trisomies and their parental origin in hyperdiploid childhood acute lymphoblastic leukemia. *Blood* 2003;102:3010-3015.

[30] Sharathkumar A, DeCamillo D, Bhambhani K, Cushing B, Thomas R, Mohamed AN, Ravindranath Y, Taub JW. Children with hyperdiploid but not triple trisomy (+4,+10,+17) acute lymphoblastic leukemia have an increased incidence of extramedullary relapse on current therapies: a single institution experience. *Am J Hematol.* 2008;83:34-40.

[31] Paulsson K, Heidenblad M, Mörse H , Borg Å, Fioretos T, Johansson B. Identification of cryptic aberrations and characterization of translocation breakpoints using array CGH in high hyperdiploid childhood acute lymphoblastic leukemia. *Leukemia* 2006; 20:2002–2007.

[32] Lilleyman J, Vora A, Goldstone AH, Franklin IM, Durrant J, Martineau M. Childhood and Adult Leukaemia Working Parties. Three distinct subgroups of hypodiploidy in acute lymphoblastic leukaemia. *Br J Haematol* 2004;125:552-559.

[33] Pui CH, Carroll AJ, Raimondi SC, Land VJ, Crist WM, Shuster JJ, Williams DL, Pullen DJ, Borowitz MJ, Behm FG, et al. Clinical presentation, karyotypic characterization, and treatment outcome of childhood acute lymphoblastic leukemia with a near-haploid or hypodiploid less than 45 line. *Blood* 1990;75:1170-1177.

[34] Arthur Zelent, Mel Greaves, Tariq Enver. Role of the *TEL-AML1* fusion gene in the molecular pathogenesis of childhood acute lymphoblastic leukaemia. *Oncogene* 2004;23,4275–4283.

[35] Shurtleff SA, Buijs A, Behm FG, et al. TEL/AML1 fusion resulting from a cryptic t(12;21) is the most common genetic lesion in pediatric ALL and defines a subgroup of patients with an excellent prognosis. *Leukemia* 1995; 9:1985-1989.

[36] McHale CM, Wiemels JL, Zhang L, Ma X, Buffler PA, Guo W, Loh ML, Smith MT. Prenatal origin of TEL-AML1-positive acute lymphoblastic leukemia in children born in California. *Genes Chromosomes Cancer* 2003;37:36-43.

[37] Wiemels JL, Hofmann J, Kang M, Selzer R, Green R, Zhou M, Zhong S, Zhang L, Smith MT, Marsit C, Loh M, Buffler P, Yeh RF. Chromosome 12p deletions in TEL-AML1 childhood acute lymphoblastic leukemia are associated with retrotransposon elements and occur postnatally. *Cancer Res* 2008;68:9935-44.

[38] Loh ML, Goldwasser MA, Silverman LB et al. Prospective analysis of *TEL/AML1*-positive patients treated on Dana-Farber Cancer Institute Consortium Protocol 95-01. *Blood* 2006; 107: 4508-4513.

[39] Johansson B, Moorman AV, Haas OA, Watmore AE, Cheung KL, Swanton S, Secker-Walker LM. Hematologic malignancies with t(4;11)(q21;q23)--a cytogenetic, morphologic, immunophenotypic and clinical study of 183 cases. European 11q23 Workshop participants. *Leukemia* 1998;12:779-787.

[40] Raimondi SC. 11q23 rearrangements in childhood acute lymphoblastic leukemia. *Atlas Genet Cytogenet Oncol Haematol*. February 2004. URL: http://AtlasGenetics Oncology.org/Anomalies/11q23ChildALLID1321.html

[41] Fu JF, Liang DC, Shih LY. Analysis of acute leukemias with MLL/ENL fusion transcripts: identification of two novel breakpoints in ENL. *Am J Clin Pathol* 2007;127:24-30.

[42] Armstrong SA, Staunton JE, Silverman LB, Pieters R, den Boer ML, Minden MD, Sallan SE, Lander ES, Golub TR, Korsmeyer SJ. MLL translocations specify a distinct gene expression profile that distinguishes a unique leukemia. *Nature genetics* 2002;30: 41-47.

[43] Bungaro S, Dell'Orto MC, Zangrando A, Basso D, Gorletta T, Lo Nigro L, Leszl A, Young BD, Basso G, Bicciato S, Biondi A, te Kronnie G, Cazzaniga G. Integration of genomic and gene expression data of childhood ALL without known aberrations identifies subgroups with specific genetic hallmarks. *Genes Chromosomes Cancer.* 2009;48:22-38.

[44] Pui CH, Raimondi SC, Hancock ML, Rivera GK, Ribeiro RC, Mahmoud HH, Sandlund JT, Crist WM, Behm FG. Immunologic, cytogenetic, and clinical characterization of childhood acute lymphoblastic leukemia with the t(1;19) (q23; p13) or its derivative. *J Clin Oncol.* 1994;12:2601-2606.

[45] Jeha S, Pei D, Raimondi SC, Onciu M, Campana D, Cheng C, Sandlund JT, Ribeiro RC, Rubnitz JE, Howard SC, Downing JR, Evans WE, Relling MV, Pui CH. Increased risk for CNS relapse in pre-B cell leukemia with the t(1;19)/TCF3-PBX1. *Leukemia* 2009;23:1406-1209.

[46] Felice MS, Gallego MS, Alonso CN, Alfaro EM, Guitter MR, Bernasconi AR, Rubio PL, Zubizarreta PA, Rossi JG. Prognostic impact of t(1;19)/ *TCF3-PBX1 in childhood acute lymphoblastic leukemia in the context of Berlin-Frankfurt-Münster-based protocols.* Posted online on May 3, 2011. (doi:10.3109/10428194.2011.565436)

[47] Aric M, Valsecchi MG, Camitta B, Schrappe M, Chessells J, Baruchel A, Gaynon P, Silverman L, Janka-Schaub G, Kamps W, Pui CH, Masera G. Outcome of treatment in children with Philadelphia chromosome-positive acute lymphoblastic leukemia. *New England J Med* 2000; 342:998-1006.

[48] Schultz KR, Bowman WP, Aledo A, Slayton WB, Sather H, Devidas M, Wang C, Davies SM, Gaynon PS, Trigg M, Rutledge R, Burden L, Jorstad D, Carroll A, Heerema NA, Winick N, Borowitz MJ, Hunger SP, Carroll WL, Camitta B. Improved early event-free survival with imatinib in Philadelphia chromosome-positive acute lymphoblastic leukemia: a children's oncology group study. *J Clin Oncol* 2009; 27:5175-5181.

[49] Kirk R Schultz, Tim Prestidge, Bruce Camitta. Philadelphia chromosome-positive acute lymphoblastic leukemia in children: new and emerging treatment options. *Expert Rev Hemat* 2010;3:731-742.

[50] Lange BJ, Raimondi SC, Heerema N, Nowell PC, Minowada J, Steinherz PE, Arenson EB, O'Connor R, Santoli D. Pediatric leukemia/lymphoma with t(8;14)(q24;q11). *Leukemia* 1992;6:613-618.

[51] Hecht JL, Aster JC. Molecular biology of Burkitt's lymphoma. *J Clinic Oncol* 2000;18: 3707-3721.
[52] Heerema NA, Sather HN, Sensel MG, Lee MK, Hutchinson R, Lange BJ, Bostrom BC, Nachman JB, Steinherz PG, Gaynon PS, Uckun FM. Clinical significance of deletions of chromosome arm 6q in childhood acute lymphoblastic leukemia: a report from the Children's Cancer Group. *Leukemia & lymphoma.* 2000; 36:467-478.
[53] Heerema NA, Nachman JB, Sather HN, La MK, Hutchinson R, Lange BJ, Bostrom B, Steinherz PG, Gaynon PS, Uckun FM. Deletion of 7p or monosomy 7 in pediatric acute lymphoblastic leukemia is an adverse prognostic factor: a report from the Children's Cancer Group. *Leukemia* 2004;18,939–947.
[54] Behrendt H, Charrin C, Gibbons B, Harrison CJ, Hawkins JM, Heerema NA, Horschler-Bˆ☐ tel B, Huret JL, LaˆØ JL, Lampert F Dicentric (9;12) in acute lymphocytic leukemia and other hematological malignancies: report from a dic(9;12) study group. *Leukemia* 1995;9:102-106.
[55] Felix CA, Lange BJ. Leukemia in Infants. *The Oncologist* 1999;225-240.
[56] Chessells JM, Harrison CJ, Kempski H, Webb DK, Wheatley K, Hann IM, Stevens RF, Harrison G, Gibson BE; MRC Childhood Leukaemia working party. Clinical features, cytogenetics and outcome in acute lymphoblastic and myeloid leukaemia of infancy: report from the MRC Childhood Leukaemia working party. *Leukemia.* 2002;16:776-784.
[57] Heerema NA, Sather HN, Ge J, Arthur DC, Hilden JM, Trigg ME, Reaman GH. Cytogenetic studies of infant acute lymphoblastic leukemia: poor prognosis of infants with t(4;11) - a report of the Children's Cancer Group. *Leukemia.* 1999;13:679-686.
[58] Heerema NA, Arthur DC, Sather H, Albo V, Feusner J, Lange BJ, Steinherz PG, Zeltzer P, Hammond D, Reaman GH. Cytogenetic features of infants less than 12 months of age at diagnosis of acute lymphoblastic leukemia: impact of the 11q23 breakpoint on outcome: a report of the Childrens Cancer Group. *Blood.* 1994;83:2274-2284.
[59] Hilden JM, Dinndorf PA, Meerbaum SO, Sather H, Villaluna D, Heerema NA, McGlennen R, Smith FO, Woods WG, Salzer WL, Johnstone HS, Dreyer Z, Reaman GH; Children's Oncology Group. Analysis of prognostic factors of acute lymphoblastic leukemia in infants: report on CCG 1953 from the Children's Oncology Group. *Blood.* 2006;108:441-451.
[60] Schneider NR, Carroll AJ, Shuster JJ, Pullen DJ, Link MP, Borowitz MJ, Camitta BM, Katz JA, Amylon MD. New recurring cytogenetic abnormalities and association of blast cell karyotypes with prognosis in childhood T-cell acute lymphoblastic leukemia: a pediatric oncology group report of 343 cases. *Blood* 2000;96:2543-2549.
[61] Graux C, J Cools, L Michaux, P Vandenberghe, A Hagemeijer. Cytogenetics and molecular genetics of T-cell acute lymphoblastic leukemia: from thymocyte to lymphoblast. *Leukemia* 2006; 20, 1496–1510.
[62] Heerema NA, Sather HN, Sensel MG, Kraft P, Nachman JB, Steinherz PG, Lange BJ, Hutchinson RS, Reaman GH, Trigg ME, Arthur DC, Gaynon PS, Uckun FM. Frequency and clinical significance of cytogenetic abnormalities in pediatric T-lineage

acute lymphoblastic leukemia: a report from the Children's Cancer Group. *J Clin Oncol* 1998;16:1270-1278.

[63] Karrman K, Forestier E, Heyman M, Andersen MK, Autio K, Blennow E, Borgström G, Ehrencrona H, Golovleva I, Heim S, Heinonen K, Hovland R, Johannsson JH, Kerndrup G, Nordgren A, Palmqvist L, Johansson B. Clinical and cytogenetic features of a population-based consecutive series of 285 pediatric T-cell acute lymphoblastic leukemias: rare T-cell receptor gene rearrangements are associated with poor outcome. *Genes Chromosomes Cancer* 2009;48:795-805.

[64] Bash RO, Hall S, Timmons CF, Crist WM, Amylon M, Smith RG, Baer R. Does activation of the TAL1 gene occur in a majority of patients with T-cell acute lymphoblastic leukemia? A pediatric oncology group study. Blood. 1995;86:666-676.

[65] Mauvieux L, Leymarie V, Helias C, Perrusson N, Falkenrodt A, Lioure B, Lutz P, Lessard M. High incidence of Hox11L2 expression in children with T-ALL. *Leukemia.* 2002;16:2417-2422.

[66] Kees UR, Heerema NA, Kumar R, Watt PM, Baker DL, La MK, Uckun FM, Sather HN. Expression of HOX11 in childhood T-lineage acute lymphoblastic leukaemia can occur in the absence of cytogenetic aberration at 10q24: a study from the Children's Cancer Group (CCG). *Leukemia* 2003;17:887-893.

[67] Graux C, Cools J, Melotte C, Quentmeier H, Ferrando A, Levine R, Vermeesch JR, Stul M, Dutta B, Boeckx N, Bosly A, Heimann P, Uyttebroeck A, Mentens N, Somers R, MacLeod RA, Drexler HG, Look AT, Gilliland DG, Michaux L, Vandenberghe P, Wlodarska I, Marynen P, Hagemeijer A. Fusion of NUP214 to ABL1 on amplified episomes in T-cell acute lymphoblastic leukemia. *Nat Genet* 2004;3:1084-1089.

[68] Lee-Sherick AB, Linger RMA, Gore Lia, Keating AK, Graham DK. Targeting paediatric acute lymphoblastic leukaemia: novel therapies currently in development. *British J Haemat* 2010;151:205-311.

[69] Felix CA, Lange BJ,. Chessells JM. Pediatric Acute Lymphoblastic Leukemia: Challenges and Controversies in 2000. *Hematology* 2000;1:285-302.

[70] Den Boer ML, van Slegtenhorst M, De Menezes RX, et al.. "A subtype of childhood acute lymphoblastic leukaemia with poor treatment outcome: a genome-wide classification study". *Lancet Oncol* 2009;10:125.

[71] Felix CA, Lange BJ, Chessells JM. Pediatric Acute Lymphoblastic Leukemia: Challenges and Controversies in 2000. *Hematology Am Soc Hematol Educ Program.* 2000:285-302.

[72] Collins-Underwood JR, Mullighan CG. Genomic profiling of high-risk acute lymphoblastic leukemia. *Leukemia.* 2010;24:1676-1685.

[73] Flotho C, Coustan-Smith E, Pei D, et al. A set of genes that regulate cell proliferation predicts treatment outcome in childhood acute lymphoblastic leukemia. *Blood* 2007;110: 1271-1277.

[74] Paulsson K, Horvat A, Strömbeck B, Nilsson F, Heldrup J, Behrendtz M, Forestier E, Andersson A, Fioretos T, Johansson B. Mutations of FLT3, NRAS, KRAS, and PTPN11 are frequent and possibly mutually exclusive in high hyperdiploid childhood acute lymphoblastic leukemia. *Genes Chromososomes Cancer* 2008;47:26-33.

[75] Mullighan CG. New strategies in acute lymphoblastic leukemia: translating advances in genomics into clinical practice. *Clin Cancer Res* 2011;17:396-400.

[76] Bungaro S, Dell'Orto MC, Zangrando A, Basso D, Gorletta T, Lo Nigro L, Leszl A, Young BD, Basso G, Bicciato S, Biondi A, te Kronnie G, Cazzaniga G. Integration of genomic and gene expression data of childhood ALL without known aberrations identifies subgroups with specific genetic hallmarks. *Genes Chromosomes Cancer.* 2009;48:22-38.

[77] Roberts KG, Mullighan CG. How new advances in genetic analysis are influencing the understanding and treatment of childhood acute leukemia. *Curr Opin Pediatr* 2011;23:34-40.

In: Acute Lymphoblastic Leukemia
Editors: Severo Vecchione and Luigi Tedesco
ISBN: 978-1-61470-872-8
©2012 Nova Science Publishers, Inc.

Chapter IV

Systems Approaches to Childhood Leukemogenesis

George I. Lambrou[1], Maria Braoudaki[1,2], Kyriaki Hatziagapiou[1], Katerina Katsibardi[1], Fotini Tzortzatou-Stathopoulou[1,2].

[1]Hematology/Oncology Unit, First Department of Pediatrics, University of Athens, «Aghia Sophia» Children's Hospital, Athens, Greece
[2]University Research Institute for the Study and Treatment of Childhood Genetic and Malignant Diseases, University of Athens, «Aghia Sophia» Children's Hospital, Athens, Greece

Abstract

The mechanisms underlying leukemogenesis in lymphocytes are hitherto poorly elucidated. Understanding those mechanisms is crucial for treatment, quality of life purposes and ethical reasons, since neoplasms in children could prove devastating.

In the advent of the 21stcentury,the trend in research has taken an interesting turn, looking for global patterns in biological systems in a holistic approach. Although this concept is not novel, it has been nowadays*baptized* as systems approach, borrowing its name from engineers. Meanwhile, additional biological principles have emerged, such as systems biology, computational biology and more lately physical biology. These disciplines aim the assistance of explaining biological phenomena with the attribution of general rules, similar to older natural sciences such as chemistry and physics. Hence, it would not be an exaggeration to state that the maturity of biological sciences would endure their "mating" with other disciplines such as mathematics and physics.

Studies concerning the etiology underlying hematological malignancies are scarce. In general, there have been several theories on oncogenesis but the mechanisms behind it remain poorly defined. Considering that even the clonal nature of leukemia is debatable, it makes leukemogenesis a challenging topic to deal with, while simultaneously attempting to explain its origin proves to be a bold effort. Starting from the common denominator that the disease is caused, by the malignant (or maybe not) hematopoietic progenitor cells, one could assume that the principles applied to other theories regarding oncogenesis should also apply in that case. Thus far, this is not very clear, since childhood malignancies have a distinctiveness that other neoplasms lack; the adequate time of development that neoplastic cells possess to deploy and grow. In particular, supposing the fact that an adult neoplasm would take years to grow due to accumulation of mutations or stress environmental factors, this time interval is simply absent in childhood malignancies. Therefore, it could be assumed that a different mechanism of oncogenesis exists. Precisely this is the fact that makes childhood malignancies further interesting, without overlooking the devastating effect of the disease in children.

The present knowledge on the theoriesof leukemogenesis, or even fragments of theories,will be reviewed. In addition, common aspects between leukemogenesis and oncogenesis, in general, will be searched. In particular, the existing systemic or even physical theories that exist on this topic will be examined and several hints to this knowledge based on studies and thoughts will be attempted.

Introduction

The Necessity of "Marriage" of Biological Sciences and the other Exact Sciences

Until recently, one of the main approaches in scientific research was the study of molecules in a sequential order. That is, we were able to discover the function and roles of genes or protein in pairs or maximal three at the same time. The last decade, this picture has changed. With the advent of high-throughput methodologies, the study of thousands of factors (and even millions meanwhile) has been plausible. Microarrays and deep-sequencing are two examples of such methodologies. Yet, we must admit that the main revolution that facilitated such discoveries was the development of the personal computer. From the time point that computational power became publicly available has revolutionized the way science has preceded with its steps. On the other hand, biology was a science that was based, and in a great extent still is, on observation. This of course was true for all natural sciences, yet other sciences such as the physical or chemical sciences were more mature since they were able to describe their phenomena through a common mathematical language. For example, it is of great certainty that an apple falling from a tree will go down towards the gravitational force of the earth and as a matter of fact we are in position, knowing the initial height of the apple, to calculate the exact velocity just before it crashes to the ground. Also, given the time interval we are able to calculate, again with great certainty, the exact position of the apple from its initial point. The amazing thing is that if we took consecutive measurements on the falling apple we would find very similar results and we would obtain for our results a very high confidence interval. On the other hand, if we have a cell population and need to know their number at a given time point, it is impossible to do so, if we know, with great certainty, the initial cell number. As in the case of the apple, if we could perform several experiments with same cells and same conditions the most probable would be that we would come up with, sometimes, very different results. The conclusion from these two examples is that physical phenomena can be described mathematically, which does not mean that these phenomena are simple but their simplified forms can be calculated with high certainty. This is not true for biological phenomena. Even the simplest observations, such as how a cell population increases in numbers, are not trivial and it is almost impossible to make predictions about a cell population.In the advent of the 21st century a new trend has emerged in biological sciences. This was a systems approach to biological phenomena. The idea was not new, since it has been described previously that there is a need for the life sciences to be integrated with the physical and mathematical sciences. The first merge occurred with the *marriage* of biology and chemistry which gave rise to biochemistry, since all life molecules are chemicals and their interactions are chemical reactions. The difficult part is the merge of the biological sciences with the physical and mathematical sciences. This has taken place from the emergence of two new disciplines namely systems biology and physical biology. Both very young and in their infancy, yet very powerful as we think it will prove to be. Systems biology has borrowed its name from the engineers and their systems theory concepts. Physical biology, on the other hand, could be mentioned that has taken its name from the merge of physics and biology and in a way it is another discipline similar to physical chemistry. This short review on biology and its branches was considered significant, since it would give us an idea why we need such ideas such as mathematical modeling of biological phenomena.

Systems biology and physical biology even more can be considered a relatively young discipline. It was in the advent of the 21st century that the first coordinated attempts became reality. However, the term had been previously mentioned both as a necessity and as a discipline. We couldn't phrase it in better words than *MihajloMesarović*in 1968:

"...in spite of the considerable interest and efforts, the application of systems theory in biology has not quite lived up to expectations...one of the main reasons for the existing lag is that systems theory has not been directly concerned with some of the problems of vital importance in biology..."

"...The real advance in the application of systems theory to biology will come about only when the biologists start asking questions which are based on the system-theoretic concepts rather than using these concepts to represent in still another way the phenomena which are already explained in terms of biophysical or biochemical principles. ...then we will not have the application of engineering principles to biological problems but rather a field of *systems biology* with its own identity and in its own right..." [1] (adapted from the book Systems Biology-Dynamic Pathway Modeling by Olaf Wolkenhauer [2]).

But in order to further define the field of systems biology we should refer to an older reference from *Henri Poincare*, who proposed a solution to the *three-body problem* in the 19th century:

"...life is a relationship among molecules and not a property of any molecule..."
"...Science is built up of facts, as a house is with stones. But a collection of facts is no more a science than a heap of stones is a house..." [2].

In general,natural sciences have matured with time especially with the integration of mathematics. For example, the disciplines of physics and chemistry have benefited from the mathematical discipline and matured enough to create a common language for describing phenomena. Similarly, biological sciences could greatly benefit by integrating knowledge from the mathematical and engineering disciplines. Today a huge amount of work is performed over the collection of data into large databases such as the *Gene Ontology* database, the *KEGG* database and others [2-11].

Theories of Carcinogenesis

In the case of cancer, tumorigenesis is the interconnection of thousands of factors acting simultaneously that brings about the malignant phenotype. A very popular theory of carcinogenesis, in general, is that the cause of the disease is the accumulation of genetic mutations throughout an individual's life. If an adequate number of such genetic mutations accumulates then there is the occurrence of cancer [12]; actually, this theory was initially proposed by *Nordling* in 1953 [13], and further on it was formulated by *Knudson,* which was called the *two-hit hypothesis*. With his hypothesis he considered that fact that several mutations are required for the immergence of cancer, also in children, and he further proposed that there is a possibility that tumorigenesis can occur in two consecutive events (hits) [14]. Initially, evidence was given for retinoblastoma, where he proposed that at least for that type of tumor (retinoblastoma) it can occur with two mutational events [14].

Yet other equally significant theories have been suggested, such as the multistage oncogenesis theory [15, 16]. Another interesting theory is that tumors are directly connected to the industrialization of modern life and it has been suggested that cancer is not actually a disease but an evolutionary adaptation of the cells in order to survive certain environmental changes/threats. In addition, it has been proposed that tumor cells are an evolution of normal cells in order to overcome environmental challenge and stress [17]. Furthermore, it has been reported that this evolutionary change might control the heterogeneity of tumor tissues. Since, genetic as well epigenetic mechanisms control the evolution of cancer then it is possible that the network of events that leads to cancer will remain unsolved due to the complexity of the phenomenon. Modeling approaches have been proposed with respect to the explanation of the evolutionary character of tumor emergence and progression [17].

Interestingly, such theories have been proposed from the beginning of the first organized observations on cancer. For example, a common characteristic of almost all types of tumors is the known *Warburg effect* described by *Otto Warburg* in 1924. This simple observation remains until today a fundamental trait of tumor biology i.e. that tumors perform a shift from oxidative phosphorylation to anaerobic glycolysis for their energy needs [18]. At the time, *Warburg* considered this as the leading etiology of cancer and of note that it was considered as such until the observation or finding that it is one of the side-effects of cancer. It is known now that the avoidance of the oxidative phosphorylation pathway, it is the one that leads to excessive lactate production causing this deteriorating effect cancerous cell have on the surrounding tissue. Yet, this property of cancer cells has been exploited and several drugs are in clinical trials functioning as inhibitors of the anaerobic fermentation of glucose. However, the origins and etiology of cancer are still being investigated.

However, a question that rises is whether these theories could be applied to childhood neoplasms, since these models/theories cannot be applied directly as the elapsed time of exposure to mutagenesis is not adequate to explain the appearance of cancer. As we will mention further on, there are several hypotheses regarding childhood neoplasms. For example, in the case of childhood leukemia it has been suggested that cytogenetic aberrations might play a role in the transformation of malignancy.

From this discussion, it is therefore evident that to be able to improve a certain condition, one first needs to understand the phenomenon or, in other words, to appreciate the governing rules of the system. Hence, returning to our previous discussion on systems biology, it works towards understanding and defining the rules governing biological phenomena.

Childhood Neoplasias and Childhood Leukemia

The question that might rise is why leukemia and especially childhood leukemia? Acute lymphoblastic leukemia (ALL) is the most frequent occurring malignancy among childhood cancers [19]. It originates in the undifferentiated lymphoblast, which abnormally ceases develop into the mature lymphoid cell giving rise to a tumor.Acute leukemia mainly appears during childhood but it can also occur in adolescence manifesting a poor prognosis regardless of age. Progress in childhood leukemia has been immense the last decades with an overall survival rate exceeding 75% [20].Still though there is an approximate 20% that relapses, which in many cases can prove fatal. Additionally, leukemia presents one of the very interesting cases of clonal expansion. As we mentioned above, until recently, scientific approaches concentrated on examining several factors simultaneouslyonly revealed part of the picture. Oncogenesis is a highly complicated process and one of the tools that current research has in its arsenal is computational and systems biology. In this respect, we are now able to investigate possible common mechanismsthat govern different neoplasms.

The prognostic factors have also been well characterized inchildhood leukemia; includingwhite blood cell count at presentation (diagnosis), age and gender, immune-phenotype, as well as the presence of CNS or certain chromosomal aberrations [20]. Treatment of childhood leukemia is successful for the majority of patients, mainly due to the use of classical chemotherapeutics. Recently, individualized treatments have also been applied, as in the case of *BCR/ABL* positive (also known as Philadelphia positive (Ph$^+$)) leukemia, using imatinibmesylate, a new agent specific for the particular gene fusion. This represents a great example of how childhood leukemia can benefit from individualized therapy.

To mention a few characteristics of ALL we should say that it comprises of cells that are undifferentiated, immortal and with the potential to divide infinitely. This means that proliferation takes place in an uncontrollable pattern. In addition, it has been reported that there is a possibility for presentation of secondary malignancy after successful treatment of a primary (therapy-related leukemia). This implies the involvement of several environmental factors (in the present case, drug administration). For example, following the successful treatment of a paravertebral embryonal rhabdomyosarcoma (ERS), a patient developed acute T-lymphoblastic leukemia [21], or therapy-related leukemia can occur inthe vast majority of myelodysplastic syndrome (MDS) treatments. The question that could be posed here is whether this development of the secondary tumor originated from cells of the primary tumor, as in the case of therapy-related leukemia, or whether there were "dormant" leukemic cells in the bone marrow, which got triggered to proliferate uncontrollably after chemotherapy. In the case where cells from one type of cancer develop into another, it probably means that the tumor cell possesses two traits: first it is able to migrate and second it is able to differentiate to another type of cell manifesting stem cell properties. This is in accordance with the stem cell theory of cancer origin, as cancer stem cells keep their ability to differentiate, migrate and even give rise to a new malignancy with almost totally new traits. Furthermore, it has been reported that therapy-related leukemia can occur due to the use of chemotherapeutics [22, 23]. This phenomenon has not been thoroughly investigated and the mechanisms underlying it are still obscure. However, it points out the fact that carcinogenesis is a complicated process, implicating a number of mechanisms and not just single events in a cell's life time. If we were to accept the hypothesis that two different tumor cells can co-exist in different locations asaccurate, then we could accept the notion that stem cells play the main role in carcinogenesis and tumor growth. On the other hand, an interesting report by *Kelly et al.*revealedthat, at least in part, the presence of cancer stem cells is not necessary for tumor growth to be sustained [24].

Progenitor hematopoietic cells originate from the embryonic mesoderm. Blood cells are derived from the *lateral mesoderm*, which gives rise to the *splachnic mesoderm* and this, in turn, to the *hemangioblastic tissue*. Further on, *paraxial mesoderm* gives rise to the un-segmented pre-somitic mesoderm, formed during *gastrulation*,and mesoderm generated from the *primitive streak*. One of the earliest genes expressed in the *paraxial mesoderm* is T (branchyury). This is also an embryonic transcription factor that is expressed in a gradient across developmental sites derived from the primitive streak and continuously expressed in the notochord [25]. The FGF (Fibroblast Growth Factor) and RA (Retinoic Acid) pathways are the main routes followed in early somatic development [25]. Another important signaling pathway that has been found to participate in developmental as well as oncogenic pathways is the NOTCH pathway. Notch genes encode transmembrane receptors. The human genome contains four NOTCH receptor homologues. In somite stage, *NOTCH1* is expressed across the presomitic mesoderm, where mutations have been found to cause defects in somatic segmentation and anterior-posterior polarity [26, 27]. On the other hand, during embryogenesis, blood cells originate from two sites: the first is thought to be the *ventral mesoderm* near the *yolk sac*, which gives rise to the intra-embryonic hematopoietic precursors, whereas the hematopoietic cells that last throughout the entire life time of an organism are derived from the mesodermal area surrounding the aorta [28]. From the point of mesoderm differentiation, strictly orchestrated regulation of various genes leads to two similar cell types with different functions and roles in the body. This is the result of a complicated network of gene regulation and expression. It is easy to assume that aberrations in the regulatory networks underlying development would lead to tumor cells. Developmentally, there are several factors that affect gene regulation in order for differentiation to take place.

An interesting reference highlights the fact that stem cells are probably found in different types of tumors, thus suggesting that stem cells are implicated in the etiology of tumor maintenance and growth [29]. However, there is evidence that even normal, already differentiated cellscan be transformed to tumorigenic [29]. Based on this observation, there was a case reporting a child manifesting four different tumor types sequentially[30]. It could be that stem cells originating from the same tissue possess similar defects but enough alterations to be able to give rise to five different types of tumor. The discovery of similar or opposing gene expression profiles may lead to the understanding of a common tumor origin, if such exists.

Another point on which attention should be drawn is the regulation of genes through transcription factors (TFs). Knowledge of gene regulatory networks is considered to be of crucial importance for the understanding of diseases such as cancer, as it may lead to new therapeutic approaches [3]. The knowledge of common transcriptional regulatory networks could potentially lead to a universal treatment for diverse diseases such as cancer, and it is through this possibility that the need for computational methods in the study of carcinogenesis becomes apparent.

Our reference to several known developmental and ontogenetic mechanisms of hematopoiesis and its aberrant function is an introduction that shows that this phenomenon is complicated. Hence, it is certain that in order to understand it better we need to formulate theories and models that would give us generalized views of the phenomenon.

Theories on Leukemogenesis

With the introduction of the basic concepts of systems approaches to biological phenomena and some developmental aspects of hematopoietic and leukemic cells we are now in position to describe the basics on the theories of leukemogenesis. We should say from the very start that this is a very complicated phenomenon and there is still an ongoing debate on the etiologies of the disease.

Chemical, Radiation and InfectiousFactors Proposed as Affecting Leukemogenesis

Mostly theories on the ontology of leukemia were based upon the characteristics that leukemic cells have as far as their cytogenetic characteristics are concerned. In the early studies on the etiology of leukemia several factors have been investigated. In several reports, it has been investigated whether environmental factors were implied in the emergence of leukemia. Such investigations included the study of electromagnetic fields, for example in the case of residency in nearby high voltage power plants [31-35]. In other cases,research was focused on whether exposure to environmental pollutants could imply a high risk for the emergence of leukemia, as in the case of exposure to benzene and its derivatives[36]. In addition, several other chemicals have been proposed as factors triggering leukemia [37, 38]. Other factors, that have been proposed as potentially leukemogenetic, include infections [39-42], autoimmunity and familial history of cancer [43, 44] among others. Hitherto, there are still under debate the reasonsunderlying leukemogenesis. The aforementioned etiologies,we already presented in the previous section, would fit in the first theories of carcinogenesis. However, a question that still rises is regarding the adequate time for mutations to occur, since the evolution of a cell to cancerous cell probably takes time and more than one step are required for a neoplasm to occur.

Cytogenetic Aberrations as Leukemogenetic Factors

Returning to the initial discussion on cytogenetic aberrations, it has been proposed that for certain leukemic types, cytogenetic aberrations are the leading effects that cause the disease. Yet, what is happening with the rest of the diseased cells that do not carry those aberrations. For example, in the case of infant acute leukemia, 80% of cases carry the *MLL* fusion gene, which is also observed in newly formed, secondary leukemia [19]. Thus, what really happens with the rest of 20%. The phenotype is the same at least as far as the disease is concerned, which means that all cells possess the ability to proliferate in an uncontrollable manner and propagate on expense of the hosting body. Moreover, in leukemia additional aberrations are found in certain percentages of diseased cells and not necessarily in all of them. Subsequently, maybe those effects observed are not the etiological grounds in leukemia but random manifestations of the same, yet another, etiology. This "dead-end" brings us to the discussion of the previous section concerning the existence of cancer stem cells (CSCs). Equally, with the existence of cancer stem cell is the existence of leukemia stem cells (LSCs).

It is meanwhile an established value that cancer tissues and in concordance leukemic cells are heterogeneous [45]. Even in the case of leukemia where, it is considered to be a clonal expansion of cells, probably it is not. It is a mixture of progenitor cells but probably with very diverse properties and genetic characteristics. Cytogenetic abnormalities and aberrant gene expression have been considered as prominent candidates for leukemogenesis such as the HOX family of proteins [46], *MEIS* and *AML* families of genes, respectively [47, 48]. Further reports on hematopoietic stem cells (HSCs) have revealed the existence of several populations among them, such as quiescent, proliferating and leukemia initializing cells [49]. Especially, as far as *MLL*-ALL is concerned there are some special issues that have to be addressed. There is a tight connection between the *MLL*/Trithorax rearrangements and the regulation of the *HOX* cluster of genes. It appears that this relation is evolutionary conserved, which gives the ability to MLL proteins to de-regulate *HOX* genes [50]. In infant leukemia, a very interesting issue is the latency of leukemia development. *MLL* leukemia occurs immediately after birth or can be delayed for years. This leads to the hypothesis that additional mutations or epigenetic transformations are required in order for leukemia to occur. The time of leukemia development is of crucial importance and the question that arises is what is the actual time that leukemia progresses from the point that an LSC or a leukemia initiating cell will appear.

The reports are numerous on leukemia cytogenetics and their causal effects on the disease. The readercould be referred to some interesting reviews for in-depth information [51-56] as the topic has been extensively covered by other chapters of our scientific group.

The Stem Cell Theories

There is a great debate on the existence of a rare cancer stem cell population in childhoodALL, which,provides a key target for novel therapeutic targets. The presence of LSCs has been clearly shown in AML by xenograft transplantation studies. It has been demonstrated that cells with the ability to initiate human leukemia in immune-deficient

NOD/*scid*mice were exclusively present within the CD34+CD38- stem cell fraction [57]. This means that in AML, such cells could provide novel targets for therapeutics as well as the evidence for changes, in the way we think of cancer biology. Immunophenotyping is a very powerful method to determine leukemic blast maturation stage and classification. Considering that the LSC exists in the very beginning as the first of its kind,consequently this would give rise to clones that would proliferate but not necessarily retain the properties of initial mother cell. This was found to be inaccurate when cells from different phenotypic maturation stages were implanted into mice, whichwere able to initiate leukemia [57]. This might imply two things: firstly, that immunophenotypic maturation is independent of the initiating LSC and maturation progresses randomly in a non-regulated pattern and secondly that during proliferation, several daughter cells retain the ability and properties of the maternal LSC. However, several studies have reported contradictory results. More specifically, in a previous report, only cells with an immature stem cell-like immunophenotype were able to initiate leukemia in nude mice [58, 59], while two other studies have suggested that more mature blast cells were able to engraft leukemia in an *in vivo* model [60, 61]. Of note, both heterogeneous reports are very interesting, since neither of them is wrongandthe existence of LSC is independent of cell maturation.

In previous considerations, childhood ALL was considered to be chemo-curable due to the fact that it was thought to originate from stem cells that were functionally transient and chemosensitive, while adult leukemia was considered to originate from a more primitive stem cell population with extensive self-renewal capabilities [62].

Evolutionary Theories of Leukemogenesis

In the previous section, we have mentioned that one of the explanations attempted to be given to tumorigenesis, is through the evolutionary processes that cells probably possess. As it has been reviewed by Greaves (2010) there are three main attributions to cancer propagation: a) a fixed and hierarchically positioned subset of stem cells resembling normal hematopoietic stem cells, b) a non-deterministic or stochastic process with plasticity of "stem-ness". At this point we would like to add another possibility that is, the existence of a deterministic yet chaotic mechanism of propagation. By saying chaotic, we do not mean the disarrangement of cell propagation but we refer to the mathematical meaning of chaos as a non-linearity. It is possible that if such phenomena occur due to evolutionary driving forces then this could be controlled by chaos i.e. non-linear dynamics and c) activity of a genetically dominant sub-clone [63]. The model of evolutionary cancer propagation is based on the idea that transformed cells pass through a series of "bottlenecks". These are selective processes that "decide" in a way, which cells will progress to a next phase ofproliferation until a final population is reached that willcause the tumor to emerge.In general, cancer cells could be considered as elements participating in a Darwinian process. The criteria of selection could be the presence or even acquisition of mutations, or even epigenetic changes. Once more, regarding childhood leukemia, and childhood neoplasms in general, the question remains on the adequate time for such phenomena to evolve. Either evolutionary processes are so rapid that the disease emerges in the early ages; that is the first years of life, or they pre-exist *in utero* as it has been previously reported for the *MLL*/ALL cases [64].

Some Physical Approaches to Leukemogenesis

To the best of our knowledge, there are no considerations concerning the merging of physical theories and applications regarding the clarification of leukemogenesis. From a single perspective, it is highly unlikely that such theory could be applied to the system called leukemogenesis. Yet, there are some physical aspects that are not taken into consideration, at least up until now. The *Warburg effect* that we mentioned in the previous section, where the current observation made, was that tumor cells had defective mitochondria, thus leading to the malfunction of oxidative phosphorylation. The net reaction for energy production in cellular metabolism gives twelve molecules of ATP for one molecule of glucose. In cancer cells this is not accurate. Each mole of glucose being consumed gives two moles of ATP and two moles of lactate. This immediately gives a hint towards the different energetic needs that each cells has, i.e. the LSC and the HSC. From the thermodynamics point of view, proliferation and survival leads to entropy minimization, while cell death leads to entropy maximization. Also, proliferating cells would produce more work than less proliferating cells. There is a clear difference between the two cell types, that is normal and tumor cells. No matter what the processes of carcinogenesis (leukemogenesis) are, those cells require energy to proliferate and they too obey to the laws of mass and energy conservation. If we represent cell proliferation as a series of equations, we would describe normal cells in a certain form and in the case of tumor cells, since the same global laws apply, we would have an imbalanced equation that should be solved.

In addition, at this point, we could combine the aspects mentioned in the previous section of evolutionary theories, which are time and stochasticity or non-determinism. Time is a physical quantity that is not irrelevant to the progress of leukemia. As we mentioned previously, there is a time interval between the point of emergence of the first cell and the presentation of the disease. This latency is probably crucial not only to understand the disease but also to cure it. A fast proliferating disease follows different biological pathways than a slow proliferating disease or even a disease that moves near a steady-state condition. Also, bearing that gene expression is a process that it is regulated very tightly even in the case of neoplasms, one might say with certainty that any details from tight regulation would lead to non-viable conditions. Since tumor cells are viable, in a contradictory sense, they do possess a tight gene regulation.

The debate becomes more interesting when it comes to the aspects of stochastic processes and non-determinism. This is a very complicated topic and we would attempt to give some thoughts on the subject. Yet, it is immensely interesting to deal with it. From the classical physics point of view, phenomena are causal. That is, for each observation there is a causal effect that brought about the phenomenon. The question now is whether this phenomenon is random or deterministic. If we consider the quantum aspect of things, this is a random process that yet with statistical certainty, will be within the limits of viability. To bring this topic to leukemogenesis, let us ask wonder what are the chances, if any, for a cell to undergo mutations that would be lethal and instead of lethality, to get exactly the opposite that is potential for infinitesimal propagation. Tumors are such an example. On one hand, the observed mutations could be random but the result is not. The regulation and biology of tumor cells implies that random phenomena could lead to non-random effects. By combining the aspects of thermodynamics on these thoughts, we could hypothesize that random phenomena usually lead to the maximization of entropy as well as increase in dispersed events, but in the case of tumors, dispersed and random events lead to entropy minimization since they lead to cell proliferation, or in other words to order. This leads to a paradox, since randomness leads to not-order but in the case of tumors randomness leads to entropy minimization, thus order. Therefore, if such phenomena i.e. leukemogenesis and tumorigenesis were purely stochastic and non-deterministic, they would contradict the physical laws to which they also obey. Therefore, it is possible that two events occursimultaneously; certainty and probability. This issue has been marvelously addressed by*Max Planck* in a lecture given at the University of Berlin in his talk entitled "*Dynamische und StatistischeGesetzmässigkeit*" ("*Dynamical andStatistical Regularity*") in 1914. In that lecture, the same example was presented in terms of fluid dynamics and energy transfer. Thus, Planck implied that the movement of a heavier fluid will move towards the gravitational forces, which is a certainty, while heat will travel upwards from the heater to the colder layers, which is a probability. This is a very complicated aspect, which has not yet been addressed in the literature as far as biological systems are concerned, and in particular tumorigenesis, while here we attempt to give some thoughts to the aspect and leave it open for future investigations.

Conclusion

Cancer is a disease of the genome, where several genetic and epigenetic changes are required in order to occur. One of the main problems with the stipulations of theories of leukemogenesis is the fact that the only hints available, at least for *in vivo* cases, are the ones at diagnosis. More specifically, at diagnosis, the observed cell population consists of a mixture of phenotypes and genotypes, which in turn represents the outcome of the events that occurred from the very first steps of leukemogenesis. Hence, we do not have any hints on what happened from the beginning of the emergence of the first leukemic cells, no matter if this was a stem cell or not, until the presentation of the disease, composing real challenge to discover what happened before the time of our observations. In general, systems and physical approaches to leukemogenesis and carcinogenesis could prove extremely useful on the elucidation of the disease and also its cure.

References

[1] Mesarovic, M, Systems Theory and Biology-The View of a Theoretician.*Systems Theory and Biology*, 1968. 351: p. 59-87.

[2] Wolkenhauer, O, *Systems Biology-Dynamic Pathway Modelling*. 2010, Rostock.

[3] Chang, L W, Nagarajan, R, Magee, J A, Milbrandt, J, and Stormo, G D, A systematic model to predict transcriptional regulatory mechanisms based on overrepresentation of transcription factor binding profiles.*Genome Res*, 2006. 16(3): p. 405-13.

[4] Chatziioannou, A, Moulos, P, and Kolisis, F N, Gene ARMADA: an integrated multianalysis platform for microarray data implemented in MATLAB.*BMC Bioinformatics*, 2009. 10: p. 354.

[5] Kanehisa, M, The KEGG database.*Novartis Found Symp*, 2002. 247: p. 91-101; discussion 101-3, 119-28, 244-52.

[6] Kanehisa, M and Goto, S, KEGG: kyoto encyclopedia of genes and genomes.*Nucleic Acids Res*, 2000. 28(1): p. 27-30.

[7] Ogata, H, Goto, S, Sato, K, Fujibuchi, W, Bono, H, and Kanehisa, M, KEGG: Kyoto Encyclopedia of Genes and Genomes.*Nucleic Acids Res*, 1999. 27(1): p. 29-34.

[8] Rubinstein, R and Simon, I, MILANO--custom annotation of microarray results using automatic literature searches.*BMC Bioinformatics*, 2005. 6: p. 12.

[9] Salwinski, L, Miller, C S, Smith, A J, Pettit, F K, Bowie, J U, and Eisenberg, D, The Database of Interacting Proteins: 2004 update.*Nucleic Acids Res*, 2004. 32(Database issue): p. D449-51.

[10] Wingender, E, Dietze, P, Karas, H, and Knuppel, R, TRANSFAC: a database on transcription factors and their DNA binding sites.*Nucleic Acids Res*, 1996. 24(1): p. 238-41.

[11] Zhang, B, Schmoyer, D, Kirov, S, and Snoddy, J, GOTree Machine (GOTM): a web-based platform for interpreting sets of interesting genes using Gene Ontology hierarchies.*BMC Bioinformatics*, 2004. 5: p. 16.

[12] Knudson, A, Alfred Knudson and his two-hit hypothesis. (Interview by Ezzie Hutchinson).*Lancet Oncol*, 2001. 2(10): p. 642-5.

[13] Nordling, C O, A new theory on cancer-inducing mechanism.*Br J Cancer*, 1953. 7(1): p. 68-72.

[14] Knudson, A G, Jr., Mutation and cancer: statistical study of retinoblastoma.*Proc Natl Acad Sci U S A*, 1971. 68(4): p. 820-3.

[15] Moolgavkar, S H, The multistage theory of carcinogenesis and the age distribution of cancer in man.*J Natl Cancer Inst*, 1978. 61(1): p. 49-52.

[16] Ritter, G, Wilson, R, Pompei, F, and Burmistrov, D, The multistage model of cancer development: some implications.*Toxicol Ind Health*, 2003. 19(7-10): p. 125-45.

[17] Iwasa, Y and Michor, F, Evolutionary dynamics of intratumor heterogeneity.*PLoS One*. 6(3): p. e17866.

[18] Warburg, O, Posener, K, and Negelein, E, Ueber den Stoffwechsel der Tumoren.*Biochemische Zeitschrift*, 1924. 152: p. 319-344.

[19] Severson, R K and Ross, J A, The causes of acute leukemia.*Curr Opin Oncol*, 1999. 11(1): p. 20-4.

[20] Carroll, W L, Bhojwani, D, Min, D J, Raetz, E, Relling, M, Davies, S, Downing, J R, Willman, C L, and Reed, J C, Pediatric acute lymphoblastic leukemia.*Hematology Am Soc Hematol Educ Program*, 2003: p. 102-31.

[21] Kaplinsky, C, Frisch, A, Cohen, I J, Goshen, Y, Jaber, L, Yaniv, I, Stark, B, Tamary, H, and Zaizov, R, T-cell acute lymphoblastic leukemia following therapy of rhabdomyosarcoma.*Med Pediatr Oncol*, 1992. 20(3): p. 229-31.

[22] Dedrick, R L and Morrison, P F, Carcinogenic potency of alkylating agents in rodents and humans.*Cancer Res*, 1992. 52(9): p. 2464-7.

[23] Park, D J and Koeffler, H P, Therapy-related myelodysplastic syndromes.*Semin Hematol*, 1996. 33(3): p. 256-73.

[24] Kelly, P N, Dakic, A, Adams, J M, Nutt, S L, and Strasser, A, Tumor growth need not be driven by rare cancer stem cells.*Science*, 2007. 317(5836): p. 337.

[25] Sewell, W and Kusumi, K, Genetic analysis of molecular oscillators in mammalian somitogenesis: clues for studies of human vertebral disorders.*Birth Defects Res C Embryo Today*, 2007. 81(2): p. 111-20.

[26] Dunwoodie, S L, Clements, M, Sparrow, D B, Sa, X, Conlon, R A, and Beddington, R S, Axial skeletal defects caused by mutation in the spondylocostal dysplasia/pudgy gene Dll3 are associated with disruption of the segmentation clock within the presomitic mesoderm.*Development*, 2002. 129(7): p. 1795-806.

[27] Kusumi, K, Sun, E S, Kerrebrock, A W, Bronson, R T, Chi, D C, Bulotsky, M S, Spencer, J B, Birren, B W, Frankel, W N, and Lander, E S, The mouse pudgy mutation disrupts Delta homologue Dll3 and initiation of early somite boundaries.*Nat Genet*, 1998. 19(3): p. 274-8.

[28] Godin, I and Cumano, A, Of birds and mice: hematopoietic stem cell development.*Int J Dev Biol*, 2005. 49(2-3): p. 251-7.

[29] Nicolis, S K, Cancer stem cells and "stemness" genes in neuro-oncology.*Neurobiol Dis*, 2007. 25(2): p. 217-29.

[30] Perilongo, G, Felix, C A, Meadows, A T, Nowell, P, Biegel, J, and Lange, B J, Sequential development of Wilms tumor, T-cell acute lymphoblastic leukemia, medulloblastoma and myeloid leukemia in a child with type 1 neurofibromatosis: a clinical and cytogenetic case report.*Leukemia*, 1993. 7(6): p. 912-5.

[31] Kleinerman, R A, Linet, M S, Hatch, E E, Wacholder, S, Tarone, R E, Severson, R K, Kaune, W T, Friedman, D R, Haines, C M, Muirhead, C R, Boice, J D, Jr., and Robison, L L, Magnetic field exposure assessment in a case-control study of childhood leukemia.*Epidemiology*, 1997. 8(5): p. 575-83.

[32] Linet, M S, Hatch, E E, Kleinerman, R A, Robison, L L, Kaune, W T, Friedman, D R, Severson, R K, Haines, C M, Hartsock, C T, Niwa, S, Wacholder, S, and Tarone, R E, Residential exposure to magnetic fields and acute lymphoblastic leukemia in children.*N Engl J Med*, 1997. 337(1): p. 1-7.

[33] Hatch, E E, Linet, M S, Kleinerman, R A, Tarone, R E, Severson, R K, Hartsock, C T, Haines, C, Kaune, W T, Friedman, D, Robison, L L, and Wacholder, S, Association between childhood acute lymphoblastic leukemia and use of electrical appliances during pregnancy and childhood.*Epidemiology*, 1998. 9(3): p. 234-45.

[34] Petridou, E, Trichopoulos, D, Kravaritis, A, Pourtsidis, A, Dessypris, N, Skalkidis, Y, Kogevinas, M, Kalmanti, M, Koliouskas, D, Kosmidis, H, Panagiotou, J P, Piperopoulou, F, Tzortzatou, F, and Kalapothaki, V, Electrical power lines and childhood leukemia: a study from Greece.*Int J Cancer*, 1997. 73(3): p. 345-8.

[35] Michaelis, J, Schuz, J, Meinert, R, Zemann, E, Grigat, J P, Kaatsch, P, Kaletsch, U, Miesner, A, Brinkmann, K, Kalkner, W, and Karner, H, Combined risk estimates for two German population-based case-control studies on residential magnetic fields and childhood acute leukemia.*Epidemiology*, 1998. 9(1): p. 92-4.

[36] Snyder, R, Xenobiotic metabolism and the mechanism(s) of benzene toxicity.*Drug Metab Rev*, 2004. 36(3-4): p. 531-47.

[37] Pyatt, D W, Aylward, L L, and Hays, S M, Is age an independent risk factor for chemically induced acute myelogenous leukemia in children? *J Toxicol Environ Health B Crit Rev*, 2007. 10(5): p. 379-400.

[38] Irons, R D and Stillman, W S, The process of leukemogenesis.*Environ Health Perspect*, 1996. 104 Suppl 6: p. 1239-46.

[39] Greaves, M F, Speculations on the cause of childhood acute lymphoblastic leukemia.*Leukemia*, 1988. 2(2): p. 120-5.

[40] Kinlen, L, Evidence for an infective cause of childhood leukaemia: comparison of a Scottish new town with nuclear reprocessing sites in Britain.*Lancet*, 1988. 2(8624): p. 1323-7.

[41] Risser, R, Horowitz, J M, and McCubrey, J, Endogenous mouse leukemia viruses.*Annu Rev Genet*, 1983. 17: p. 85-121.

[42] Hehlmann, R, Schetters, H, Kreeb, G, Erfle, V, Schmidt, J, and Luz, A, RNA-tumorviruses, oncogenes, and their possible role in human carcinogenesis.*Klin Wochenschr*, 1983. 61(24): p. 1217-31.

[43] Sandler, D P and Ross, J A, Epidemiology of acute leukemia in children and adults.*Semin Oncol*, 1997. 24(1): p. 3-16.

[44] Hayes, R B, Yin, S N, Dosemeci, M, Li, G L, Wacholder, S, Travis, L B, Li, C Y, Rothman, N, Hoover, R N, and Linet, M S, Benzene and the dose-related incidence of hematologic neoplasms in China. Chinese Academy of Preventive Medicine--National Cancer Institute Benzene Study Group.*J Natl Cancer Inst*, 1997. 89(14): p. 1065-71.

[45] Dick, J E, Stem cell concepts renew cancer research.*Blood*, 2008. 112(13): p. 4793-807.

[46] Sitwala, K V, Dandekar, M N, and Hess, J L, HOX proteins and leukemia.*Int J Clin Exp Pathol*, 2008. 1(6): p. 461-74.

[47] Mikhail, F M, Serry, K A, Hatem, N, Mourad, Z I, Farawela, H M, El Kaffash, D M, Coignet, L, and Nucifora, G, AML1 gene over-expression in childhood acute lymphoblastic leukemia.*Leukemia*, 2002. 16(4): p. 658-68.

[48] Zeisig, B B, Milne, T, Garcia-Cuellar, M P, Schreiner, S, Martin, M E, Fuchs, U, Borkhardt, A, Chanda, S K, Walker, J, Soden, R, Hess, J L, and Slany, R K, Hoxa9 and Meis1 are key targets for MLL-ENL-mediated cellular immortalization.*Mol Cell Biol*, 2004. 24(2): p. 617-28.

[49] Forsberg, E C, Passegue, E, Prohaska, S S, Wagers, A J, Koeva, M, Stuart, J M, and Weissman, I L, Molecular signatures of quiescent, mobilized and leukemia-initiating hematopoietic stem cells.*PLoS One*. 5(1): p. e8785.

[50] Marschalek, R, Mechanisms of leukemogenesis by MLL fusion proteins.*Br J Haematol*. 152(2): p. 141-54.

[51] Hunger, S P, Raetz, E A, Loh, M L, and Mullighan, C G, Improving outcomes for high-risk ALL: translating new discoveries into clinical care. *Pediatr Blood Cancer.* 56(6): p. 984-93.

[52] Bacher, U, Haferlach, T, Fehse, B, Schnittger, S, and Kroger, N, Minimal residual disease diagnostics and chimerism in the post-transplant period in acute myeloid leukemia. *ScientificWorldJournal.* 11: p. 310-9.

[53] Marcucci, G, Haferlach, T, and Dohner, H, Molecular genetics of adult acute myeloid leukemia: prognostic and therapeutic implications. *J Clin Oncol.* 29(5): p. 475-86.

[54] Bassan, R and Hoelzer, D, Modern therapy of acute lymphoblastic leukemia. *J Clin Oncol.* 29(5): p. 532-43.

[55] Bejar, R, Levine, R, and Ebert, B L, Unraveling the molecular pathophysiology of myelodysplastic syndromes. *J Clin Oncol.* 29(5): p. 504-15.

[56] Ebert, B L, Genetic deletions in AML and MDS. *Best Pract Res Clin Haematol.* 23(4): p. 457-61.

[57] le Viseur, C, Hotfilder, M, Bomken, S, Wilson, K, Rottgers, S, Schrauder, A, Rosemann, A, Irving, J, Stam, R W, Shultz, L D, Harbott, J, Jurgens, H, Schrappe, M, Pieters, R, and Vormoor, J, In childhood acute lymphoblastic leukemia, blasts at different stages of immunophenotypic maturation have stem cell properties. *Cancer Cell*, 2008. 14(1): p. 47-58.

[58] Cobaleda, C, Gutierrez-Cianca, N, Perez-Losada, J, Flores, T, Garcia-Sanz, R, Gonzalez, M, and Sanchez-Garcia, I, A primitive hematopoietic cell is the target for the leukemic transformation in human philadelphia-positive acute lymphoblastic leukemia. *Blood*, 2000. 95(3): p. 1007-13.

[59] Cox, C V, Evely, R S, Oakhill, A, Pamphilon, D H, Goulden, N J, and Blair, A, Characterization of acute lymphoblastic leukemia progenitor cells. *Blood*, 2004. 104(9): p. 2919-25.

[60] Castor, A, Nilsson, L, Astrand-Grundstrom, I, Buitenhuis, M, Ramirez, C, Anderson, K, Strombeck, B, Garwicz, S, Bekassy, A N, Schmiegelow, K, Lausen, B, Hokland, P, Lehmann, S, Juliusson, G, Johansson, B, and Jacobsen, S E, Distinct patterns of hematopoietic stem cell involvement in acute lymphoblastic leukemia. *Nat Med*, 2005. 11(6): p. 630-7.

[61] Hong, D, Gupta, R, Ancliff, P, Atzberger, A, Brown, J, Soneji, S, Green, J, Colman, S, Piacibello, W, Buckle, V, Tsuzuki, S, Greaves, M, and Enver, T, Initiating and cancer-propagating cells in TEL-AML1-associated childhood leukemia. *Science*, 2008. 319(5861): p. 336-9.

[62] Greaves, M F, Stem cell origins of leukaemia and curability. *Br J Cancer*, 1993. 67(3): p. 413-23.

[63] Greaves, M, Cancer stem cells: back to Darwin? *Semin Cancer Biol.* 20(2): p. 65-70.

[64] Greaves, M, In utero origins of childhood leukaemia. *Early Hum Dev*, 2005. 81(1): p. 123-9.

In: Acute Lymphoblastic Leukemia
Editors: Severo Vecchione and Luigi Tedesco

ISBN: 978-1-61470-872-8
©2012 Nova Science Publishers, Inc.

Chapter V

Histone Deacetylase Inhibitors: Pre-clinical and Clinical Evidence in Treating Acute Lymphoblastic Leukemia

Ana Lucia Abujamra
Children's Cancer Institute
Cancer Research Laboratory, University Hospital Research Center (HCPA)
Federal University of Rio Grande do Sul
National Institute for Translational Medicine (INCT-TM) Porto Alegre,
Rio Grande do Sul, Brazil

1. Overview

Acute lymphoblastic leukemia is the most common type of cancer in the pediatric population. In spite of recent reports stating that standard treatment may yield 5-year event-free survival rates of approximately 80%, and 5-year survival rates approaching 90%, a significant subset of pediatric leukemia patients either relapse or fail to ever achieve a complete remission. Moreover, there have been increasing incidences of late therapy-related effects, warranting a need for new therapies which prove to be effective for high-risk patients, all the while decreasing the incidence of long-term sequelae. Histone deacetylase inhibitors (HDIs) promote or enhance several different anticancer mechanisms and therefore are in evidence as potential antileukemia agents. Studies on leukemia have provided examples for their functional implications in cancer development and progression, as well as their relevance for therapeutic targeting. A number of HDIs have been tested in clinical trials, and most studies have shown that they are safe, all the while demonstrating significant clinical activity. The use of HDIs in association with other molecules, such as classical chemotherapeutic drugs and DNA demethylating agents, has been implied as a promising treatment alternative for leukemia patients. Taking into consideration the process of leukemogenesis and the clinical course of acute lymphoblastic leukemia, this chapter will focus on the pre-clinical and clinical results of histone deacetylase inhibitors as single-agent or in combination with other drugs for the treatment of this disease.

Table 1. Classical drugs currently in use to treat leukemia and their mechanism of action. Drug class is listed in italics, followed by the medication name in bold

Mechanism of Action			Classical drugs to treat leukemia
Spindle Poison / Mitotic Inhibitor (M phase)	Block microtubule assembly		*Vinca alkaloids*: Vincristine
DNA replication inhibitor	DNA precursors/ antimetabolites (S phase)	Folic acid	*Dihydrofolate reductase inhibitor*: Methotrexate
		Purine	*Thiopurine*: Mercaptopurine
			Halogenated/ribonucleotide reductase inhibitors: Cladribine, Clofarabine, Fludarabine
			Thiopurine: Thioguanine
		Pyrimidine	*DNA polymerase inhibitor*: Cytarabine
		Deoxyribonucleotide	*Ribonucleotide reductase inhibitor*: Hydroxyurea
	Topoisomerase inhibitor (S phase)	II	*Podophyllum*: Etoposide, Teniposide
		II+Intercalation	*Anthracyclines*: Daunorubicin, Doxorubicin, Idarubicin
			Anthracenediones: Mitoxantrone
	Crosslinking of DNA (CCNS)	Alkylating	*Nitrogen mustards*: Mechlorethamine, Cyclophosphamide, Chlorambucil.
			Alkyl sulfonates: Busulfan
		Alkylating-like	*Platinum*: Carboplatin, Cisplatin
Other	Enzyme inhibitors		*PrI*: Bortezomib
	Other/ungrouped		*Retinoids:* Tretinoin
			Asparagine depleter: Asparaginase
			Vorinostat

2. Treatment Options for Leukemia

Leukemia is a malignant cancer of the bone marrow and blood that affects both children and adults, and is commonly divided into four categories: acute myelogenous (AML) or chronic myelogenous (CML), involving the myeloid elements of the bone marrow (leukocytes, erithrocytes and megakaryocytes) and acute lymphoblastic (ALL) or chronic lymphoblastic (CLL), involving the cells of the lymphoid lineage. Standard treatment for all types of leukemia usually involves chemotherapy and/or bone marrow transplantation and/or radiation therapy. The classical drugs currently in use to treat leukemia were initially developed and tested between the 1950s and 1970s (Pui et al., 2008). The main classical drugs that are now being used in the clinic are asparaginase, cyclophosphamide, cytarabine, daunorubicin, doxorubicin, etoposide, mercaptopurine, methotrexate, mitoxantrone, thioguanine and vincristine (Table 1), being that treatment usually involves a combination of two or more anticancer drugs.

Based on the signaling pathways known to be dysregulated in ALL (PI3-kinase, AKT, MAPK/ERK and mTOR, to name a few) targeted therapies, mainly those that explore kinase inhibitors, have been developed (Table 2). However, despite their promise in being more efficient in eliminating the transformed cell, all the while sparing the normal, functional cell, it was soon observed that they had insufficient sustained effect as single agents (Ottmann et al., 2002) or that the patients invariably developed resistance to such therapies.

Table 2. Established and experimental targeted therapy molecules for the treatment of leukemia

Description	Name	Mechanism of Action
Kinase Inhibitors	Imatinib	ABL1 Inhibitor
	Dasatinib	ABL1 Inhibitor
	Nilotinib	ABL1 Inhibitor
	Lestaurtinib	FLT-3 Inhibitor
	Midostaurin	FLT-3 Inhibitor
	Rapamycin	mTOR inhibitor
	Temsirolimus	mTOR inhibitor
	MLN8237	Aurora kinase inhibitor
	Sorafenib	Multi-kinase inhibitor
	Ruxolitinib	JAK1/2 inhibitor
	MK-2206	Allosteric Akt inhibitor
Other Inhibitors	Bortezomib	Proteasome inhibitor
	Marizomib	Proteasome inhibitor
	Tipifarnib	Farnesyltransferase inhibitor
Apoptosis Pathway Agonists /antagonists	Obatoclax	Pan-apoptotic BCL2 antagonist
	Mapatumumab	TRAIL receptor agonist
	Lexatumumab	TRAIL receptor agonist
Monoclonal Antibodies to Surface Receptors	Epratuzumab	Monoclonal antibody to CD-22
	Rituximab	Monoclonal antibody to CD-20
	Alemtuzumab	Monoclonal antibody to CD-52

Acute lymphoblastic leukemia responds very well to either classical drugs or targeted therapy, with an 80% 5-year event-free survival. However, a significant subset of ALL patients either relapses or fails to ever achieve a complete remission. Owing to the tremendous clinical variability among remissions observed in leukemia patients, the treatment for ALL is very complex. Patients who are resistant to therapy have very short survival times, regardless of when the resistance occurs. Moreover, the drugs most frequently used to treat this malignancy are often administered in high doses, causing several toxic side effects. There have also been increasing incidences of late therapy-related effects, the main one being cognitive impairment (Temming and Jenney, 2010). Therefore, despite improvements in outcome with current treatment programs, efforts to identify new chemotherapeutic or adjuvant agents for the treatment of leukemia are still warranted.

3. Histone Deacetylases (HDACs) and Histone Deacetylase Inhibitors (HDIs)

Chromatin organization is crucial for the regulation of gene expression. In particular, both the nucleosome properties and its positioning influence promoter-specific transcription in response to extracellular or intracellular signals. The acetylation and deacetylation of histones play significant roles in transcriptional regulation of eukaryotic cells, and are catalyzed by specific enzyme families: histone acetyl-transferases (HATs) and histone deacetylases (HDACs), respectively. HATs were originally identified as transcriptional co-activators and HDACs as yeast transcriptional regulators (Kourkalis and Theocharis, 2006). HDACs are a family of enzymes present in bacteria, fungi, plants, and animals that remove the acetyl moiety from the ϵ-amino groups of the lysine residues present within the N-terminal extension of the core histones. Consequently, the positive charge density on the N-termini of the core histones increases, strengthening the interaction with the negatively charged DNA and blocking the access of the transcriptional machinery to the DNA template (Paris et al., 2008).

The balance between acetylation and deacetylation is an important factor in regulating gene expression, and is thus linked to the control of cell fate. Disruption of HAT or HDAC activity is possibly associated with cancer development (Timmerman et al., 2001), and if so the molecular processes leading to the activation or repression of transcription are possible targets for anticancer therapy. HDACs have been implicated for the first time in cancer while studying acute promyelocytic leukemia (Warrell et al., 1998). Since then, HDAC silencing or inhibition has been shown to have an impact on cell cycle, cell growth, chromatin decondensation, cell differentiation, apoptosis, and angiogenesis in several cancer cell types (Paris et al., 2008).

Since inhibition of HDAC activity reverses the epigenetic silencing frequently observed in cancer, various HDAC inhibitors (HDIs) have been developed for therapeutic purposes (Table 2). These include short-chain fatty acids, such as valproic acid and butyrates (Jeong et al., 2003); hydroxamic acids, such as Vorinostat (Bouchain et al., 2003); Trichostatin A (Van Ommeslaeghe et al., 2003), Panobinostat (LBH-589), Belinostat (PXD101), tubacin, benzamides (MS-275), cyclic tetrapeptides, such as trapoxin, apicidin and depsipeptide (Piekarz and Bates, 2004), and a variety of other chemical compounds (Carew et al., 2008; Kourkalis and Theocharis, 2006). HDAC inhibitors also have varying degrees of specificity, although the molecular anticancer mechanism of each specific agent is not completely clear. The creation of inhibitors with greater specificity will enable each HDAC function to be more fully elucidated, besides yielding improved efficacy and reduced toxicity (Carew et al.,

2008). Current research in cancer therapy focuses on the design of drugs that are specific against molecular alterations found only in the transformed cell. The aim is to associate a specific tumor type with a specific gene expression profile, thus defining the alteration responsible for each cancer (Paris et al., 2008)

HDIs have been used as a new class of anticancer agents in clinical trials, and have been studied extensively in the laboratory. Clinical studies have shown that histone hyperacetylation can be achieved safely in humans, and that treatment with such agents is plausible (Kourkalis and Theocharis, 2006). Many HDIs, including Vorinostat (SAHA), depsipeptide, MS-275, and TSA have a synergistic effect in enhancing the anticancer activity of a large number of conventional chemotherapeutic drugs (Bolden et al., 2006; Glaser, 2007). These include gemcitabine, paclitaxel, cisplatin, etoposide, and doxorubicin, which target malignant cells through different mechanisms (Arnold et al., 2007; Dowdy et al., 2006; Fuino et al., 2003; Kim et al., 2003; Rikiishi et al., 2007). A large amount of work has been carried out in the past 5 years in the field of HDIs, and more than 100 patents claiming new chemical series have been published (Paris et al., 2008).

Table 3. Main histone deacetylase inhibitors evaluated as adjuvants for the treatment of leukemia

Class	Compound	IUPAC Name
Short-chain fatty acids	Valproic acid	2-propylpentanoic acid
	Butyrates	Butanoate
Hydroxamic acids	Vorinostat (SAHA)	N'-hydroxy-N-phenyloctanediamide
	Trichostatin A (TSA)	(2E,4E)-7-(4-dimethylaminophenyl)-N-hydroxy-4,6-dimethyl-7-oxohepta-2,4-dienamide
	Panobinostat (LBH-589)	(E)-N-hydroxy-3-[4-[[2-(2-methyl-1H-indol-3-yl)ethylamino]methyl]phenyl]prop-2-enamide
	Belinostat (PXD101)	(E)-N-hydroxy-3-[3 (phenylsulfamoyl) phenyl]prop-2-enamide
Benzamides	MS-275	Pyridin-3-ylmethyl N-[[4-[(2-aminophenyl) carbamoyl]phenyl] methyl] carbamate
Cyclic tetrapeptide	Romidepsin or depsipeptide (FK-228)	(1S,4S,7Z,10S,16E,21R)-7-ethylidene-4,21-di(propan-2-yl)-2-oxa-12,13-dithia-5,8,20,23-tetrazabicyclo[8.7.6]tricos-16-ene-3,6,9,19, 22-pentone

4. Evidence for HDIs as a Therapeutic Strategy in Acute Lymphocytic Leukemia

It was soon established that HDIs were not as effective as single agents as they were when combined with other drugs already established in the clinic. In many cases, HDIs alone could only induce growth arrest or differentiation, with unremarkable cytotoxic effects (Villar-Garea and Esteller, 2004). On the other hand, it was soon noted that HDIs could potentiate the effects of classic chemotherapeutic drugs. One example was the combination treatment with butyrate and antineoplastic agents such as cytarabine (Ara-C), etoposide and vincristine on the leukemic cell line THP-1. Butyrate increased apoptosis induced by the three agents as seen by measurement of DNA content, annexin exposure and morphological characteristics. This study concluded that butyrate could be a promising adjuvant for treating leukemia in combination with other antineoplastic drugs (Ramos et al., 2004). In another study, Sanchez-Gonzalez et al. (2006) studied the cellular and molecular effects of combining the anthracycline idarubicin with two different HDIs: vorinostat (SAHA) and valproic acid (VPA). Their results indicate that the combination of an anthracycline with an HDI displays a synergistic effect *in vitro*.

The fact that HDIs potentiated the effects of nearly all chemotherapeutic agents studied hinted at the fact that their mechanisms of action were rather broad – an assumption that hindered their use in pre-clinical and phase I clinical trials. It was not until later that studies indicated that some, but not all chemotherapeutic drugs synergized with HDIs. One study investigated the effects on *in vitro* cellular proliferation when combining sodium butyrate (NaB) with antineoplastic drugs commonly used to treat leukemias. NaB increased the cytotoxic effects of Ara-C and etoposide, but not of bleomycin, doxorubicin, vincristine or methotrexate (dos Santos et al., 2009). In another study, valproic acid (VPA) was shown to increase the efficiency of etoposide, doxorubicin and cisplatin, and to restore cells' sensitivity to imatinib (Hrebackova et al., 2010). These data suggested that NaB could be a promising adjuvant therapeutic agent for the treatment of lymphoblastic leukemias, and provides a basis for further studies detailing the specificity of these synergistic effects. In fact, many other studies indicated that HDIs could act in a more specific manner.

Their broad synergistic capacity indicates that HDIs are likely to lower the threshold for tumor cells to undergo apoptotic cell death triggered by other agents. This can explain how one class of agents triggers cell death synergistically with such a wide array of other anticancer drugs. Consistent with this idea, the HDAC inhibitor MS-275 has been reported to decrease the levels of anti-apoptotic molecules and increase the levels of pro-apoptotic molecules, promoting differentiation or apoptosis in leukemia cells of human origin (Rosato et al., 2003). One study explored the effect of MS-275 against a panel of leukemia cells of human origin, each with defined genetic alterations. With an IC_{50} of less than 1μM, as measured by 3-(4,5-dimethylthiazol-2-yl)-2,5-diphenyltetrazolium bromide assay, MS-275 significantly induced growth arrest in the AML cell line, MOLM13, and in the biphenotypic leukemia cell line, MV4-11, which both possess an internal tandem duplication mutation in the fms-like tyrosine kinase 3 (FLT3) gene (FLT3-ITD). Exposure of these cells to MS-275 decreased total and phosphorylated levels of FLT3 protein, resulting in inactivation of its downstream signaling pathways (Akt, ERK, and STAT5). Further studies found that MS-275 induced acetylation of heat shock protein 90 (HSP90) in conjunction with ubiquitination of FLT3, leading to degradation of FLT3 proteins in these cells. This was abrogated by treatment with the proteasome inhibitor bortezomib, confirming that FLT3 was degraded via the ubiquitin/proteasome pathway. Moreover, this study found that further inhibition of MEK/ERK signaling potentiated the effects of MS-275 in these cells. Altogether, these results suggest that MS-275 may be useful in treating individuals who carry a mutation on the FLT3 gene (Nishioka et al., 2008).

Enhanced anticancer activity has been observed with various HDIs in combination with other transcriptional modulators. This synergistic approach has shown to reactivate epigenetically silenced genes, such as CDKN1A (p21) and CDKN2B (p15). On the flip side, a potential caveat of HDI combinations is their ability to induce the cdk inhibitor, p21. While induction of p21 is critical for HDI-mediated cell-cycle arrest, it may also interfere with the efficient execution of the apoptotic cascade (Warrell et al., 1998). Therefore, agents that suppress the induction of p21 and that are stimulated by HDIs are highly desired, and several have been identified to date. Flavopiridol, LY294002, PKC412, and sorafenib have been reported to block HDI-mediated induction of p21, which increases the overall apoptotic capacity and therefore contributes to their enhanced anticancer activity in human leukemia cells (Bali et al., 2004; Dasmahapatra et al., 2007; Rahmani et al., 2003b; Rosato et al., 2004). In addition to decreasing the levels of these anti-apoptotic proteins, several HDIs may also increase the expression of death receptors, such as DR5, and enhance the formation of the death-inducing signaling complex (DISC). In human acute leukemia cells, co-treatment with the HDI LAQ824, a cinnamic acid hydroxamate, enhances Apo-2L/TRAIL-induced death by enhancing several signaling cascades and apoptosis (Guo et al., 2004). The HDIs SAHA and butyrate induce apoptosis synergistically with the proteasome inhibitor bortezomib. The combination proteasome/HDI may represent a novel strategy for treating leukemias, including those that are apoptosis-resistant and Bcr/Abl-positive (Yu et al., 2003a). Dai et al. (2008a) characterized the interactions between bortezomib and the clinically relevant HDIs romidepsin or belinostat in leukemia cell lines. Co-administration of romidepsin or belinostat with bortezomib induced cell death synergistically, likely through mechanisms involving, among other factors, NF-κB inactivation and changes in the expression levels of pro-apoptotic and anti-apoptotic proteins. This study calls further attention to the strategy of combining HDI with proteasome inhibitors.

A number of combination strategies with targeted agents in leukemia cells, either *in-vitro* or *ex-vivo* have been proposed, such as treatment with SAHA and imatinib (Nimmanapalli et al., 2003), *in vitro* treatment with SAHA and desatinib in primary imatinib-sensitive or imatinib-resistant cells (Fiskus et al., 2006a), *in vitro* treatment with the nucleoside analogue fludarabine (Maggio et al., 2004), *in vitro* treatment with the proteasome inhibitor bortezomib combined with SAHA (Yu et al., 2003a and 2003b) and *in vitro* treatment with SAHA and an HSP90 antagonist (Rahmani et al., 2003a). The HDIs SAHA, LBH-589 and butyrate also appear to enhance the anticancer activity of targeted agents, including imatinib (a protein-tyrosine kinase inhibitor that targets the Bcr-Abl tyrosine kinase, which is created by the Philadelphia chromosome abnormality) and the HSP90 antagonist 17-allylamino-17-demethoxygeldanamycin (17-AAG) in human leukemia cells (Yu et al., 2003b; George et al., 2005). The HDI depsipeptide (FK228) may mediate its effects on imatinib-resistant leukemia cells (Okabe et al., 2007).

Interactions between the Bcr/Abl and aurora kinase inhibitor, MK-0457, and the HDI vorinostat were examined in Bcr/Abl(+) leukemia cells resistant to imatinib mesylate (IM), particularly those with the T315I mutation. Co-administration of vorinostat dramatically increased MK-0457-induced lethality in the K562 and LAMA84 cell lines. Notably, the MK-0457/vorinostat regimen was highly active against primary CD34(+) CML cells and against Ba/F3 cells bearing various Bcr/Abl mutations, such as T315I, E255K, and M351T, and against IM-resistant K562 cells exhibiting Bcr/Abl-independent, Lyn-dependent resistance. These events were associated with inactivation and down-regulation of wild-type (wt) and mutated Bcr/Abl, particularly T315I. Treatment with MK-0457 resulted in an accumulation of cells with a DNA content of 4n or more. Co-administration of vorinostat and MK-0457, nonetheless, preferentially killed polyploid cells and markedly enhanced aurora kinase inhibition. Furthermore, vorinostat interacted with a selective inhibitor of aurora kinase A and B to potentiate apoptosis without modifying Bcr/Abl activity. Finally, vorinostat induced Bcl-2-interacting mediator of cell death (Bim) expression significantly, while blockade of Bim induction by siRNA dramatically diminished vorinostat´s ability to potentiate MK-0457-induced cell death. Together, these findings indicate that vorinostat strikingly increases MK-0457 activity against IM-sensitive and -resistant cells through inactivation of Bcr/Abl and aurora kinases, as well as by induction of Bim (Dai et al., 2008b).

Fiskus et al. (2006b) evaluated the combined effects of the novel tyrosine kinase inhibitor, AMN107, and the HDI LBH589 against human leukemia cells that are sensitive or not to IM and that express Bcr/Abl. As compared with either agent alone, co-treatment with AMN107 and LBH589 induced a pronounced reduction of viable cells in primary IM-resistant cells (Fiskus et al., 2006b). The mechanism by which LBH589 functions was investigated in Philadelphia chromosome-negative (Ph(-)) ALL. Two human Ph(-) ALL cell lines (T-cell MOLT-4 and pre-B-cell Reh) were treated with LBH589 and evaluated for biologic and gene expression responses. Nanomolar concentrations (IC_{50}: 5-20nM) of LBH589 induced cell-cycle arrest, apoptosis, and histone (H3K9 and H4K8) hyperacetylation. LBH589 treatment also increased mRNA levels of pro-apoptotic, growth arrest, and DNA damage repair genes such as FANCG, FOXO3A, GADD45A, GADD45B, and GADD45G, being that the latter was the most over-expressed gene (up to a 45-fold induction) post-treatment. LBH589 treatment was associated with increased histone acetylation at the GADD45G promoter and with phosphorylation of histone H2A.X. This treatment was active against cultured primary Ph(-) ALL cells, including those from a relapsed patient, inducing a decrease in cell viability of up to 70% and increasing GADD45G mRNA expression up to 35-fold. Thus, LBH589 demonstrates considerable growth inhibitory activity against Ph(-) ALL cells, which is associated with up-regulation of genes that are critical for DNA damage response and growth arrest, and provides a rationale for exploring the clinical activity of LBH589 in treating patients with Ph(-) ALL (Scuto et al., 2008).

The cytotoxic interaction of the HDI Romidepsin (FK228) in combination with conventional antileukemic agents was evaluated using several human leukemia cell lines. FK228 demonstrated an additive effect with Ara-C, carboplatin, doxorubicin, etoposide, 4-hydroperoxy-cyclophosphamide, 6-mercaptopurine and SN-38 (an active metabolite of irinotecan) in all the cell lines studied. FK228 in combination with methotrexate had an antagonistic effect in three of the four cells lines, whereas the combination of FK228 and vincristine behaved similarly in only one of the four cell lines. An additive effect was observed when FK228 was co-administered with imatinib in all three Ph(+) leukemia cell lines. These findings suggest that FK228 is a promising adjuvant candidate, except when co-administered with methotrexate and vincristine (Kano et al., 2007)

Antileukemia activity has also been evaluated with HDIs that are administered in combination hypomethylating agents. The combination of 5-aza-2'-deoxycytidine (DAC), a hypomethylating agent with significant antileukemia activity in humans, with VPA had a synergistic effect in growth inhibition, induction of apoptosis, and reactivation of p57KIP2 and p21CIP1 on human leukemia cell lines, suggesting that the combination of DAC and VPA could have significant antileukemia activity *in vivo* (Yang et al., 2005).

The use of HDIs alone has also been evaluated. FR235222, a novel HDI, triggered accumulation of acetylated histone H4, inhibition of cellular proliferation and G1 cell-cycle arrest, accompanied by an increase in p21 protein levels and a down-regulation of cyclin E in the human promyelocytic leukemia cell line, U937. At a concentration of 50nM, the compound was also able to increase both mRNA and protein levels of annexin A1 (ANXA1) without affecting apoptosis. Similar effects were observed in the human CML cell line, K562, and in the human T-cell leukemia cell line, Jurkat. Cell-cycle arrest and ANXA1 expression were also induced by different HDIs like suberoylanilide hydroxamic acid (SAHA) and trichostatin-A (TSA). FR235222, when used at 0.5µM, triggered apoptosis in all leukemia cell lines, an event associated with an increased expression of the full-length (37kDa) ANXA1 protein and the appearance of a 33kDa N-terminal cleavage product in both the cytosol and membrane. These results suggest that ANXA1 expression may mediate cell-cycle arrest induced by low doses of FR235222, whereas apoptosis induced by high doses of FR235222 is associated with ANXA1 processing (Petrella et al., 2008).

5. Preclinical and Clinical Trials of HDIs in Patients with Acute Lymphocytic Leukemia

Most clinical trials to this date have accrued adult patients to evaluate maximum tolerated dose (MTD) and dose-related toxicities resulting from treatments with HDIs and other cytotoxic drugs. Byrd et al. (2005) carried out a phase 1 and pharmacodynamic study of depsipeptide (FK228), in which patients with CLL or AML were treated with depsipeptide intravenously. Neither life-threatening toxicities nor cardiac toxicities were noted, although the majority of patients experienced progressive fatigue, nausea, and other constitutional symptoms that prevented repeated dosing. Several patients had evidence of antitumor activity following treatment, but no partial or complete responses were noted. An increase in HDAC inhibition and histone acetylation of at least 100% was noted, as well as an increase in p21 promoter H4 acetylation, p21 protein levels, and 1D10 antigen expression. The researchers concluded that depsipeptide effectively inhibits HDAC *in vivo* in patients with CLL and AML, but its use in the current schedule of administration is limited by progressive constitutional symptoms. Another study evaluated the toxicity, pharmacokinetic profile, and selected pharmacodynamic properties of depsipeptide in patients with AML or MDS. The most common grade 3/4 toxicities were febrile neutropenia/infection, neutropenia/ thrombocytopenia, nausea, and asymptomatic hypophosphatemia. No clinically significant cardiac toxicity was observed. The responses seen in all eleven examined patients were: one patient with complete remission, six patients with stable disease, and progression of disease in four patients. Exploratory laboratory studies showed modest but rapid increases in apoptosis and changes in myeloid maturation marker expression. The authors concluded that depsipeptide therapy can be administered with acceptable short-term toxicity. However, gastrointestinal symptoms and fatigue seem to be treatment-limiting after multiple cycles (Klimek et al., 2008).

In a phase I study, LBH589 was administered intravenously in patients with AML, ALL, or MDS. The levels of histone acetylation were measured using quantitative flow cytometry, and plasma LBH589 concentrations were also assayed. Four dose-limiting toxicities were observed. Other potentially LBH589-related toxicities included nausea (40%), diarrhea (33%), vomiting (33%), hypokalemia (27%), loss of appetite (13%), and thrombocytopenia (13%). The area under the curve increased proportionally with the dose and exhibited a terminal half-life of approximately 11 hours. The intravenous administration of LBH589 was well tolerated at doses below 11.5 mg/m^2, with consistent transient biological and anti-tumor effects (Giles et al., 2006).

A pilot study was designed to target DNA methylation and histone deacetylation through the sequential administration of 5-azacytidine followed by sodium phenylbutyrate (PB) in patients with AML or MDS. Fifty percent of patients were able to achieve a beneficial clinical response (partial remission or stable disease). The combination regimen was well tolerated, with common toxicities of injection site skin reaction (90% of the patients) from 5-azacytidine, and somnolence/fatigue from the sodium PB infusion (80% of the patients). Correlative laboratory studies demonstrated the consistent reacetylation of histone H4, although no relationship with the clinical response could be demonstrated. Results from this pilot study demonstrate that a combination approach targeting different mechanisms of transcriptional modulation is clinically feasible with acceptable toxicity and measurable biologic and clinical outcomes (Maslak et al., 2006).

Garcia-Manero et al. (2006) conducted a phase 1/2 study to evaluate the combination of 5-aza-2'-deoxycytidine (decitabine) and VPA in patients with leukemia, including untreated patients. The patients were treated with decitabine administered concomitantly with escalating doses of VPA. Twelve (22%) patients had objective responses, including ten (19%) complete remissions (CRs) and two (3%) CRs with incomplete platelet recovery (CRp). Among ten patients, five (50%) responded (4CRs, 1CRp's). Induction mortality was observed in one (2%) patient. Major cytogenetic responses were documented in six of eight responders. Remission duration was of 7.2 months (range, 1.3-12.6+ months). Overall survival was of 15.3 months (range, 4.6-20.2+ months) in responders. Transient DNA hypomethylation and global histone H3 and H4 acetylation were induced, and were associated with p15 reactivation. Patients with lower pre-treatment levels of p15 methylation had a significantly higher response rate. In this work, the combination of epigenetic therapy was safe and active for treating leukemia, and was associated with transient reversal of aberrant epigenetic marks (Garcia-Manero et al., 2006). Another phase I study of decitabine alone or in combination with VPA in AML determined an optimal biologic dose (OBD) of decitabine as a single agent and then the maximum-tolerated dose (MTD) of VPA combined with decitabine. Clinical responses were similar for decitabine alone or with VPA. Low-dose decitabine was safe and showed encouraging clinical and biologic activity in AML, but the addition of VPA led to encephalopathy at relatively low doses. The authors suggest that additional studies of decitabine alone or with an alternative deacetylating agent are warranted (Blum et al., 2007).

MS-275 is a benzamide derivative with potent HDAC inhibitory and anti-tumor activity in preclinical models. A phase 1 and pharmacologic study of MS-275 was carried out in patients with refractory and relapsed acute leukemias. Dose-limiting toxicities (DLTs) included infections and neurologic toxicity manifesting as unsteady gait and somnolence. Other frequent non-DLTs were fatigue, anorexia, nausea, vomiting, hypoalbuminemia, and hypocalcemia. Treatment with MS-275 also increased total and acetylated histone H3 and H4, p21 expression, and caspase-3 activation in bone marrow mononuclear cells. No responses by classical criteria were seen. The results demonstrated that MS-275 effectively inhibits HDAC *in vivo* in patients with advanced myeloid leukemias and should be further tested, preferably in patients with less advanced disease (Gojo et al., 2007).

In a phase 1 study in patients with leukemia, MGCD0103, an isotype-selective inhibitor of histone deacetylases targeted to isoforms 1, 2, 3, and 11, was administered orally three times weekly without interruption. The maximum tolerated dose was established at 60 mg/m^2, with dose-limiting toxicities (DLTs) presenting as fatigue, nausea, vomiting, and diarrhea at higher doses. Three patients achieved a complete bone marrow response (blasts below or equal to 5%). Pharmacokinetic analysis indicated absorption of MGCD0103 within one hour and an elimination half-life in plasma of 9 (+/- 2) hours. Exposure to MGCD0103 was proportional to doses up to 60 mg/m^2. Analysis of peripheral white cells demonstrated induction of histone acetylation and dose-dependent inhibition of HDAC enzyme activity. In summary, MGCD0103 is safe and demonstrates mechanism-based anti-tumor activity in patients with advanced leukemia (Garcia-Manero., 2008). MGCD-0103 is currently undergoing phase II clinical trials in patients with lymphoma, leukemia, myelodysplastic syndromes and solid tumors (Kell, 2007).

Gimsing et al. (2008) evaluated the safety, dose-limiting toxicity and maximum tolerated dose (MTD) of the novel hydroxamate histone deacetylase inhibitor belinostat (PXD101) in patients with advanced hematological neoplasms. The most common treatment-related adverse events (all grades) were nausea (50%), vomiting (31%), fatigue (31%) and flushing (31%). No grade 3 or 4 hematological toxicity as compared with baseline occurred, with the exception of grade 3 lymphopenia. The only related grade 3 events noticed in more than one patient were fatigue and neurological symptoms, being that one patient had status epilepticus in association with uremia and the other had paresthesia. All other related grade 3 events occurred as single events in patients, and no cardiac events were noted. No complete or partial remissions were noted in these heavily pre-treated (average of four prior regimens) patients. However, five patients, including two patients with diffuse large-cell lymphoma (including one patient with transformed CML, two patients with CLL, and one patient with multiple myeloma), achieved disease stabilization in two to nine treatment cycles. Therefore, intravenous belinostat at 600, 900 and 1000 mg/m^2/d is well tolerated by patients with hematological malignancies. The study was carried out in parallel to a similar dose-finding study in patients with solid tumors, in which the MTD was determined to be 1000 mg/m^2/d days 1-5 in a 21-d cycle. This dose can also be recommended for phase II studies in patients with hematological neoplasms (Gimsing et al., 2008)

Recently Fouladi et al. (2010) conducted a study to determine the maximum-tolerated dose (MTD), dose-limiting toxicities (DLT), and pharmacokinetics of vorinostat administered as a single agent and in combination 13-cis retinoic acid (13cRA) in children with refractory solid tumors, and to evaluate the tolerability of the solid tumor MTD in children with refractory leukemias. The MTD was 230 mg/m(2)/d with dose-limiting neutropenia, thrombocytopenia, and hypokalemia at 300 mg/m(2)/d. A mild dose reduction was required when combining vorinostat with 13cRA, but even then significant accumulation of acetylated H3 histone in peripheral blood mononuclear cells was observed after administration of vorinostat (Fouladi et al., 2010). It was concluded that the drug disposition was similar to that observed in adults.

Conclusion

In vitro and *in vivo* studies have been carried out in recent years to evaluate the use of HDIs on leukemia treatments. A number of HDIs have been tested in clinical trials, demonstrating safe and significant clinical activity. The use of HDIs in association with others molecules, such as classical chemotherapeutic drugs and DNA demethylating agents, may be promising alternatives for treating patients with leukemia. The great potential of these epigenetic modulators for treating leukemia has provided the basis for many studies, including those designed to identify HDAC variants in order to predict drug response and composition, to identify new methods of use, and to determine the efficacy of treatments with HDIs alone or in combination with other molecules.

So far, molecular studies have identified new HDIs, and combinations of these with other classical agents have been proposed. Since SAHA was approved by the FDA for the treatment of cutaneous T-cell lymphoma in 2006, the clinical use of HDIs in patients with leukemia will be a reality in a short time. Further clinical trials involving a number of HDIs, used either alone or in combination with other antileukemia agents, are needed to consolidate the clinical use of these epigenetics modulators.

Acknowledgment

This work was supported in part by the Children's Cancer Institute (ICI-RS, Porto Alegre, Brazil), the Academic Research Hospital (HCPA-FIPE, Porto Alegre, Brazil), and the National Institute for Translational Medicine (INCT program), all of which pose no conflicts of interest pertaining the author.

References

Arnold NB, Arkus N, Gunn J, Korc M. The histone deacetylase inhibitor suberoylanilide hydroxamic acid induces growth inhibition and enhances gemcitabine-induced cell death in pancreatic cancer. *Clin Cancer Res* 2007;13:18–26.

Bali P, George P, Cohen P, Tao J, Guo F, Sigua C, Vishvanath A, Scuto A, Annavarapu S, Fiskus W, Moscinski L, Atadja P, Bhalla K. Superior activity of the combination of histone deacetylase inhibitor LAQ824 and the FLT-3 kinase inhibitor PKC412 against human acute myelogenous leukemia cells with mutant FLT-3. *Clin Cancer Res* 2004;10:4991–4997.

Blum W, Klisovic RB, Hackanson B, Liu Z, Liu S, Devine H, Vukosavljevic T, Huynh L, Lozanski G, Kefauver C, Plass C, Devine SM, Heerema NA, Murgo A, Chan KK, Grever MR, Byrd JC, Marcucci G. Phase I study of decitabine alone or in combination with valproic acid in acute myeloid leukemia. *J Clin Oncol* 2007;25(25):3884-91.

Bolden JE, Peart MJ, Johnstone RW. Anticancer activities of histone deacetylase inhibitors. *Nat Rev Drug Discov* 2006;5:769–784.

Bouchain G, Leit S, Frechette S, Khalil EA, Lavoie R, Moradei O, Woo SH, Fournel M, Yan PT, Kalita A, Trachy-Bourget MC, Beaulieu C, Li Z, Robert MF, MacLeod AR, Besterman JM, Delorme D. Development of potential antitumor agents. Synthesis and biological evaluation of a new set of sulfonamide derivatives as histone deacetylase inhibitors. *J Med Chem.* 2003;46(5):820-30.

Byrd JC, Marcucci G, Parthun MR, Xiao JJ, Klisovic RB, Moran M, Lin TS, Liu S, Sklenar AR, Davis ME, Lucas DM, Fischer B, Shank R, Tejaswi SL, Binkley P, Wright J, Chan KK, Grever MR. A phase 1 and pharmacodynamic study of depsipeptide (FK228) in chronic lymphocytic leukemia and acute myeloid leukemia. *Blood* 2005;105(3):959-67.

Carew JS, Giles FJ, Nawrocki ST. Histone deacetylase inhibitors: Mechanisms of cell death and promise in combination cancer therapy. *Cancer Lett* 2008;269(1):7-17

Chuang DM. Valproic acid, a mood stabilizer and anticonvulsant, protects rat cerebral cortical neurons from spontaneous cell death: a role of histone deacetylase inhibition. *FEBS Lett* 2003;542: 74-78.

Dai Y, Chen S, Kramer LB, Funk VL, Dent P, Grant S. Interactions between bortezomib and romidepsin and belinostat in chronic lymphocytic leukemia cells. *Clin Cancer Res* 2008a;14(2):549-58.

Dai Y, Chen S, Venditti CA, Pei XY, Nguyen TK, Dent P, Grant S. Vorinostat synergistically potentiates MK-0457 lethality in chronic myelogenous leukemia cells sensitive and resistant to imatinib mesylate. *Blood.* 2008b;112(3):793-804.

Dasmahapatra G, Yerram N, Dai Y, Dent P, Grant S. Synergistic interactions between vorinostat and sorafenib in chronic myelogenous leukemia cells involve Mcl-1 and p21CIP1 down-regulation. *Clin Cancer Res* 2007;13:4280–4290.

Dos Santos MP, Schwartsmann G, Roesler R, Brunetto AL, Abujamra AL. Sodium butyrate enhances the cytotoxic effect of antineoplastic drugs in human lymphoblastic T-cells. *Leuk Res.* 2009;33(2):218-21.

Dowdy SC, Jiang S, Zhou XC, Hou X, Jin F, Podratz KC, Jiang SW. Histone deacetylase inhibitors and paclitaxel cause synergistic effects on apoptosis and microtubule stabilization in papillary serous endometrial cancer cells. *Mol Cancer Ther* 2006;5:2767–2776.

Fiskus W, Pranpat M, Balasis M, Bali P, Estrella V, Kumaraswamy S, Rao R, Rocha K, Herger B, Lee F, Richon V, Bhalla K. Cotreatment with vorinostat (suberoyl hydroxamic acid) enhances activity of dasatinib (BMS-354825) against imatinib mesylate-sensitive or imatinib mesylate-resistant chronic myelogenous leukemia cells. *Clin Cancer Res* 2006a;12:5869–5878.

Fiskus W, Pranpat M, Bali P, Balasis M, Kumaraswamy S, Boyapalle S, Rocha K, Wu J, Giles F, Manley PW, Atadja P, Bhalla K. Combined effects of novel tyrosine kinase inhibitor AMN107 and histone deacetylase inhibitor LBH589 against Bcr-Abl-expressing human leukemia cells. *Blood* 2006b;108(2):645-52.

Fouladi M, Park JR, Stewart CF, Gilbertson RJ, Schaiquevich P, Sun J, Reid JM, Ames MM, Speights R, Ingle AM, Zwiebel J, Blaney SM, Adamson PC. Pediatric phase I trial and pharmacokinetic study of vorinostat: a Children's Oncology Group phase I consortium report. *J Clin Oncol.* 2010;28(22):3623-9.

Fuino L, Bali P, Wittmann S, Donapaty S, Guo F, Yamaguchi H, Wang HG, Atadja P, Bhalla K. Histone deacetylase inhibitor LAQ824 down-regulates Her-2 and sensitizes human breast cancer cells to trastuzumab, taxotere, gemcitabine, and epothilone B. *Mol Cancer Ther* 2003;2:971–984.

Garcia-Manero G, Kantarjian HM, Sanchez-Gonzalez B, Yang H, Rosner G, Verstovsek S, Rytting M, Wierda WG, Ravandi F, Koller C, Xiao L, Faderl S, Estrov Z, Cortes J, O'brien S, Estey E, Bueso-Ramos C, Fiorentino J, Jabbour E, Issa JP. Phase 1/2 study of the combination of 5-aza-2'-deoxycytidine with valproic acid in patients with leukemia. *Blood* 2006;108(10):3271-9.

Garcia-Manero G, Assouline S, Cortes J, Estrov Z, Kantarjian H, Yang H, Newsome WM, Miller WH Jr, Rousseau C, Kalita A, Bonfils C, Dubay M, Patterson TA, Li Z, Besterman JM, Reid G, Laille E, Martell RE, Minden M. Phase 1 study of the oral isotype specific histone deacetylase inhibitor MGCD0103 in leukemia. *Blood.* 2008;112(4):981-9.

George P, Bali P, Annavarapu S, Scuto A, Fiskus W, Guo F, Sigua C, Sondarva G, Moscinski L, Atadja P, Bhalla K. Combination of the histone deacetylase inhibitor LBH589 and the hsp90 inhibitor 17-AAG is highly active against human CML-BC cells and AML cells with activating mutation of FLT-3. *Blood* 2005;105(4):1768-76.

Giles F, Fischer T, Cortes J, Garcia-Manero G, Beck J, Ravandi F, Masson E, Rae P, Laird G, Sharma S, Kantarjian H, Dugan M, Albitar M, Bhalla K. A phase I study of intravenous LBH589, a novel cinnamic hydroxamic acid analogue histone deacetylase inhibitor, in patients with refractory hematologic malignancies. *Clin Cancer Res* 2006;12(15):4628-35.

Gimsing P, Hansen M, Knudsen LM, Knoblauch P, Christensen IJ, Ooi CE, Buhl-Jensen P. A phase I clinical trial of the histone deacetylase inhibitor belinostat in patients with advanced hematological neoplasia. *Eur J Haematol.* 2008;81(3):170-6.

Glaser KB. HDAC inhibitors: clinical update and mechanism-based potential. *Biochem Pharmacol* 2007;74:659–671.

Gojo I, Jiemjit A, Trepel JB, Sparreboom A, Figg WD, Rollins S, Tidwell ML, Greer J, Chung EJ, Lee MJ, Gore SD, Sausville EA, Zwiebel J, Karp JE. Phase 1 and pharmacologic study of MS-275, a histone deacetylase inhibitor, in adults with refractory and relapsed acute leukemias. *Blood* 2007;109(7):2781-90.

Guo F, Sigua C, Tao J, Bali P, George P, Li Y, Wittmann S, Moscinski L, Atadja P, Bhalla K. Cotreatment with histone deacetylase inhibitor LAQ824 enhances Apo-2L/tumor necrosis factor-related apoptosis inducing ligandinduced death inducing signaling complex activity and apoptosis of human acute leukemia cells. *Cancer Res* 2004;64:2580–2589.

Hrebackova J, Hrabeta J, Eckschlager T. Valproic acid in the complex therapy of malignant tumors. *Curr Drug Targets*. 2010;11(3):361-79.

Jeong MR, Hashimoto R, Senatorov VV, Fujimaki K, Ren M, Lee MS and Kim MS, Blake M, Baek JH, Kohlhagen G, Pommier Y, Carrier F. Inhibition of histone deacetylase increases cytotoxicity to anticancer drugs targeting DNA. *Cancer Res* 2003;63:7291–7300.

Kano Y, Akutsu M, Tsunoda S, Izumi T, Kobayashi H, Mano H, Furukawa Y. Cytotoxic effects of histone deacetylase inhibitor FK228 (depsipeptide, formally named FR901228) in combination with conventional anti-leukemia/lymphoma agents against human leukemia/lymphoma cell lines. *Invest New Drugs* 2007;25(1):31-40.

Kell J. Drug evaluation: MGCD-0103, a histone deacetylase inhibitor for the treatment of cancer. *Curr Opin Investig Drugs* 2007;8(6):485-92.

Klimek VM, Fircanis S, Maslak P, Guernah I, Baum M, Wu N, Panageas K, Wright JJ, Pandolfi PP, Nimer SD. Tolerability, pharmacodynamics, and pharmacokinetics studies of depsipeptide (romidepsin) in patients with acute myelogenous leukemia or advanced myelodysplastic syndromes. *Clin Cancer Res* 2008;14(3):826-32.

Kouraklis G, Theocharis S. Histone deacetylase inhibitors: a novel target of anticancer therapy (review). *Oncol Rep* 2006;15:489-94.

Maggio SC, Rosato RR, Kramer LB, Dai Y, Rahamani M, Paik DS, Czarnik AC, Payne SG, Spiegel S, Grant S. The histone deacetylase inhibitor MS-275 interacts synergistically with fludarabine to induce apoptosis in human leukemia cells. *Cancer Res* 2004;64:2590–2600.

Maslak P, Chanel S, Camacho LH, Soignet S, Pandolfi PP, Guernah I, Warrell R, Nimer S. Pilot study of combination transcriptional modulation therapy with sodium phenylbutyrate and 5-azacytidine in patients with acute myeloid leukemia or myelodysplastic syndrome. *Leukemia* 2006;20(2):212-7.

Nimmanapalli R, Fuino L, Stobaugh C, Richon V, Bhalla K. Cotreatment with the histone deacetylase inhibitor suberoylanilide hydroxamic acid (SAHA) enhances imatinib-induced apoptosis of Bcr-Abl-positive human acute leukemia cells. *Blood* 2003;101:3236–3239.

Nishioka C, Ikezoe T, Yang J, Takeuchi S, Koeffler HP, Yokoyama A. MS-275, a novel histone deacetylase inhibitor with selectivity against HDAC1, induces degradation of FLT3 via inhibition of chaperone function of heat shock protein 90 in AML cells. *Leuk Res*. 2008;32(9):1382-92.

Okabe S, Tauchi T, Nakajima A, Sashida G, Gotoh A, Broxmeyer HE, Ohyashiki JH, Ohyashiki K. Depsipeptide (FK228) preferentially induces apoptosis in BCR/ABL-expressing cell lines and cells from patients with chronic myelogenous leukemia in blast crisis. *Stem Cells Dev* 2007;16(3):503-14.

Ottmann OG, Wassmann B, Hoelzer D. Imatinib for relapsed BCR/ABL positive leukemias. *Ann Hematol*. 2002;81 Suppl 2:S36-7.

Paris M, Porcelloni M, Binaschi M, Fattori D. Histone deacetylase inhibitors: from bench to clinic. *J Med Chem* 2008;51(6):1505-29.

Petrella A, D'Acunto CW, Rodriquez M, Festa M, Tosco A, Bruno I, Terracciano S, Taddei M, Paloma LG, Parente L. Effects of FR235222, a novel HDAC inhibitor, in proliferation and apoptosis of human leukaemia cell lines: role of annexin A1. *Eur J Cancer.* 2008;44(5):740-9.

Piekarz R and Bates S. A review of depsipeptide and other histone deacetylase inhibitors in clinical trials. *Curr Pharm Des* 2004;10: 2289-2298.

Pui CH, Robison LL, Look AT. Acute lymphoblastic leukaemia. *Lancet* 2008;371:1030-43.

Rahmani M, Yu C, Dai Y, Reese E, Ahmed W, Dent P, Grant S. Coadministration of heat shock protein 90 antagonist 17-allyamino-17-demethoxygeladnamycin with suberoylanilide hydroxamic acid or sodium butyrate synergistically induces apoptosis in human leukemia cells. *Cancer Res* 2003a;63:8420–8427.

Rahmani M, Yu C, Reese E, Ahmed W, Hirsch K, Dent P, Grant S. Inhibition of PI-3 kinase sensitizes human leukemic cells to histone deacetylase inhibitor-mediated apoptosis through p44/42 MAP kinase inactivation and abrogation of p21(CIP1/WAF1) induction rather than AKT inhibition. *Oncogene* 2003b;22:6231–6242.

Ramos MG, Rabelo FL, Brumatti G, Bueno-da-Silva AE, Amarante-Mendes GP, Alvarez-Leite JI. Butyrate increases apoptosis induced by different antineoplastic drugs in monocytic leukemia cells. *Chemotherapy* 2004;5:221-8.

Rikiishi H, Shinohara F, Sato T, Sato Y, Suzuki M, Echigo S. Chemosensitization of oral squamous cell carcinoma cells to cisplatin by histone deacetylase inhibitor, suberoylanilide hydroxamic acid. *Int J Oncol* 2007;30: 1181–1188.

Rosato RR, Almenara JA, Grant S. The histone deacetylase inhibitor MS-275 promotes differentiation or apoptosis in human leukemia cells through a process regulated by generation of reactive oxygen species and induction of p21CIP1/WAF1 1. *Cancer Res* 2003;63:3637–3645.

Rosato RR, Almenara JA, Yu C, Grant S. Evidence of a functional role for p21WAF1/CIP1 down-regulation in synergistic antileukemic interactions between the histone deacetylase inhibitor sodium butyrate and flavopiridol. *Mol Pharmacol* 2004;65:571–581.

Sanchez-Gonzalez B, Yang H, Bueso-Ramos C, Hoshino K, Quintas-Cardama A, Richon VM, Garcia-Manero G. Antileukemia activity of the combination of an anthracycline with a histone deacetylase inhibitor. *Blood* 2006;108(4):1174-82.

Scuto A, Kirschbaum M, Kowolik C, Kretzner L, Juhasz A, Atadja P, Pullarkat V, Bhatia R, Forman S, Yen Y, Jove R. The novel histone deacetylase inhibitor, LBH589, induces expression of DNA damage response genes and apoptosis in Ph- acute lymphoblastic leukemia cells. *Blood.* 2008;111(10):5093-100.

Temming P, Jenney ME. The neurodevelopmental sequelae of childhood leukaemia and its treatment. *Arch Dis Child.* 2010;95(11):936-40.

Timmerman S, Lehrmann H, Popesskaya A and Harel-Bellan A. Histone acetylation and disease. *Cell Mol Life Sci* 2001;58: 728-736.

Van Ommeslaeghe KEG, Brecx V, Papeleu P, Iterbeke K, Geerlings P, Tourwe D and Rogiers V. Amide analogues of TSA: synthesis, binding mode analysis and HDAC inhibition. *Bioorg Med Chem Lett* 2003;13: 1861-1864.

Villar-Garea A and Esteller M. Histone deacetylase inhibitors: understanding a new wave of anticancer agents. *Int J Cancer* 2004;112: 171-178.

Warrell RP Jr, He L, Richon V, Calleja E, Pandolfi P. Therapeutic targeting of transcription in acute promyelocytic leukemia by use of an inhibitor of histone deacetylase. *J Natl Cancer Inst* 1998;90: 1621-1625.

Yang H, Hoshino K, Sanchez-Gonzalez B, Kantarjian H, Garcia-Manero G. Antileukemia activity of the combination of 5-aza-2'-deoxycytidine with valproic acid. *Leuk Res* 2005;29(7):739-48.

Yu C, Rahamani M, Conrad D, Subler M, Dent P, Grant S. The proteasome inhibitor bortezomib interacts synergistically with histone deacetylase inhibitors to induce apoptosis in Bcr/Abl+ cells sensitive and resistant to STI571. *Blood* 2003a;102:3765–3774.

Yu C, Rahmani M, Almenara J, Subler M, Krystal G, Conrad D, Varticovski L, Dent P, Grant S. Histone deacetylase inhibitors promote STI571-mediated apoptosis in STI571-sensitive and -resistant Bcr/Abl+ human myeloid leukemia cells. *Cancer Res* 2003b;63:2118–2126.

In: Acute Lymphoblastic Leukemia
Editors: Severo Vecchione and Luigi Tedesco

ISBN: 978-1-61470-872-8
©2012 Nova Science Publishers, Inc.

Chapter VI

A Therapeutic Target in Leukemia: The NK-1 Receptor

Miguel Muñoz[1,*]*, Ana González-Ortega*[1] *and Rafael Coveñas*[2]

[1] Research Laboratory on Neuropeptides, Virgen del Rocío University Hospital, Sevilla, Spain

[2] Institute of Neurosciences of Castilla y León, Laboratory of Neuroanatomy of the Peptidergic Systems, Salamanca, Spain

Abstract

Acute lymphoblastic leukemia (ALL) is the most common malignancy in children and represents approximately 75% of all leukemias. Despite the advances in the treatment of the disease achieved over the past years, the five-year event-free survival rate is nearly 80% for children with ALL and approximately 40% for adults. Thus, there is an urgent need to improve therapy in leukemia patients. In recent years, the expression and secretion of peptides by tumors has attracted increasing interest and, in particular, it is known that the substance P (SP)/neurokinin (NK)-1 receptor system plays an important role in the development of cancer (SP, after binding to the NK-1 receptor, induces mitogenesis in tumor cells). It is also known that after binding to NK-1 receptors NK-1 receptor antagonists (aprepitant, L-733,060, L-732,138) inhibit cancer cell proliferation and that tumor cells die by apoptosis and that NK-1 receptor expression is significantly increased in cancer cells in comparison with normal cells. This means that the NK-1 receptor is a promising new target in human cancer treatment. Here, we review the data currently available concerning the involvement of the SP/NK-1 receptor system in human ALL: 1) SP is expressed in blast cells; 2) SP induces the proliferation of ALL cells; 3) NK-1 receptors are expressed in such cells; 4) Isoforms of the NK-1 receptor of about

---

[*] Full Address: Dr. Miguel Muñoz; Hospital Infantil Universitario Virgen del Rocío, Unidad de Cuidados Intensivos Pediátricos, Avda. Manuel Siurot s/n, 41013-Sevilla, Spain. Phone number: 34-955012965; E-mail: mmunoz@cica.es; Fax number: 34-955012921.

33, 58 and 75 kDa have been reported in ALL cells; 5) ALL cells express mRNA for the tachykinin NK-1 receptor; 6) The tachykinin 1 (*TAC1*) gene is overexpressed in ALL cells; 7) NK-1 receptors are involved in the viability of ALL cells; 8) NK-1 receptor antagonists elicit the inhibition of ALL cell growth; 9) The specific antitumor action of NK-1 receptor antagonists on ALL cells occurs through the NK-1 receptor; and 10) ALL cell death is due to apoptosis. These findings suggest that NK-1 receptor antagonists could be considered as new antitumor drugs for the treatment of human ALL.

Keywords: Acute lymphoblastic leukemia; Apoptosis; Aprepitant; L-733,060; L-732,138; NK-1 receptor antagonist; Substance P

Introduction

In the United States, leukemias are the most common forms of childhood cancer, representing approximately 31% of all cancer cases occurring in children under the age of 15 [42]. Acute lymphoblastic leukemia (ALL) is the most common malignancy in children, representing approximately 75% of all leukemias, the five-year event-free survival rate being nearly 80% for children with ALL and approximately 40% for adults [41]. No effective treatment exists and ALL will continue to be a major problem in oncology over the next decades despite the availability of treatment with cytotoxic chemotherapeutic agents and/or radiotherapy. Accordingly, new and effective therapeutic interventions are urgently required to improve therapy in ALL. The ultimate goal of cancer therapy is to cure the disease with no side effects, but the antitumor agents currently used in clinical practice - the so-called cytostatic drugs - are compounds that show a very low safety profile and very severe side effects, these effects being due to the fact that cytostatic drugs are not specific against tumor cells and hence the research accent has always been on the search for a drug with the same or greater antitumor potential but with fewer side effects. This can only be achieved if the drug used is specific against tumor cells and hence it is of huge importance to identify novel molecular targets for blocking tumor growth. One of the targets could be the neurokinin (NK)-1 receptor, since there are numerous data suggesting that the substance P (SP)/NK-1 receptor system plays an important role in the development of cancer [25, 27, 36].

The undecapeptide SP belongs to the tachykinin family of peptides; it is derived from the preprotachykinin A gene; it is widely distributed throughout the body, and it has been implicated in tumor cell proliferation, neoangiogenesis and metastasis [27]. SP is a major mediator in the growth of capillary vessels and in the proliferation of cultured endothelial cells, and it has also been demonstrated that NK-1 receptor agonists induce neoangiogenesis [49]. Moreover, the active migration of tumor cells is regulated by SP signals [15]; SP induces mitogenesis in several tumor cell lines [16, 23, 24, 29-31, 33, 44]; the expression of preprotachykinin A is increased in cancer cells in comparison with normal cells [see 27, 32], and SP is expressed in tumor cells [3]. The biological actions of SP, NKA and NKB are mediated by three receptors, named NK-1, NK-2 and NK-3, the NK-1 receptor showing preferential affinity for SP. It is known that NK-1 receptors are overexpressed in tumors; that tumor cells express several isoforms of this receptor, and that the NK-1 receptor is involved in the viability of tumor cells [19, 23, 24, 32, 44]. Moreover, it has been demonstrated that

NK-1 receptor antagonists exert antitumor activity and that this antiproliferative action is due to the fact that these antagonists induce cancer cells to die by apoptosis [19, 27-29, 32, 44].

All the data reported above indicate that SP is a mitogen in NK-1 receptor-expressing cancer cells, and that NK-1 receptor antagonists could offer a promising therapeutic strategy for the treatment of human cancer. Accordingly, here we review the latest data published about the involvement of the SP/NK-1 receptor system in ALL.

Leukemia and the Substance P/Neurokinin-1 Receptor System

In recent years, the expression and secretion of peptides by tumors has gained increasing interest since these peptides have been shown to influence tumor proliferation. In addition, the number of NK-1 receptors expressed by tumor cells is an important point to be taken into account, since it has been reported that the number of NK-1 receptors expressed in normal human cells is lower than that expressed in human tumoral cells (e.g., the NK-1 receptor expression is increased 25-36-fold in human pancreatic cancer cell lines in comparison with normal controls); that tumor samples from patients with advanced tumor stages exhibit significantly higher NK-1 receptor levels (e.g., astrocytoma and glioblastoma tumors possessing the most malignant phenotypes show an increased percentage of NK-1 receptor expression) [6, 7], and that in comparison with benign tissues mRNA NK-1 receptor expression is increased in all malignant tissues studied [see 26, 27]. All these data indicate that the expression of NK-1 receptors is correlated with the degree of malignancy.

It has been reported that human blood T-lymphocytes and human IM-9 B-lymphoblasts cell express 7,000-10,000 and 25,000-30,000 NK-1 receptors per cell, respectively [40] and that SP is expressed in human blast cells in ALL [35]. In human acute lymphoblastic leukemia cell lines (T-ALL BE-13 and B-ALL SD-1), the presence of NK-1 receptors has been reported using Western blot analysis [19]. Two bands (isoforms of about 33 and 58 kDa) were observed in the human T-ALL BE-13 cell line, whereas the B-ALL SD-1 cells expressed isoforms of 33, 58 and 75 kDa. Using Polymerase Chain Reaction analyses, it has been demonstrated that the BE-13 and SD-1 tumor cell lines also express mRNA for the tachykinin NK-1 receptor [19]. Moreover, real-time quantitative RT-PCR has been also performed to analyze NK-1 receptor expression in both cell lines using beta-actin as a control: the mean NK-1 receptor/beta-actin ratio was 1.23 ± 4.2 for the BE-13 tumor cell line and 3.2 ± 0.8 for the SD-1 tumor cell line, whereas the ratio was 0.01 ± 3.9 in the HEK 293 normal cell line. This means that the NK-1 receptor mRNA level is approximately 30-fold higher in leukemia cell lines than in that normal cell line [19]. Moreover, with a knockdown gene-silencing method (siRNA), it has been demonstrated that NK-1 receptors play an important role in the viability of T-ALL BE-13 and B-ALL SD-1 cells [19]. After the administration of the siRNA Tachykinin 1 gene receptor (*TAC 1R*) to both cultured cell lines, many more apoptotic cells were found in siRNA cells than in siRNA-negative control cells [19]. Thus, after 72 h 9.7 x 10^5 siRNA-negative control BE-13 cells and 5.4 x 10^5 siRNA *TAC 1R* cells were found, and regarding SD-1 cells, 5 x 10^5 siRNA-negative control cells and 2 x 10^5 siRNA *TAC 1R* cells were found (Figure 1).

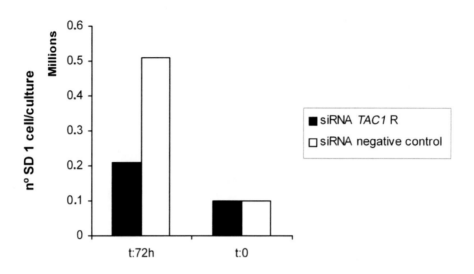

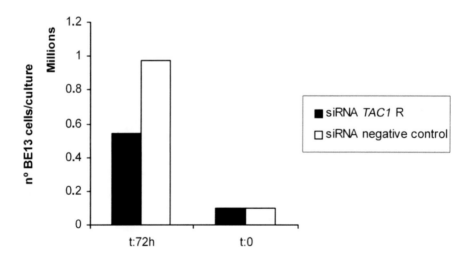

Figure 1. Viability of SD-1 and BE-13 leukemia cells. The number of siRNA-negative control cells is compared with the number of siRNA *TAC1R* cells. At 72 h the decrease in the number of siRNA *TAC1R* cells was significant in comparison with the number of siRNA-negative control cells.

The presence of isoforms of the NK-1 receptor in the BE-13 (33 and 58 kDa) and SD-1 (33, 58 and 75 kDa) ALL cell lines is in agreement with previous studies in which the presence of isoforms of the NK-1 receptor in neuroblastoma, glioma, retinoblastoma, melanoma, pancreatic, larynx, colon and gastric carcinoma cell lines was reported [23, 24, 28, 31, 32, 44]. Moreover, it has been demonstrated that *TAC1R* cDNA is present in human ALL cell lines with the highest levels in ALL cells and the lowest ones in normal cells. This is in agreement with previous findings, since it is known that NK-1 receptors are overexpressed in primary glioblastomas, breast cancer and its metastasis, retinoblastoma, and larynx, pancreatic, gastric and colon carcinomas [3, 7, 11, 28, 44, 46] and, as mentioned above, it is also known that NK-1 receptor expression is increased 25-36-fold in human pancreatic cancer cell lines in comparison with normal controls and that tumor samples from patients with advanced tumor stages exhibit significantly higher NK-1 receptor levels [7].

The growth of the BE-13 and SD-1 ALL cell lines after the addition of SP has also been reported: nanomolar concentrations of SP were seen to induce cell proliferation as compared to the controls [19]. This indicates that the activation of SP receptors leads to mitogenesis in the BE-13 and SD-1 human ALL cell lines: the percentage of cell proliferation of both cell lines increased from 14.5% to 77.5% in BE-13 and from 17.25% to 49.30% in SD-1, depending on the dose of SP administered [19]. It should be noted that endogenous SP is widely distributed in the body. The demonstration that SP stimulates tumor cell proliferation suggests a new mechanism for the regulation of local tumor activity through sensory nerves containing SP. Thus, SP could modulate the growth of tumor cells, exerting a direct interaction between the neural system and the tumor cells [see 26]. In this sense, SP stimulates mitogenesis by activating NK-1 receptors expressed in tumor cells (as mentioned, this expression is increased in tumor cells in comparison with normal cells), probably via four mechanisms: 1) through an autocrine mechanism, in which SP is secreted from primary tumors (e.g., neuroblastoma, keratocystic odontogenic tumors, oral squamous cell carcinoma, larynx carcinoma, melanoma...); 2) through a paracrine mechanism, in which the SP released from tumor cells and acting on other surrounding cells elicits cancer progression; 3) through the peripheral nervous system, since SP is released from peripheral nerve terminals; and 4) through an endocrine mechanism, related to emotional behavior, in which SP reaches the whole body through the blood stream [see 26].

The induction of mitogenesis by SP in human ALL cell lines is in agreement with previous studies in which it has been reported that SP exerts a mitogenic action on several other cancer cell lines [16, 23, 24, 26, 29-31, 33, 44]. It is known that in ALL SP is expressed in the cytoplasm of human blast cells [35]. This means that SP could be released from these cells, stimulating their own mitogenesis via an autocrine/paracrine mechanism, although the peptide could also be released from nerve terminals and a potential role of bone marrow stroma cells as a potential source of SP should not be discarded. As mentioned, the demonstration that SP stimulates ALL cell proliferation at low (nanomolar) concentrations suggests a new mechanism for the regulation of ALL activity through SP and that a direct interaction between the nervous system and leukemia cells might occur, through the SP/NK-1 receptor system.

Moreover, it is known that upon exposure to the agonist SP, this peptide and its receptor are internalized into early endosomes within minutes of binding (SP induces a clathrin-dependent internalization of the NK-1 receptor) after which SP is degraded, whereas the NK-1 receptor recycles at the cell surface [9, 17]. The stimulation of NK-1 receptors by SP can generate several second messengers (cAMP accumulation via stimulation of adenylate cyclase; arachidonic acid mobilization via phospholipase A2; stimulation, via phospholipase C, of phosphatidyl inositol turnover, leading to calcium mobilization), which in turn can trigger a broad range of effector mechanisms responsible for regulating cellular excitability and function [26, 27]. In fact, as mentioned above, at nanomolar concentration SP stimulates mitogenesis by activating NK-1 receptors in human ALL cell lines and in several normal and cancer cell lines [20, 21, 23, 24, 28, 30-32, 44]. Via the NK-1 receptor, SP could activate members of the mitogen-activated protein kinase (MAPK) pathway, including extracellular signal-regulated kinases 1 and 2 (ERK1/2) and p38MAPK. Once activated, ERK1/2 could be translocated into the nucleus, inducing proliferation and protecting the cell from apoptosis [see 26, 27]. Moreover, it is known that SP-induced MAPK activation requires the presence of a functional EGFRkinase domain and that stimulation by SP of the NK-1 receptor increases the phosphorylation and activity of Akt or protein kinase B, a serine-threonine protein kinase that becomes activated via phosphatidyl-3-kinase (PI3K) [see 26, 27]. The activation of Akt suppresses apoptosis [see 26, 27]. In addition, it has been suggested that the expression of c-myc protein would also be involved in the mitogenic effect [see 26, 27].

SP has been found in human neuroblastoma cells of the parotid gland, in human malignant glioma and retinoblastoma, and it is expressed in metastatic neuroblastoma cells in the bone marrow; in primary invasive malignant melanomas; in metastatic melanomas; in *in situ* melanomas; in atypical nevi; and in spindle and epithelioid nevi [14, 37, 48] and in glioma. SP has been reported in the cytoplasm and in the nucleus of tumor cells in keratocystic odontogenic tumors, oral squamous cell carcinoma and larynx carcinoma tissues [1, 3, 8]. However, to date the presence of SP in the BE-13 and SD-1 ALL cell lines is unknown.

The NK-1 receptor has been reported to be expressed in many human cancer cell lines (glioma, neuroblastoma, retinoblastoma, melanoma, pancreatic, gastric and colon carcinomas...), and NK-1 receptors have been localized in human primary retinoblastoma and neoplastic cells [11, 13, 23, 24, 26, 28, 31, 32, 37, 38, 44]. Moreover, keratocystic odontogenic tumors, oral squamous cell carcinoma and larynx carcinoma tissues express NK-1 receptors in the cytoplasm of the tumor cells [1, 3, 8], although in general immunoreactive NK-1 receptors are clearly confined to the plasma membrane of such cells [see 44]. Recently, in several human tumor cell lines the presence of four more abundant isoforms (75, 54-58, 46, 33-38 kDa) of the NK-1 receptor has been described [7, 23, 28, 31, 32, 44], but the functional roles of the different isoforms of the NK-1 receptor observed in human cancer cells are currently unknown. Moreover, it seems that tumor cells express more different isoforms of the NK-1 receptor than normal cells due to their proliferative-malignancy characteristics or due to other unknown reasons that make tumor cells overexpress more different isoforms. It should be noted that tumor cell lines as different as human ALL, retinoblastoma, neuroblastoma, glioma, melanoma, larynx and pancreas carcinomas, and gastric and colon adenocarcinomas express the same isoforms of the NK-1 receptor.

Table 1. Maximum (IC_{100}) and half (IC_{50}) inhibitions in ALL cell lines following the administration of NK-1 receptor antagonists

ALL cell lines	L-733,060 IC_{100} μM	IC_{50} μM	Aprepitant IC_{100} μM	IC_{50} μM	L-732,138 IC_{100} μM	IC_{50} μM
SD-1	45.7	18.4	59.2	29.4	103.5	49.7
BE-13	36.3	15.4	45.6	19.5	124	63.9

Leukemia and Neurokinin-1 Receptor Antagonists

The development of molecules as antagonists of the NK-1 receptor (e.g. WIN- 51,708 (a steroid); RP-67,580 and RP-73,467 (perhydroisoindolones); CP-96,345 and L-709,210 (benzylamino and benzylether quinuclidine); CP-99,994 and GR-203,040 (benzylamino piperidines); L-733,060 and L-741,671 (benzylether piperidines); L-732,138 (tryptophan-based)) has represented an important opportunity to further exploit compounds that are active against this receptor as novel therapeutic agents. There are two NK-1 receptor antagonist types: peptide NK-1 receptor antagonists (also called SP analogue antagonists, SP antagonists and SP receptor antagonists) and non-peptide NK-1 receptor antagonists. The binding sites for non-peptide NK-1 receptor antagonists, SP and peptide NK-1 receptor antagonists are different. Thus, SP and peptide NK-1 receptor antagonists bind to the extracellular ends of the transmembrane helices and especially to the extracellular loops of the receptor, whereas non-peptide NK-1 receptor antagonists bind more deeply between the transmembrane segments [12]. After binding to the NK-1 receptor NK-1 receptor antagonists block the effect of SP. It has been reported that the NK-1 receptor antagonists L-733,060, L-732,138 and the drug aprepitant (MK-869) exert dose-dependent antitumoral activity against several human cancer cell lines [19-24, 28-32, 44]. This means that these antagonists are broad-spectrum antitumor drugs and that the structurally very different molecules piperidine (L-733,060), L-tryptophan (L-732,138), and morpholine (aprepitant) exert the same effect: an antitumor action. These molecules only have their specificity for the NK-1 receptor in common. The data also suggest a common mechanism for cancer cell proliferation mediated by SP and NK-1 receptors [26, 27]. It has also been reported that the anti-tumoral action of L-733,060 against human cancer cell lines is more potent than that of aprepitant, and that the anti-tumoral action of aprepitant is more potent than that of L-732,138 [21, 29, 32]. This is in agreement with the results found for the antitumoral action exerted by the three NK-1 receptor antagonists against both T-ALL BE-13 and B-ALL SD-1 cell lines [19] (Table 1).

Growth inhibition of the BE-13 and SD-1 cell lines by the NK-1 receptor antagonists L-733,060, L-732,138 and aprepitant (Figure 2) was observed after the addition of increasing concentrations of these [19]. It has been reported that the concentrations required for a 50% reduction in optical density (IC$_{50}$) with L-733,060 are 15.4 µM for BE-13, and 18.4 µM for SD-1; with L-732,138, they are 63.9 µM for BE-13, and 49.7 µM for SD-1, and with aprepitant they are 19.5 µM for BE-13, and 29.4 µM for SD-1 (Table 1). Maximum inhibition was observed when the drug was present at a concentration of 36.3 µM L-733,060; 124 µM L-732,138 or 45.6 µM aprepitant (BE-13), and 45.7 µM L-733,060; 103.5 µM L-732,138 or 59.2 µM aprepitant (SD-1) during the culture periods (Table 1). With the maximum concentration, no remaining living cells were observed (Figure 2). After the administration of NK-1 receptor antagonists (L-733,060, L-732,138 or aprepitant), many apoptotic cells were found in both the BE-13 and the SD-1 ALL cell lines (Figure 3). This means that NK-1 receptor antagonists exert an antitumor action and that this action is because these antagonists induce the apoptosis of the tumor cells. Thus, the induction of apoptosis represents one of the most appropriate methods for cancer treatment, although at molecular level we have little knowledge about which mechanisms are responsible for inducing apoptosis in ALL cell lines [27]. The induction of apoptosis by NK-1 receptor antagonists is not exclusive to ALL cells; this effect has also been reported in many other cancer cells (e.g., retinoblastoma, melanoma, larynx, gastric and colon carcinomas) [23, 28, 32, 44]. It is also known that the same NK-1 receptor antagonist inhibits the growth of a large number of tumor cell types in which NK-1 receptors are expressed [26, 27]. It should be noted that in cell lines as different as human ALL, neuroblastoma, glioma, retinoblastoma, melanoma and pancreatic, larynx, gastric and colon carcinomas the same NK-1 receptor antagonist elicits growth inhibition. This means that a common mechanism for cancer cell proliferation mediated by SP and the NK-1 receptor occurs; that NK-1 receptor antagonists could inhibit a large number of tumor cell types in which NK-1 receptors are expressed [7, 15, 24, 28, 31, 32, 46], and that NK-1 receptor antagonists could be candidates as broad-spectrum antineoplastic drugs. Treatment with NK-1 receptor antagonists leads to apoptosis because the increase in phosphorylation due to SP is blocked by them. It is also known that the blockade of NK-1 receptors by NK-1 receptor antagonists inhibits the basal kinase activity of Akt. This is important, since in tumor cells the basal activity of Akt is linked to a poor prognosis. It should be remarked that the induction of apoptosis in cancer cells is not exclusively mediated by NK-1 receptor antagonists, since the COX2-selective inhibitor NS398 and the TRAIL (tumor necrosis factor-related apoptosis-inducing ligand) also induce apoptosis in several tumor cells [45]. It is known that a number of genes, molecules or signals are often changed in cancer, some of them are key regulators of apoptosis, and it has been suggested that any cellular genetic damage would activate one or more of the programmed cell death pathways [4]. ALL and tumor cells in general need to exploit strategies to neutralize the multiple pathways leading to cell death, and it may be proposed that at least one of the most important strategies is the activation and/or increase of the phenotypic expression of the NK-1 receptor [see 4]. Overexpression of the NK-1 receptor renders tumor cells highly dependent on the SP stimulus, a potent mitotic signal. This increased mitogenic signal could counteract the different death signal pathways activated in each tumor cell by its own genetic damage, oncogene activation, and others, and it is independent of the particular genetic profile of each tumor. Lack of these signals after the receptor has been blocked with the NK-1 receptor antagonist could render the balance inside the cell favourable to apoptotic/death signals, and hence the cell will die. Each tumor harbours a different set of mutations, oncogene activation and/or suppressor gene losses, and a number of different death signals are overriden by the SP-mediated mitotic stimulus. Accordingly, by cutting only the potent mitotic signal induced by SP, NK-1 receptor antagonists leave the cell alone with its death load, or at least render the balance between life and death signals favourable to the latter [4]. This is in agreement with the findings that demonstrated, after application of the small interfering RNA gene-silencing method (siRNA), that the NK-1 receptor plays an important role in the viability of melanoma and ALL cells [19, 32]. In those studies apoptosis was higher in siRNA melanoma/ALL cells than in siRNA-negative ones and hence the number of siRNA melanoma/ALL cells was significantly decreased in comparison with the number of siRNA-negative control cells found [19, 32].

In order to demonstrate that NK-1 receptor antagonists inhibit ALL cell proliferation via an interaction with the NK-1 receptor, the NK-1 receptor agonist SP has been tested in competition experiments [19]. The results showed that L-733,060, L-732,138 and aprepitant block SP mitogen stimulation, since NK-1 receptor antagonist-induced growth inhibition was partially reversed by the administration of a nanomolar dose of exogenous SP. This indicates the specificity of tachykinin NK-1 receptor activation in the growth of the human T-ALL and B-ALL cell lines, since an increase in the cellular concentration (47.50% and 34.60% in the case of L-733,060, for example) was respectively observed in the BE-13 and SD-1 cell lines with respect to the values found when the antagonist was administered alone [19].

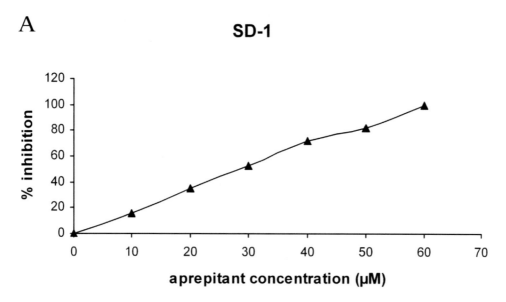

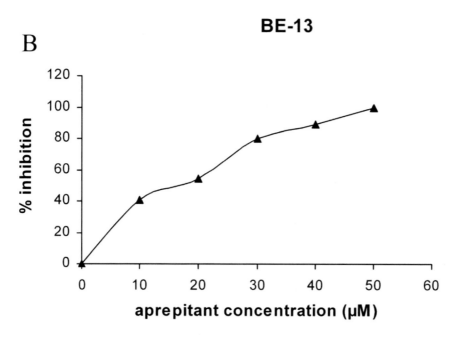

Figure 2. Percentage of growth inhibition of SD-1 (A) and BE-13 (B) cells, at 32 h and 48 h respectively, in *in vitro* cultures following the addition of increasing concentrations of aprepitant.

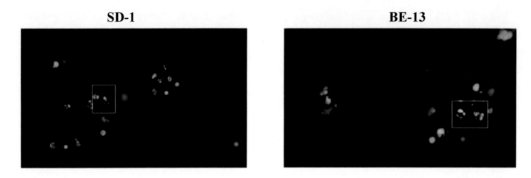

Figure 3. SD-1 and BE-13 culture cells treated with aprepitant. The delimited regions show apoptotic figures: chromatin condensation and nuclear fragmentation.

It is known that angiogenesis (a sequential process, with early endothelial proliferation followed by new vessel formation and increased blood flow), a hallmark of tumor development, is associated with increased tissue innervation and the expression of NK-1 receptors; that SP and NK-1 receptors are found in both intra- and peri-tumoral blood vessels; that SP stimulates vessel growth, enhancing endothelial cell proliferation, and that NK-1 receptor antagonists block the endothelial proliferative action of SP, markedly reducing tumor-associated angiogenesis [10, 11, 49]. All these data suggest that the NK-1 receptor target could be used for the inhibition of angiogenesis by using NK-1 receptor antagonists, which exert an antiangiogenic action, since NK-1 receptor agonists can directly stimulate the process of neovascularization, probably through the induction of endothelial cell proliferation [49]. Thus, through NK-1 receptors found at high density in blood vessels SP may strongly influence vascular structure and function inside and around tumors by increasing tumoral blood flow and by fostering stromal development. Moreover, the active migration of tumor cells is a crucial requirement for the development of infiltration and cancer progression. It is known that SP induces the migration of tumor cells to specific organs by binding to NK-1 receptors in cancer cells, where it can be blocked by NK-1 receptor antagonists [15], and that membrane blebbing is important in cell movement, cell spreading, and cancer cell infiltration [5]. It has been reported that the activation of NK-1 receptors by SP induces a rapid change in cellular shape (including blebbing), this not being associated with apoptosis but with the Rho-activated ROCK system [18]. It is known that aprepitant crosses the blood-brain barrier and that it blocks SP-induced changes in cellular shape, including blebbing [18]. This is quite important for the possible treatment of infiltration in the central nervous system. Treatment failure in children with ALL has been reported to be closely related to the expression of SP observed at the start of treatment, and a connection between the presence of SP-positive blasts and leukemia relapse has been suggested [34].

Future Research and Conclusions

The past two decades have witnessed an exponential increase in research into cancer. This has led to a considerable increase in investment in the field, reflected in the scientific literature through the publication of articles (1,400,000) in all types of journals, including those with the highest impact factors. However, this effort has not afforded in better perspectives as regards the problem, although several fields of research have been promising, such as the human genome project, gene therapy, the search for new cytostatic agents, and stem cell research. The short- and medium-term perspectives are not very promising, such that new pathways must now be opened up to offer future hope to oncologic patients. It is also necessary to search in other different directions because, unfortunately, the discoveries in the above-mentioned fields have not been fully successful. In this sense, it is expected that in the near future newer, more effective and safer anticancer drugs will become available for the treatment of tumors, and in this sense researchers are seeking to identify novel molecular targets for blocking tumor growth. One of these treatments could involve NK-1 receptor antagonists. Currently, there are more than thirty compounds that act as NK-1 receptor antagonists, and hence the development of antagonist molecules of the NK-1 receptor represents an important opportunity for exploiting these molecules as novel therapeutic agents for the treatment of cancer. There are many data suggesting that NK-1 receptor antagonists may offer a new and promising generation of anticancer drugs.

In addition to their antitumor action, NK-1 receptor antagonists display other beneficial actions such as anti-inflammatory, analgesic, anxiolytic, antiemetic, neuroprotector and hepatoprotector effects [26, 27]. Thus, for example, aprepitant is currently used for the treatment of emesis. It has been reported that in general the administration of NK-1 receptor antagonists does not cause serious side effects (e.g., headache, hiccup, vertigo and drowsiness) [2, 39, 43, 47] and that the NK-1 receptor antagonist L-733,060 does not cause adverse cardiovascular effects [see 27]. Moreover, the safety of aprepitant has been reported: at dose of 300 mg/day was well tolerated and no statistically significant differences in the frequency of adverse events was observed as compared to placebo [see 27]. It is also known that the IC_{50} of aprepitant for fibroblast cells is approximately three times higher than the IC_{50} for tumor cells [22].

Summing up the data, the following key points emerge (Figure 4): 1) SP is expressed in blast cells; 2) Human BE-13 and SD-1 ALL cell lines express NK-1 receptors; 3) The presence of different NK-1 receptor complex isoforms (33, 58, 75 kDa) has been reported in ALL cells; 4) ALL cells express mRNA for the tachykinin NK-1 receptor; 5) The tachykinin 1 receptor (*TAC1R*) gene is overexpressed in ALL cell lines; 6) The NK-1 receptor is involved in the viability of ALL cells; 7) After binding to the NK-1 receptor, SP induces tumor cell proliferation in ALL cells; 8) SP induces the migration of tumor cells, a crucial requirement for the development of metastasis and the progression of cancer; 9) Neoangiogenesis, a hallmark of tumor development, is stimulated by SP; 10) In most tumors investigated, NK-1 receptors are found in the intra- and peritumoral blood vessels; 11) NK-1 receptor antagonists (L-733,060, L-732,138 and aprepitant) block the substance P-induced mitogen stimulation of ALL cells; 12) NK-1 receptor antagonists inhibit both SP-induced rapid changes in cellular shape and the SP-mediated increased migratory activity of tumor cells; 13) NK-1 receptor antagonists exert antiangiogenic properties; 14) NK-1 receptor antagonists elicit the inhibition of ALL cell growth in a dose-dependent manner; 15) The specific antitumor action of NK-1 receptor antagonists on ALL cells occurs through the NK-1 receptor; and 16) ALL cell death is due to apoptosis.

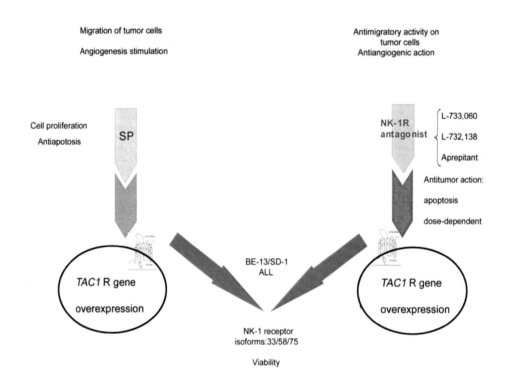

Figure 4. Involvement of the SP/NK-1 system in human BE-13 and SD-1 ALL cells.

All these data support the notion that the NK-1 receptor could be a new target candidate in the treatment of human ALL, and that NK-1 receptor antagonists (e.g., aprepitant) could be considered as promising new antitumor drugs for the treatment of human ALL. Thus, the ultimate goal in this field is to demonstrate that NK-1 receptor antagonists improve prognosis and decrease morbidity and mortality in ALL patients. However, it should be noted that the main limitation of the findings reported above regarding the involvement of the SP/NK-1 receptor system in ALL is that the research is currently in preclinical phase and most of the data obtained are from *in vitro* studies. Thus, before developing clinical trials in humans, *in vivo* studies must be carried out in depth. In this sense, the involvement of the SP/NK-1 receptor system in ALL should be tested in experimental animal models, as should the antitumor action of the NK-1 receptor antagonists. In ALL cells, it is also necessary to determine the cellular signaling pathways downstream from the NK-1 receptor, which after binding to SP lead to cell proliferation and antiapoptotic effects, whereas after binding to NK-1 receptor antagonists inhibit tumor cell proliferation and exert an apoptotic effect. In addition, new NK-1 receptor antagonists should be designed as novel therapeutic agents.

Once new *in vitro* and *in vivo* preclinical studies have been completed and have confirmed the key points reported above, the greatest challenge in this research line will be to develop clinical trials in order to verify the beneficial actions of NK-1 receptor antagonists in ALL patients, since in many cases the results of encouraging initial preclinical studies are followed by a lack of effectiveness in human trials. In order to enhance the therapeutic effects and to minimize side effects, in these clinical trials the concomitant use of the NK-1 receptor antagonists (e.g., aprepitant) with classic chemotherapy should be also tested. Aprepitant is an excellent candidate for testing in human trials since it is currently used in clinical practice and is well tolerated. Aprepitant shows no statistically significant difference in the frequency of adverse events as compared to placebo and, in general, NK-1 receptor antagonists exert beneficial effects in the host (antiemetic, anti-inflammatory, analgesic, anxyolitic...) and do not cause serious side effects. Finally, the findings described are not exclusive to ALL, since there are sufficient data to suggest that a common mechanism for cancer cell proliferation mediated by SP and the NK-1 receptor occurs, and that NK-1 receptor antagonists might be considered to be broad-spectrum antineoplastic drugs. This should be confirmed definitively in the coming years.

Acknowledgment

This work was supported by the "Sandra Ibarra de Solidaridad Contra el Cancer" foundation and by the Consejería de Innovacion, Ciencia y Empresa of the Junta de Andalucía (CTS-2247, Spain). The authors thank N. Skinner (University of Salamanca, Spain) for stylistic revision of the English text. The technical assistance of Dr. Manuel Lisardo Sánchez is gratefully acknowledged.

References

[1] Brener, S; González-Moles, MA; Tostes, D; Esteban, F; Gil-Montoya, JA; Ruiz-Avila, I; Bravo, M; Muñoz, M. A role for the substance P/NK-1 receptor complex in cell proliferation in oral squamous cell carcinoma. *Anticancer Res.* 2009; 29, 2323-2329.

[2] Choi, MR; Jiles, C; Seibel, NL. Aprepitant use in children, adolescents, and young adults for the control of chemotherapy-induced nausea and vomiting (CINV). *J. Pediatr. Hematol. Oncol.* 2010; 32, e268-271.

[3] Esteban, F; González-Moles, MA; Castro, D; Martín-Jaén, MM; Redondo, M; Ruiz-Avila, I; Muñoz, M. Expression of substance P and neurokinin-1-receptor in laryngeal cancer: linking chronic inflammation to cancer promotion and progression. *Histopathology* 2009; 54, 258-260.

[4] Esteban, F; Muñoz, M; González-Moles, MA; Rosso, M. A role for substance P in cancer promotion and progression: a mechanism to counteract intracellular death signals following oncogene activation or DNA damage. *Cancer Metast. Rev.* 2006; 25, 137-145.

[5] Fackler, OT; Grosse, R. Cell motility through plasma membrane blebbing. *J. Cell Biol.* 2008; 181, 879-884.

[6] Fowler, CJ; Brannstrom, G. Substance P enhances forskolin-stimulated cyclic AMP production in human UC11MG astrocytoma cells. *Methods. Find. Exp. Clin. Pharmacol.* 1994; 16, 21-28.

[7] Friess, H; Zhu, Z; Liard, V; Shi, X; Shrikhande, SV; Wang, L; Lieb, K; Korc, M; Palma, C; Zimmermann, A; Reubi, JC; Buchler, MW. Neurokinin-1 receptor

[8] expression and its potential effects on tumor growth in human pancreatic cancer. *Lab. Invest.* 2003; 83, 731-742.
[8] González-Moles, MA; Mosqueda-Taylor, A; Esteban, F; Gil-Montoya, JA; Díaz-Franco, MA; Delgado, M; Muñoz, M. Cell proliferation associated with actions of the substance P/NK-1 receptor complex in keratocystic odontogenic tumours. *Oral. Oncol.* 2008; 44, 1127-1133.
[9] Grady, EF; Garland, AM; Gamp, PD; Lovett, M; Payan, DG; Bunnett, NW. Delineation of the endocytic pathway of substance P and its seven transmembrane domains NK1 receptor. *Mol. Biol. Cell.* 1995; 6, 509-524.
[10] Guha, S; Eibl, G; Kisfalvi, K; Fan, RS; Burdick, M; Reber, H; Hines, OJ; Strieter, R; Rozengurt, E. Broad-spectrum G protein–coupled receptor antagonist, [D-Arg1,DTrp5,7,9,Leu11]SP: a dual inhibitor of growth and angiogenesis in pancreatic cancer. *Cancer Res.* 2005; 65, 2738-2745.
[11] Hennig, IM; Laissue, JA; Horisberger, U; Reubi, JC. Substance-P receptors in human primary neoplasms: tumoral and vascular localization. *Int. J. Cancer* 1995; 61, 786-792.
[12] Hökfelt, T; Pernow, B; Wahren, J. Substance P: a pioneer amongst neuropeptides. *J. Intern. Med.* 2001; 249, 27-40.
[13] Johnson, CL; Johnson, CG; Stauderman, KA; Buck, SH. Characterization of substance receptors in human astrocytoma cells. *Ann. NY. Acad. Sci.* 1991; 632, 410-412.
[14] Khare, VK; Albino, AP; Reed, JA. The neuropeptide/mast cell secretagogue substance P is expressed in cutaneus melanocytic lesions. *J. Cutan. Pathol.* 1998; 25, 2-10.
[15] Lang, K; Drell, TL; Lindecke, A; Niggemann, B; Kaltschmidt, C; Zaenker, KS; Entschladen, F. Induction of a metastatogenic tumor cell type by neurotransmitters and its pharmacological inhibition by established drugs. *Int. J. Cancer* 2004; 112, 231-238.
[16] Luo, W; Sharif, TR; Sharif, M. Substance P-induced mitogenesis in human astrocytoma cells correlates with activation of the mitogen-activated protein kinase signalling pathway. *Cancer Res.* 1996; 56, 4983-4991.
[17] Mantyh, PW; Allen, CJ; Ghilardi, JR; Rogers, SD; Mantyh, CR; Liu, H; Basbaum, AI; Vigna, SR; Maggio, JE. Rapid endocytosis of a G protein-coupled receptor: substance P evoked internalization of its receptor in the rat striatum *in vivo*. *Proc. Natl. Acad. Sci, USA* 1995; 92, 2622-2626.
[18] Meshki, J; Douglas, SD; Lai, JP; Schwartz, L; Kilpatrick, LE; Tuluc, F. Neurokinin 1 receptor mediates membrane blebbing in HEK293 cells through a Rho/Rho-associated coiled-coil kinase-dependent mechanism. *J. Biol. Chem.* 2009; 284, 9280-9289.
[19] Muñoz, M; González-Ortega, A; Coveñas, R. The NK-1 receptor is expressed in human leukemia and is involved in the antitumor action of aprepitant and other NK-1 receptor antagonists on acute lumphoblastic leukemia cell lines. *Invest. New Drugs* 2011 DOI 10.1007/s10637-010-9594-0.
[20] Muñoz, M; Pérez, A; Coveñas, R; Rosso, M; Castro, E. Antitumoural action of L-733,060 on neuroblastoma and glioma cell lines. *Arch. Ital. Biol.* 2004; 142, 105- 112.
[21] Muñoz, M; Pérez, A; Rosso, M; Zamarriego, C; Rosso, R. Antitumoral action of the neurokinin-1 receptor antagonist L-733,060 on human melanoma cell lines. *Melanoma Res.* 2004; 14, 183-188.

[22] Muñoz, M; Rosso, M. The NK-1 receptor antagonist aprepitant as a broad spectrum antitumor drug. *Invest. New Drugs* 2010; 28, 187-193.
[23] Muñoz, M; Rosso, M; Aguilar, FJ; González-Moles, MA; Redondo, M; Esteban, F. NK-1 receptor antagonists induce apoptosis and counteract substance P- related mitogenesis in human laryngeal cancer cell line HEp-2. *Invest. New Drugs* 2008; 26, 111-118.
[24] Muñoz, M; Rosso, M; Coveñas, R. The NK-1 receptor is involved in the antitumoural action of L-733,060 and in the mitogenic action of substance P on human pancreatic cancer cell lines. *Lett. Drug Des. Discovery* 2006; 3, 323-329.
[25] Muñoz, M; Rosso, M; Coveñas, R. NK-1 receptor antagonists as new anti- tumoural agents: action on human neuroblastoma cell lines. In: Fernandes JA, editor. *Focus on Neuroblastoma Research.* New York: Nova Science Publishers; 2007; pp. 31-56.
[26] Muñoz, M; Rosso, M; Coveñas, R. A new frontier in the treatment of cancer: NK-1 receptor antagonists. *Curr. Med. Chem.* 2010; 17, 504-516.
[27] Muñoz, M; Rosso, M; Coveñas, R. The NK-1 receptor: a new target in cancer therapy. *Curr. Drug Targets* 2011; 12, 909-921.
[28] Muñoz, M; Rosso, M; Coveñas, R; Montero, I; González-Moles, MA; Robles, MJ. Neurokinin-1 receptors located in human retinoblastoma cell lines: antitumor action of its antagonist, L-732,138. *Invest. Ophthalmol. Vis. Sci.* 2007; 48, 2775-2781.
[29] Muñoz, M; Rosso, M; González-Ortega, A; Coveñas, R. The NK-1 receptor antagonist L-732,138 induces apoptosis and counteracts substance P-related mitogenesis in human melanoma cell lines. *Cancers* 2010; 2, 611-623.
[30] Muñoz, M; Rosso, M; Pérez, A; Coveñas, R; Rosso, R; Zamarriego, C; Soult, JA; Montero, I. Antitumoral action of the neurokinin-1-receptor antagonist L- 733,060 and mitogenic action of substance P on human retinoblastoma cell lines. *Invest. Ophthalmol. Vis. Sci.* 2005; 46, 2567-2570.
[31] Muñoz, M; Rosso, M; Pérez, A; Coveñas, R; Zamarriego, C; Piruat, JI. The NK1 receptor is involved in the antitumoural action of L-733,060 and the mitogenic action of substance P on neuroblastoma and glioma cell lines. *Neuropeptides* 2005; 39, 427-432.
[32] Muñoz, M; Rosso, M; Robles-Frías, MJ; Salinas-Martín, MV; Coveñas, R. The NK-1 receptor is expressed in human melanoma and is involved in the antitumor action of the NK-1 receptor antagonist aprepitant on melanoma cell lines. *Lab. Invest.* 2010; 90, 1259-1269.
[33] Muñoz, M; Rosso, M; Soult, JA; Coveñas, R. Antitumoural action of neurokinin- 1 receptor antagonists on human brain cancer cell lines. In: Yang AV, editor. *Brain Cancer: Therapy and Surgical Intervention.* New York: Nova Science Publishers; 2006; pp. 45-75.
[34] Nowicki, M; Miskowiak, B. Substance P - a potent risk factor in childhood lymphoblastic leukaemia. *Leukemia* 2003; 17, 1096-1099.
[35] Nowicki, M; Miskowiak, B; Ostalska-Nowicka, D. Detection of substance P and its mRNA in human blast cells in childhood lymphoblastic leukaemia using immunocytochemistry and in situ hybridisation. *Folia Histochem. Cytobiol.* 2003; 41, 33-36.

[36] Palma, C. Tachykinins and their receptors in human malignancies. *Curr. Drug Targets* 2006; 7, 1043-1052.

[37] Palma, C; Bigioni, M; Irrissuto, C; Nardelli, F; Maggi, CA; Manzini, S. Anti- tumour activity of tachykinin NK1 receptor antagonists on human glioma U373 MG xenograft. *Br. J. Cancer* 2000; 82, 480-487.

[38] Palma, C, Nardelli, F; Manzini, S; Maggi, CA. Substance P activates responses correlated with tumour growth in human glioma cells line bearing tachykinin NK1 receptors. *Br. J. Cancer* 1999; 79, 236-243.

[39] Paul, B; Trovato, JA; Thompson, J; Badros, AZ; Goloubeva, O. Efficacy of aprepitant in patients receiving high-dose chemotherapy with hematopoietic stem cell support. *J. Oncol. Pharm. Pract.* 2010; 16, 45-51.

[40] Payan, DG; McGillis, JP; Organist, ML. Binding characteristics and affinity labeling of protein constituents of the human IM-9 lymphoblast receptor for substance P. *J. Biol. Chem.* 1986; 261, 14321-14329.

[41] Pui, CH; Relling, MV; Downing, JR. Acute lymphoblastic leukemia. *N. Engl. J. Med.* 2004; 350, 1535-1548.

[42] Ries, LA; Kosary, CL; Hankey, BF; Miller, BA; Clegg, L; Edwards, BK. SEER cancer statistics review, 1973-1996. Bethesda: National Cancer Institute; 1999.

[43] Roila, F; Rolski, J; Ramlau, R; Dediu, M; Russo, MW; Bandekar, RR; Grunberg, SM. Randomized, double-blind, dose-ranging trial of the oral neurokinin-1 receptor antagonist casopitant mesylate for the prevention of cisplatin-induced nausea and vomiting. *Ann. Oncol.* 2009; 20, 1867-1873.

[44] Rosso, M; Robles-Frías, M; Coveñas, R; Salinas-Martín, MV; Muñoz, M. The NK-1 receptor is involved in the antitumor action of L-733,060 and in the mitogenic action of substance P on human gastrointestinal cancer cell lines. *Tumor Biol.* 2008; 29, 245-254.

[45] Shi, J; Zheng, D; Liu, Y; Sham, MH; Tam, P; Farzaneh, F; Xu, R. Over-expression of soluble TRAIL induces apoptosis in human lung adenocarcinoma and inhibits growth of tumor xenografts in nude mice. *Cancer Res.* 2005; 65, 1687-1692.

[46] Singh, D; Joshi, DD; Hameed, M; Qian, J; Gascón, P; Maloof, PB; Mosenthal, A; Rameshwar, P. Increased expression of preprotachykinin-I and neurokinin receptors in human breast cancer cells: Implications for bone marrow metastasis. *Proc. Natl. Acad. Sci. USA* 2000; 97, 1388-1393.

[47] Ständer, S; Siepmann, D; Herrgott, I; Sunderkötter, C; Luger, TA. Targeting the neurokinin receptor 1 with aprepitant: a novel antipruritic strategy. *PLoS One* 2010; 5, e10968.

[48] Tarkkanen, A; Tervo, T; Tervo, K; Eranko, L; Eranko, O; Cuello, AC. Substance P immunoreactivity in normal human retina and in retinoblastoma. *Ophthalmic. Res.* 1983; 15, 300-306.

[49] Ziche, M; Morbidelli, L; Pacini, M; Gepetti, P; Alessandri, G; Maggi, CA. Substance P stimulates neovascularization *in vivo* and proliferation of cultured endothelial cells. *Microvas. Res.* 1990; 40, 264-278.

In: Acute Lymphoblastic Leukemia
Editors: Severo Vecchione and Luigi Tedesco

ISBN: 978-1-61470-872-8
©2012 Nova Science Publishers, Inc.

Chapter VII

Minimal Residual Disease Monitoring in Childhood Acute Lymphoblastic Leukemia

Katerina Katsibardi[1], Maria Braoudaki[1,2], George I. Lambrou[1], Kyriaki Hatziagapiou[1], Fotini Tzortzatou-Stathopoulou[1,2].

[1]Hematology/Oncology Unit, First Department of Pediatrics, University of Athens, «Aghia Sophia» Children's Hospital, Athens, Greece
[2]University Research Institute for the Study and Treatment of Childhood Genetic and Malignant Diseases, University of Athens, «Aghia Sophia» Children's Hospital, Athens, Greece

Summary

Minimal residual disease (MRD) is a powerful prognostic indicator which might be used to adjust treatment intensity in childhood acute lymphoblastic leukemia (ALL). Assays measuring MRD are capable to determine the treatment response in children with ALL much more precisely than morphologic screening of bone marrow. Minimal residual disease monitoring is performed through cytogenetic, immunologic and molecular information obtained from fluorescence in situ hybridization (FISH), flow cytometry (FC) and polymerase chain reaction (PCR) techniques, respectively. Specifically, PCR techniques use either patient specific junctional regions of immunoglobulin and T-cell receptor genes or chromosome aberrations which result in fusion genes or aberrant expression of transcripts. These techniques illustrate particular advantages and disadvantages while considering specificity, sensitivity, applicability, feasibility and precise MRD quantification. The incorporation of modern applications of PCR techniques, such as real time quantitative PCR (RQ-PCR), permits the accurate quantification of MRD levels. The clinical significance of MRD detected either by FC or PCR-based methods in childhood ALL has been evaluated during the last years. Both techniques have been incorporated in multicenter treatment protocols. However, it still remains open to discussion which is the appropriate and whether there is a universal technique to investigate MRD among different diagnostic laboratories. Issues related to MRD techniques and the evidence supporting the use of MRD for risk assignment in childhood ALL will be discussed in this chapter.

Introduction

Remarkable progress has been seen considering the diagnosis, treatment and outcome of pediatric acute lymphoblastic leukemia (ALL) during the last decades. Nowadays, the five-year event-free survival in childhood ALL approaches 80-85% [1,2]. The application of modern molecular techniques contributed in the precise risk-group classification of ALL patients, which in addition to morphological features (WBC at diagnosis, patient's age, immunophenotype, CNS involvement, prednisone response), embraces molecular characteristics, such as gene rearrangements of immunoglobulin heavy chain and T-cell receptor, as well as, chromosomal aberrations [3].

The majority of the leukemic cells are characterized by particular clonal rearrangements and chromosomal abnormalities. This means that each leukemic clone at diagnosis comprises specific genetic traits. Molecular detection and assessment of these genetic characteristics allows the discovery of leukemic cells even at a very low rate, which is defined as minimal residual disease (MRD). Estimation of the leukemic cells by conventional morphologic techniques has low sensitivity, since they can be detected in bone marrow with certainty only when they constitute 5% or more of the total cell population. Assessment of MRD by the employment of molecular methods can be 100 times more sensitive than morphologic examination and permits a more objective evaluation of treatment response [4].

The incorporation of MRD in the study of ALL has been proved valuable. First of all, sequential monitoring of MRD has been adapted into the definition of complete remission in ALL patients [5]. In addition, monitoring of patients' response to treatment protocol has become possible, whereas prompt and precise potential risk of relapse can be predicted [6,7].

Over the last decade, assessment of MRD has been a challenge for investigators, who attempted to point up its prognostic value, as well as, the most suitable approaches of detecting MRD. Several techniques have been developed, based on immunologic or molecular markers: polymerase chain reaction (PCR) amplification of breakpoint fusion genes, PCR amplification of antigen-receptor genes and flow cytometric profiling of aberrant immunophenotypes.

Techniques for MRD Monitoring

Optimal techniques for the evaluation of MRD should be characterized by sensitivity of at least 10^{-4} (one malignant cell within 10000 normal cells), applicability for the vast majority of patients under the study, leukemia-specificity (ability to discriminate between malignant and normal lymphoblasts, without false-positive results), feasibility (easy standardization and rapid collection of results for clinical application) and quantification (possibility of precise quantification of MRD levels) [8].

Minimal residual disease monitoring is generally obtained through cytogenetic, immunologic and molecular information. Cytogenetic methods use karyotypic abnormalities at diagnosis or at follow-up, which are identified either after cell culture or by fluorescence in situ hybridization (FISH). Cytogenetic methodology is not considered of first choice in the evaluation of MRD, since its sensitivity is very low [9].

At present, three different techniques are used for the detection of MRD in ALL patients: a) multiparameter flow cytometric immunophenotyping based on leukemia associated aberrant phenotypes b) PCR analysis of patient-specific junctional regions of immunoglobulin and T-cell receptor genes c) PCR analysis of fusion gene transcripts associated with chromosomal aberrations [10].

MRD Monitoring by Multiparameter Flow Cytometric Immunophenotyping

Flow cytometric immunophenotypic detection is based on the fact that leukemic cells express cell markers which divulge their origin as B- or T-lymphoid precursors. It is considered a fast, applicable in most patients and relatively cheap technique, which is based on the identification of phenotypes in leukemic cells at diagnosis that are not detected in normal bone marrow cells of the same lineage.

Specifically, leukemic cells display an unusual antigen expression as a result either of cross-lineage antigen expression, expression of asynchronous antigen maturation, antigen over-expression or ectopic antigen expression [11]. Furthermore, in order to recognize immunophenotypes for effective MRD estimation, one must regard the variations in the composition and immunophenotype of bone marrow cell populations which occur with age and exposure to drugs. For instance, early lymphoid progenitors (hematogones) may be abundant particularly in the bone marrow of young children and of patients with malignancy after transplantation or chemotherapy completion [12]. In these cases, normal cells expressing phenotypes that are undetectable in samples obtained from healthy individuals may be revealed. Therefore, aberrant or "leukemia"-associated" immunophenotypes (LAIPS) principally constitute the targets which are used in flow cytometric analysis of MRD [9]. An additional advantage of flow cytometric MRD detection is the recognition of intact blood cells, in contrast to PCR techniques in which contaminating nucleic acid material from dead cells can complicate the result of the analysis. In Table 1 are summarized the LAIPS which are used as for markers for MRD assessment in ALL patients.

Leukemia-associated immunophenotypes must be identified at diagnosis by comparing the cell marker profile of leukemic blasts to that of reference bone marrow samples, including those from patients receiving or recovering from chemotherapy. Transient fluctuations in cell marker profile may occur during chemotherapy in each leukemic clone, however, a confounding result may be diminished by using multiple sets of markers [13]. The use of at least two LAIPS is necessary in each patient in order to prevent false negative results [10].

Table 1. Leukemia-associated immunophenotypes used as markers of MRD assessment in ALL patients

Marker	Frequency (%)
B-lineage ALL	
CD19/CD34/CD10/CD58	40-60
CD19/CD34/CD10/CD38	30-50
CD19/CD34/CD10/CD45	30-50
CD19/CD34/CD10/anti-TdT	30-50
CD19/CD34/CD10/CD22	20-30
CD19/CD34/CD10/CD13	10-20
CD19/CD34/anti-TdT/anti-IgM	10-20
CD19/CD34/CD10/CD66c	10-20
CD19/CD34/CD10/CD33	5-10
CD19/CD34/CD10/CD65	5-10
CD19/CD34/CD10/CD15	5-10
CD19/CD34/CD10/CD21	5-10
T-lineage ALL	
Anti-TdT/CD5/CD3	90-95
CD34/CD5/CD3	30-50

MRD: minimal residual disease; ALL: acute lymphoblastic leukemia.

Until the late nineties, the flow cytometric MRD analysis was based on 3 or 4 markers [14]. However, current methodology extended this range to eight or even more markers. This enhanced the capability of discrimination between normal and leukemic cells, increased the sensitivity of MRD detection and allowed the study of biologic features of leukemic cells, such as expression of molecules related to proliferation, signaling, and drug resistance [13]. The sensitivity of flow cytometric MRD analysis remains unclear, though most centers report that the detection limit varies between 10^{-3} and 10^{-4}. In conditions, such as using distinct phenotypic target cells and in availability of a large number of cells ($\geq 10^7$) for analysis, the sensitivity of flow cytometry is comparable to that of PCR. However, the number of cells that can be analyzed for each set of markers is usually less than 1×10^6.

Considering that a distinct cluster of at least 10 to 20 dots is necessary to construe flow cytometric events, the maximum sensitivity achievable turns into 1 in 10^5 cells. Furthermore, the phenotype of primary leukemic cells might not be as distinct as that of cell lines used in an experimental setting and the sensitivity of detection may be influenced by the treatment interval at which the sample is obtained because of the variable proportion of normal B-cell precursors. Therefore, a sensitivity of 1 in 10^4 is probably the maximum that can be achieved consistently during routine MRD testing [15]. In general, the technique allows the detection of leukemia-associated phenotypes in the majority (60-98%) of B-precursor ALL and in nearly all T-ALL because of their specific thymocytic phenotype [16].

A main advantage of flow cytometry over PCR-based assays is the permission of direct quantitation of MRD, rather than extrapolating it from PCR products. This aspect makes quantitation easier and probably more accurate. In addition, it is possible to identify dying cells and cellular debris and to evaluate the status of normal hematopoietic cells. On the other hand, flow cytometry has some limitations, the most important of them being that lower sensitivity than PCR can be reached. Specifically, detection of 1 leukemic cell among 10^5 or more normal cells is difficult to be achieved usually by flow cytometry. Another limitation is that the immunophenotype of leukemic cells might change during the progression of the disease, therefore, resulting in false-negative findings. The potential adverse effect of this phenomenon is inversely related to the number of marker combinations that can be applied in each case [17].

Comparison between flow cytometry and PCR MRD detection within the same study group of ALL patients yielded concordant results in the vast majority of cases, even though the estimated levels of MRD varied. Out of the 190 B-lineage ALL cases that have been studied using flow cytometry and PCR in tandem to monitor MRD, most of them (96%) had proper immunophenotypes for flow cytometric monitoring of MRD and (89%) had rearrangements of heavy chain immunoglobulin and *TCR* genes. Thus, by combining the 2 methods the majority (99.5%) of patients were amenable to MRD studies. Therefore, the employment of both techniques in tandem ensures MRD monitoring in all patients [18].

MRD Monitoring by PCR Analysis of Fusion Gene Transcripts

Leukemic cells bear genetic abnormalities which can be used to distinguish them from normal blood cells. These structural chromosomal aberrations remain stable during the course of the disease and therefore represent significant clone-specific markers. The detection of chromosomal aberrations is feasible with the use of PCR amplification of mRNA transcripts. The targets used more commonly for MRD detection, by real time PCR (RT-PCR), are fusion gene transcripts, such as *ETV6-RUNX1* result of t(12;21)(p13;q22), *BCR-ABL1* including the two main types of t[9;22)(q34;q11), *MLL-AF4* result of t(4;11)(q21;q23) and the *TCF3-PBX1* coming from the fusion of *TCF3 (E2A)* at 19p13 with *PBX1* at 1q23. These fusion genes are identified in about 40% of cases of childhood ALL [19,20]. The most commonly fusion genes transcripts used for MRD analysis in ALL patients are presented in Table 2.

Among the recently abnormalities used for MRD monitoring are gene fusions involving *CRLF2* (translocation of the immunoglobulin heavy chain gene *IGH@* on 14q32 to *CRLF2; IGH@-CRLF2,* or an interstitial deletion centromeric of *CRLF2* resulting in a *P2RY8-CRLF2* fusion). Both fusion genes are principally present in high-risk B-lineage ALL children that lack traditional fusion rearrangements such as *MLL, TCF3, TEL/AML1* and *BCR/ABL* [21,22]. Fusion genes related to *CRLF2* are identified in approximately half of ALL patients with Down syndrome [23].

In principle, RT-PCR analysis of fusion gene transcripts can reach sensitivities of 10^{-4} up to 10^{-6}. The main advantage of the technique is that patient-specific primer synthesis, as well as, standardization steps during the procedure are not required, since fixed set of primers are used in each fusion gene [19]. An additional advantage of the technique is the steady connection between the fusion gene and the leukemic clone, with a potential for detecting preleukemic cells.

Table 2. Most commonly fusion genes for MRD analysis in ALL patients

Chromosomal aberration	Molecular target	Frequency (%)
B-lineage ALL		
t(12;21)(p13;q22)	*TEL-AML1*	25
t(1;19)(q23;p13.3)	*E2A-PBX1*	6
t(9;22)(q34;q11)	*BCR-ABL*	4
t(4;11)(q21;q23)	*MLL-AF4*	2
T-lineage ALL		
	TAL (DNA) or SIL-TAL (RNA)	15-25
t(5;14)(q35;q32)	*HOX11L2 (RNA)*	20

MRD: minimal residual disease; ALL: acute lymphoblastic leukemia.

To the contrary, a major pitfall of the RT-PCR analysis of fusion gene transcripts is that, due to its high sensitivity, there is an increased risk of false positive results via cross-contamination of RT-PCR products between patient samples. It is rather difficult to recognize such a contamination because, though fusion gene transcript targets are leukemia specific, they are not patient-specific markers. This is in contrast to PCR studies with antigen receptor genes, which can be carried out by the use of patient-specific oligonucleotide probes. In addition, RNA is rather unstable and it is more prone to degradation than DNA. The reason that RT-PCR is used, instead of PCR, in gene fusion transcript analysis is that for most translocations the breakpoints are scattered over much large DNA segments. This means that, chimeric messenger RNA and the resulting complementary DNA (cDNA) after reverse transcription are the preferred targets for PCR analysis [19]. Therefore, quantitation of MRD by RT-PCR fusion genes lacks the precision achieved when antigen receptor genes are used as targets. However, in breakpoints that occur in relatively small areas, such as less than 2 kb, amplification is feasible with PCR using DNA as a starting material. This is the case of T-cell acute lymphocytic leukemia 1 (*TAL1*) on chromosome 1p32 deletions, which is found in 5% to 15% of patients with T-lineage acute lymphoblastic leukemia (T-ALL) [24].

An alternative method of monitoring MRD by detecting chromosomal aberrations is fluorescence in situ hybridization (FISH). However, it has been reported that the use of FISH is not the optimal choice in MRD study, due to its low sensitivity (10^{-3}). Furthermore, its employability in the follow up of clonal persistence is limited, taking into consideration that the possibility of a novel aberration cannot be ruled out in cases of relapse. Thus, however, FISH may be used even in combination with comparative genomic hybridization (CGH), it is not generally applied in MRD assessment [25].

MRD Monitoring by PCR Analysis of Immunoglobulin and T-cell Receptor Gene Rearrangements

During the maturation of B-cell, clonal rearrangements occur that involve the V (variable), D (diverse) and J (junctional) segments of immunoglobulin (Ig) genes which generate a unique sequence (VDJ) for its cell and its progeny. In the same way, the genes encoding the T-cell receptor (TCR) undergo rearrangements during the development of T-cell precursors. Furthermore, the random insertion and deletion of nucleotides at the junctional regions increases the diversity of the rearranged region [26]. Therefore, the Ig/TCR clonal gene rearrangements outline "fingerprint-like" sequences, which differ in length and composition in each lymphocyte, as well as, in each lymphoid malignancy and constitute significant tumor-specific targets for MRD analysis. It is noteworthy, that such targets are able to be identified in the vast majority of precursor-ALL and T-ALL.

Immunoglobulin gene rearrangements are predominant in childhood B-lineage ALL, found in more than 95% of cases, while most of them contain immunoglobulin κ gene rearrangements (30%) or deletions (50%). Additionally, in 20% of B-lineage ALL cases immunoglobulin λ gene rearrangements are identified. However, considering that leukemic cells uphold recombination activity, *TCR* gene rearrangements also occur in B-lineage ALL. Specifically, *TCRβ*, *TCRγ*, and *TCRδ* gene rearrangements and/or deletions are found in 35%, 60%, and 90% of cases, respectively. On the hand, TCR rearrangements prevail in T-lineage ALL. Immunoglobulin gene rearrangements occur in approximately 20% of T-ALL cases and involve virtually only genes of heavy chain [27].

The most common approach to the clonal gene rearrangements is the use of PCR with primers matched to the V and J regions of the various antigen-receptor genes. Heteroduplex analysis or GeneScan analysis is applied in order to establish the clonality in almost 98% of cases at diagnosis. When clonality is identified, the PCR product is sequenced to define the precise junctional region of the rearranged gene and the sequence constitutes the template to design allele-specific oligonucleotides [28]. The application of region-specific oligonucleotides increases the detection of malignant cells at low frequencies. Quantitation of MRD is most commonly performed by using "real-time" quantitative PCR (RQ-PCR) and generally reaches sensitivities of 10^{-4} up to 10^{-5}). It is important to keep in mind that, parallel tests with mixtures of leukemic and normal DNA are necessary in order to determine the sensitivity of the assay.

The sensitivity of MRD-PCR analysis of clonal gene rearrangements is dependent on several factors, including the type of rearrangement, the size of the junctional region and the amount of the leukemic population. Therefore, in case that a relatively high proportion of leukemic cells is present, the level of MRD can be reliably quantified, however in case of very low amount of leukemic cells the identification of MRD levels becomes less accurate. Additionally, the sensitivity depends on the presence of normal lymphoid cells with comparable immunoglobulin or *TCR* gene rearrangements. For example, Vγl-Jγ1.3 and Vγl-Jγ2.3 joinings are found in a large fraction of normal T-lymphocytes, limiting the sensitivity and applicability of MRD assays based on *TCRγ* gene rearrangements [29].

Table 3. Characteristics of the techniques used for MRD monitoring in childhood ALL

Method	Target	Applicability	Sensitivity	Advantages	Disadvantages
Flow cytometry	Leukemic immuno-phenotypes	60-98%: B-ALL 90-95%: T-ALL	0.01%	• widely applicable • rapid-relatively cheap • accurate quantification • provides overview of hematopoiesis	• limited sensitivity • lack of expertise may lead to false-positive and false-negative results • need for multiple aberrant immunophenotypic markers per patient due to phenotypic shifts
RQ-PCR	Fusion gene transcripts	40%	0.01%-0.001%	• rapid-relatively cheap • suitable for monitoring uniform patient groups (Ph-ALL) • leukemia specific • stable target during disease	• applicable in a minority of patients • uncertain quantification Because of unknown number of transcripts per cell • RNA degradation may produce results false-negative • cross-contamination false positive results
RQ-PCR	IG/TCR rearrangements	90-95%	0.01%-0.001%	• high sensitivity • patient specific • generally accurate quantification	• laborious at diagnosis; identification of the junctional regions and sensitivity testing • relatively expensive • need for two PCR targets, due to chance of clonal evolution • false-negative results due to clonal evolution and oligoclonality • requirement for more than one target reduces applicability to 30% of patients

MRD: minimal residual disease; ALL: acute lymphoblastic leukemia; IG: Immunoglobulin; TCR: T-cell receptor.

Some critical points that should be taken into consideration when studying MRD by PCR studies, is that in oligoclonality (identification of three or more unrelated rearrangements within one locus), monitoring of all the identified rearrangements should be performed with the aim of increasing the chance that even the slowest-responding leukemic subclone will be followed [30]. In 30% to 40% of B-lineage ALL at diagnosis, the leukemic cell population consists of two or more subclones in which the immunoglobulin gene rearrangements may differ. To the contrary, *TCR* gene oligoclonality is rarely seen at diagnosis in T-ALL [31]. Clonal evolution affecting immunoglobulin and *TCR* gene rearrangements can be another source of false-negative results. Though, despite the high frequency of immunogenotypic changes in childhood ALL at relapse, at least one rearranged heavy chain of Ig, *TCR*γ, and/or *TCR*δ allele remains stable in 75% to 90% of B-lineage ALL and in 90% of T-ALL cases [32].

However, it is not known at diagnosis which subclone may eventually cause a relapse and which rearrangements should preferably be used as distinct MRD-PCR targets. Thus, in order to limit the risk of false-negative MRD results due to clonal evolution phenomena (ongoing rearrangements, loss of subclones), it has been suggested to monitor at least two different rearrangements at diagnosis [28]. The obligation of monitoring two or even more clonal rearrangements has the major disadvantage, that it reduces the number of patients amenable to MRD monitoring. In the AIEOP-BFM ALL 2000 study, (Associazione Italiana Ematologia Oncologia Pediatrica (AIEOP) and Berlin-Frankfurt-Munster (BFM) groups), 71% of patients had two sensitive targets [33]. Therefore, the use of an additional MRD technique, such as flow cytometry or PCR gene fusion analysis, may help to reduce the risk of false-negative results. This means that in many cases the combination of two molecular assays gives the optimal result in the study of MRD. The principal characteristics of the techniques used for MRD monitoring in childhood ALL are summarized in Table 3.

Prognostic Value of Minimal Residual Disease

Several prospective studies have demonstrated that fundamental information are drawn from the detection of MRD in bone marrow, inciting the design of clinical trials in which MRD is used for risk assignment and treatment selection. Results from the majority of trials indicate the prognostic impact of MRD monitoring at the early phases of treatment, particularly at the end of induction treatment. Patients with undetectable MRD at the end of induction have excellent prognosis and usually do not need further treatment intensification or hematopoietic stem cell transplantation [33-35]. In contrast, children with high MRD levels at the end induction treatment are in urgent need for treatment intensification, particularly when such high MRD levels persist into the consolidation treatment [10]. Groups collaborating in the International BFM Study Group have pioneered the evaluation of MRD by PCR in childhood ALL, at two time points, using 2 clonal Ig/TCR markers. MRD-based stratification was superior to that based on other clinically relevant risk factors [36].

Investigators in the Children's Oncology Group measured MRD in bone marrow, at the end of induction treatment, in 2086 patients with B-lineage ALL, found that 0.01% or more MRD by flow cytometry was significantly associated with a worse outcome [15]. Besides, the

Italian cooperative group (AIEOP) studied bone marrow samples from 830 patients by flow cytometry on day 15 of treatment and identified three risk groups according to MRD level: standard (MRD < 0.1%, 42%), intermediate (MRD 0.1%–<10%, 47%), and high (MRD ≥10%, 11%). The 5-year incidence of relapse in these groups was 7.5%, 17.5%, and 47.2%, respectively [36].

In a study by the Dana-Farber Cancer Institute ALL Consortium, in 284 patients with B-lineage ALL, the 5-year risk of relapse was 44% in patients with detectable MRD at the end of remission induction therapy and only 5% in patients with undetectable MRD. Furthermore, it was reported that even the use of only one MRD target was sufficient to identify patients at high risk of relapse in order to merit change in treatment [34]. In a study by the St Jude Children's Research Hospital, in 455 patients with B-lineage ALL, the adverse prognostic impact of MRD as detected by PCR amplification of immunoglobulin and TCR genes at the end of remission induction therapy was confirmed. They reported that patients with levels of MRD (0.001% to <0.01%) had significantly higher risk of relapse in comparison to those with findings below 0.001% [37]. In a recent study of our laboratory, 792 bone marrow samples were analyzed in 91 patients with ALL and PCR amplification of immunoglobulin and TCR gene rearrangements was performed in order to monitor MRD. It was demonstrated that identification of MRD on day 28 was strongly predictive for patients' outcome, since it was significantly associated with higher incidence of relapse at 5 years compared to patients with undetectable MRD at the same time point ($P=0.0002$). Furthermore, it was verified that the 5-year event free-survival was associated to MRD positivity at the end of induction and not to patients' risk group, as defined clinically at diagnosis [6].

Conclusion

Monitoring of MRD has been proved an essential parameter that accurately gauges treatment response and allows estimation of the residual leukemic cell burden during clinical remission in ALL patients. MRD stratification can be used as an independent parameter in patients' risk classification. In this manner, it has a vital role in the selection of the appropriate therapeutic strategy in each patient. The most useful MRD assays that are currently available are PCR amplification of fusion transcripts and rearranged antigen-receptor genes, as well as, flow cytometric detection of aberrant immunophenotypes.

Each of the mentioned methods for studying MRD in childhood ALL has relative advantages and disadvantages. The choice of the appropriate MRD methodology in childhood ALL depends principally on the plan of the study and the available facilities in each laboratory. By some investigators, the detection and quantification of clonal immunoglobulin and TCR rearrangements is considered the most widely employed approach of MRD monitoring. Even though this MRD strategy is laborious, expensive and time consuming, it can be performed in the vast majority of patients and it is the most reproducible approach between the different laboratories. However, flow cytometry could be used in a complementary fashion for different aims within the same population. In this regard, a prospect strategy may be to adopt more extensively the concept of MRD early response and to combine it with flow cytometry in MRD evaluation.

In general, the use of multiple approaches simultaneously can increase the number of patients who can be studied and offset the limitations of individual methods. However, the main challenge for MRD investigators is to identify novel vigorous leukemic markers that will allow the simplification of the current methodology, while maintaining or even increasing their reliability. The most significant benefit would be the dissemination of the potential advantages of MRD monitoring in childhood ALL.

References

[1] Pui CH, Evans WE. Treatment of acute lymphoblastic leukemia. *N Engl J Med.* 2006;354:166-78.

[2] Pulte D, Gondos A, Brenner H. Trends in 5- and 10-year survival after diagnosis with childhood hematologic malignancies in the United States, 1990-2004. *J Natl Cancer Inst.* 2008;100:1301-9.

[3] Smith M, Arthur D, Camitta B, et al. Uniform approach to risk classification and treatment assignment for children with acute lymphoblastic leukemia. *J Clin Oncol.* 1996;14:18-24.

[4] Campana D. Determination of minimal residual disease in leukemia patients. *Br J Haematol.* 2003;121:823-38.

[5] Arico M, Baruchel A, Bertrand Y, et al. *The seventh international childhood acute lymphoblastic leukemia workshop report:* Palermo, Italy, January 29-30, 2005. Leukemia 2005;19:1145-52.

[6] Katsibardi K, Moschovi MA, Braoudaki M, et al. Sequential monitoring of minimal residual disease in acute lymphoblastic leukemia: 7-year experience in a pediatric hematology/oncology unit. *Leuk Lymphoma* 2010;51:846-52.

[7] Escherich G, Horstmann MA, Zimmermann M, et al. COALL study group. Cooperative study group for childhood acute lymphoblastic leukaemia (COALL): long-term results of trials 82,85,89,92 and 97. *Leukemia* 2010;24:298-308.

[8] Hoelzer D, Gökbuget N, Ottmann O, Pui CH, et al. *Acute Lymphoblastic Leukemia Hematology* 2002;162-92.

[9] Basso G, Buldini B, De Zen L, et al. New methodologic approaches for immunophenotyping acute leukemias. *Haematologica* 2001;86:675-92.

[10] Szczepański T. Why and how to quantify minimal residual disease in acute lymphoblastic leukemia? *Leukemia.* 2007;21:622-6.

[11] van der Velden VH, Boeckx N, van Wering ER, et al. Detection of minimal residual disease in acute leukemia. *J Biol Regul Homeost Agents.* 2004;18:146-54.

[12] McKenna RW, Washington LT, Aquino DB, et al. Immunophenotypic analysis of hematogones (B-lymphocyte precursors) in 662 consecutive bone marrow specimens by 4-color flow cytometry. *Blood.* 2001;98:2498-2507.

[13] Campana D. Role of minimal residual disease monitoring in adult and pediatric acute lymphoblastic leukemia. *Hematol Oncol Clin North Am* 2009;23:1083-98.

[14] Dworzak MN, Fröschl G, Printz D, et al. Prognostic significance and modalities of flow cytometric minimal residual disease detection in childhood acute lymphoblastic leukemia. *Blood* 2002;99:1952-8.
[15] Borowitz MJ, Devidas M, Hunger SP, et al.: Clinical significance of minimal residual disease in childhood acute lymphoblastic leukemia and its relationship to other prognostic factors. a Children's Oncology Group study. *Blood* 2008;111:5477-85.
[16] Dworzak MN. Immunological detection of minimal residual disease in acute lymphoblastic leukemia. *Onkologie.* 2001;24:442-8.
[17] Oelschlagel U, Nowak R, Schaub A, et al. Shift of aberrant antigen expression at relapse or at treatment failure in acute leukemia. *Cytometry.* 2000;42:247-53.
[18] Neale GA, Coustan-Smith E, Stow P, et al. Comparative analysis of flow cytometry and polymerase chain reaction for the detection of minimal residual disease in childhood acute lymphoblastic leukemia. *Leukemia.* 2004;18:934-8.
[19] Gabert J, Beillard E, van der Velden VH, et al. Standardization and quality control studies of 'real-time' quantitative reverse transcriptase polymerase chain reaction of fusion gene transcripts for residual disease detection in leukemia - a Europe Against Cancer program. *Leukemia.* 2003;17:2318-57.
[20] Campana D: Molecular determinants of treatment response in acute lymphoblastic leukemia. *Hematology Am Soc Hematol Educ Program* 2008. 2008:366-373.
[21] Harvey RC, Mullighan CG, Chen IM, et al. Rearrangement of CRLF2 is associated with mutation of JAK kinases, alteration of IKZF1, Hispanic/Latino ethnicity, and a poor outcome in pediatric B-progenitor acute lymphoblastic leukemia. *Blood* 2010;115:5312-21.
[22] Yoda A, Yoda Y, Chiaretti S, et al. Functional screening identifies CRLF2 in precursor B-cell acute lymphoblastic leukemia. *Proc Natl Acad Sci* U S A. 2010;107:252-7.
[23] Mullighan CG, Collins-Underwood JR, Phillips LA. Rearrangement of CRLF2 in B-progenitor– and Down syndrome–associated acute lymphoblastic leukemia. *Nat Genet.* 2009;41:1243-6.
[24] Pongers-Willemse MJ, Seriu T, Stolz F, et al. Primers and protocols for standardized detection of minimal residual disease in acute lymphoblastic leukemia using immunoglobulin and T cell receptor gene rearrangements and TAL1 deletions as PCR targets. *Leukemia* 1999;13:110-8.
[25] Kanerva J, Vettenranta K, Autio K, et al. Minimal residual disease by metaphase FISH in children with ALL: clonal cells during or after chemotherapy may not predict relapse. *Leuk Res.* 2002;26:545-50.
[26] Sanz I. Multiple mechanisms participate in the generation of diversity of human H chain CDR3 regions. *J Immunol.* 1991;147:1720-9.
[27] Brüggemann M, Schrauder A, Raff T, et al. Standardized MRD quantification in European ALL trials: proceedings of the Second International Symposium on MRD assessment in Kiel, Germany, 18-20 September 2008. *Leukemia.* 2010;24:521-35.
[28] van der Velden V, Cazzaniga G, Schrauder A, et al. Analysis of minimal residual disease by Ig/TCR gene rearrangements: guidelines for interpretation of real-time quantitative PCR data. *Leukemia* 2007;21:604-11.

[29] van der Velden VH, Wijkhuijs JM, Jacobs DC, et al. T cell receptor gamma gene rearrangements as targets for detection of minimal residual disease in acute lymphoblastic leukemia by real-time quantitative PCR analysis. *Leukemia.* 2002;16:1372-80.

[30] Meleshko AN, Lipay NV, Stasevich IV, et al. Rearrangements of IgH, TCRD and TCRG genes as clonality marker of childhood acute lymphoblastic leukemia. *Exp Oncol.* 2005;27:319-24.

[31] Beishuizen A, Verhoeven MA, Van Wering ER, et al. Analysis of Ig and T-cell receptor genes in 40 childhood acute lymphoblastic leukemias at diagnosis and subsequent relapse: implications for the detection of minimal residual disease by polymerase chain reaction analysis. *Blood* 1994;83:2238-47.

[32] Szczepanski T, van der Velden VH, Raff T, et al. Comparative analysis of T-cell receptor gene rearrangements at diagnosis and relapse of T-cell acute lymphoblastic leukemia (T-ALL) shows high stability of clonal markers for monitoring of minimal residual disease and reveals the occurrence of second T-ALL. *Leukemia.* 2003;17:2149-56.

[33] Flohr T, Schrauder A, Cazzaniga G, et al. International BFM Study Group (I-BFM-SG). Minimal residual disease-directed risk stratification using real-time quantitative PCR analysis of immunoglobulin and T-cell receptor gene rearrangements in the international multicenter trial AIEOP-BFM ALL 2000 for childhood acute lymphoblastic leukemia. *Leukemia.* 2000;22:771-82.

[34] Zhou J, Goldwasser MA, Li A, et al.: Quantitative analysis of minimal residual disease predicts relapse in children with Blineage acute lymphoblastic leukemia in DFCI ALL Consortium Protocol 95-01. *Blood* 2007;110:1607–11.

[35] Schultz KR, Pullen DJ, Sather HN, et al. Risk- and response-based classification of childhood B-precursor acute lymphoblastic leukemia: a combined analysis of prognostic markers from the Pediatric Oncology Group (POG) and Children's Cancer Group (CCG). *Blood.* 2007;109:926-35.

[36] Basso G, Veltroni M, Valsecchi MG, et al. Risk of relapse of childhood acute lymphoblastic leukemia is predicted by flow cytometric measurement of residual disease on day 15 bone marrow. *J Clin Oncol* 2009;27:5168–74.

[37] Stow P, Key L, Cjen X, et al.: Clinical significance of low levels of minimal residual disease at the end of remission induction therapy in childhood acute lymphoblastic leukemia. *Blood.* 2010;115:4657-63.

In: Acute Lymphoblastic Leukemia
Editors: Severo Vecchione and Luigi Tedesco

ISBN: 978-1-61470-872-8
©2012 Nova Science Publishers, Inc.

Chapter VIII

Clinical Relevance and Application of Cytogenetic Approaches in Pediatric Acute Lymphoblastic Leukaemia

Maria Braoudaki[1,2], Katerina Katsibardi[2], George I. Lambrou[2], Kyriaki Hatziagapiou[2], Fotini Tzortzatou-Stathopoulou[1,2].

[1]University Research Institute for the Study and Treatment of Childhood Genetic and Malignant Diseases, University of Athens, «Aghia Sophia» Children's Hospital, Athens, Greece

[2]Hematology/Oncology Unit, First Department of Pediatrics, University of Athens, «Aghia Sophia» Children's Hospital, Athens, Greece

Summary

Childhood acute lymphoblastic leukaemia (ALL) is commonly characterized by specific and non-random chromosomal abnormalities, which might play a vital role in the etiology and pathogenesis of the disease. The majority of patients with ALL demonstrate an abnormal karyotype, either in chromosome number (ploidy) or as structural changes often translocations, inversions, or deletions. Translocations fuse oncogenes with other gene loci leading to the production of chimeric fusion genes and the activation of oncogenes under specific regulatory genes that are responsible for malignant transformation. A number of these cytogenetic abnormalities are associated with distinct immunologic phenotypes of ALL and characteristic outcomes. The detection of precise prognostic cytogenetic markers in ALL is necessitated to guide diagnosis and the choice of treatment. For this purpose, several molecular approaches have been described, which can provide high through-put including conventional cytogenetics, real-time quantitative polymerase chain reaction (RQ-PCR), fluorescence in situ hybridization (FISH), comparative genome hybridization (CGH) and array-based CGH. These techniques, although useful, include several limitations. In the current review the application of major cytogenetic aberrations as prognostic, diagnostic and therapeutic markers and the clinical relevance of current approaches were recapitulated.

Introduction

Pediatric acute lymphoblastic leukemia (ALL) is a malignancy that represents around 25-35% of all cancer cases among pediatric patients and is generally favorable with cure rates presently exceeding 80%, due to effective treatment regimens. However, hitherto, despite the incremental anticancer therapeutic improvements, significant subsets of children, systematically relapse, carrying a dismal prognosis.

Novel therapeutic interventions are focused on tailoring therapy to the predicted risk of relapse that can be achieved through the precise risk stratification, based on the additionally important patient's structural and numerical chromosomal abnormalities. The identification of recurrent chromosomal abnormalities present in the malignant cells is essential to guide optimal therapy in the individual patient with ALL [1]. Importantly, patients harboring fusion genes associated with inferior prognosis are candidates for more intensive treatment protocols or for bone marrow transplantation.

However, considering that ALL risk stratification is based partially on cytogenetic analyses, both undetected poor risk aberrations and insufficient knowledge of molecular events underlying leukemogenesis may contribute to therapy failures. Subsequently, the use of reliable laboratory methods is essential for the precise determination of the childhood ALL-associated cytogenetic alterations.

Molecular Approaches

Significant advances in molecular biology have provided several procedures for the detection and characterization of chromosomal abnormalities in pediatric ALL. These include: metaphase cytogenetics, polymerase chain reaction (PCR) techniques; reverse transcriptase PCR (RT-PCR) and real-time quantitative PCR (RQ-PCR), Southern blotting, loss of heterozygosity (LOH), fluorescence in situ hybridization (FISH) based karyotyping, such as interphase FISH (iFISH) and multiple colour FISH in the form of multiplex FISH (M-FISH), spectral karyotyping (SKY) and combinatorial binary ratio labeling (COBRA)-FISH, as well as comparative genome hybridization (CGH) and array-based CGH (aCGH). These molecular approaches, although useful, include several limitations; consequently they have been routinely employed in a complementary fashion to accurately detect genetic abnormalities.

Conventional Cytogenetics

Conventional cytogenetic analysis initially identified changes in chromosome number [2]. It has enabled the description of the majority of recurrent cytogenetic abnormalities identified in childhood ALL. However, there are several limitations associated with the poor *in vitro* growth of leukemic cells and insufficient chromosome morphology in this disease, which might prevent a reliable characterization of chromosomal breakpoints [3, 4, 5].

RT-PCR & RQ-PCR

PCR analysis is considered extremely sensitive with ablity to detect one leukemic cell in 10^5-10^6 normal bone marrow cells [6]. The identification of chromosomal aberrations is complemented by RT-PCR analysis of molecular equivalents of structural chromosomal aberrations [4]. There have been established RT-PCR procedures and primer sets for the reliable detection of well defined chromosomal aberrations [6]. RQ-PCR is able to quantify a PCR product and confirm the presence and number of copies in a sample. It is generally based on the detection of fluorescent dyes or fluorescence tagged DNA probes [1]. RQ-PCR is extremely sensitive in identifying rare abnormal cells and in achieving results in a short time. One disadvantage relies on the fact that this technique is specific for only one individual genetic rearrangement and subsequently numerous RQ-PCR reactions are necessitated to effectively screen all ALL-associated rearrangements [7]. In addition, with the usage of RQ-PCR technique, information on genetic abnormalities in transcriptionally inactive cells cannot be obtained [3,6].

Southern Blotting

Southern blotting allows genetic rearrangements to be identified in a malignant tissue. This technique is no longer extensively used in clinical diagnostic laboratories for the identification of cytogenetic abnormalities. The majority of earlier analyses were based on Southern blotting, which although proved to be reliable, it can be laborious and requires large amounts of patients' samples, which are not always available [8]. In general, RT-PCR is considered 400-4000 times more sensitive than Southern blotting [6].

FISH

FISH is considered a high valuable technique for the analysis of chromosomal rearrangements due to its elevated sensitivity, rapidity, specificity and most importantly due to its potential to simultaneously detect multiple target regions [3]. However, FISH analysis is limited to the genomic regions covered by the probes, therefore deletions not covering these specific regions remain undetected. Regarding the metaphase FISH, it allows visualization of addition or deletion of chromosomal material as well as the position of the probe in the genome. Nonetheless, frequently the number of the malignant metaphases is insufficient to allow a proper evaluation of the chromosomal changes [5]. As far as it concerns the iFISH, it enables the analysis of samples that may fail conventional cytogenetics due to lack of metaphases [9]. iFISH is usually the method of choice for the quick detection of specific numerical aberrations, gene rearrangements, deletions and amplifications [5,7,10] In general, iFISH is considered robust and easy to perform, requiring only smears from diagnostic bone marrow samples with small demands in their storage [10].

Multicolor Whole Chromosome Painting (M-FISH, SKY and COBRA-FISH)

Multicolor FISH offers the ability to identify several targets simultaneously using different colors. The application of multicolor FISH techniques has highlighted a number of novel chromosomal abnormalities and elucidated complex karyotypes. The major multicolor FISH techniques include M-FISH and SKY, which use degenerate oligonucleotide PCR amplification of flow sorted chromosomes and a combinational labeling approach [9]. These procedures are based on the hybridization of 24 differentially labeled human chromosome painting probes, which allow simultaneous identification of the 22 pairs of autosomes and the sex chromosomes each in a different color in a single metaphase [6]. More specifically, the M-FISH captures the separate fluorochrome images for each of the five fluorochromes using specifically selected narrow bandpass filter sets, whereas SKY uses a single exposure of the image and a combination of cooled charge coupled device imaging and Fourier transform spectrometry to analyze the spectral signature of the fluorochrome combinations. An additional multicolor FISH technique affords the COBRA-FISH, which utilizes both combinatorial and ratio labeling achieving 24 colors using four fluorochromes [9, 11].

CGH and aCGH

CGH is considered a valuable tool for the assessment of chromosomal imbalances. It provides genome-wide screening for copy number changes without preliminary knowledge of the chromosomal aberrations [4]. More specifically, CGH determines the copy number gains and losses between two samples, by competitively hybridizing differentially labeled DNA to metaphase chromosomes [12]. However, CGH to metaphase chromosomes can provide a limited resolution of 3-10 Mb for detection of copy number losses and gains and 2Mb for amplifications [4, 13]. Arrays based CGH can be applied to both detection and mapping of amplified genes and homozygous deletions when chromosomal targets are placed by arrays consisting of genomic clones or cosmids that have been spotted onto glass microscope slides using robotic devices. In general, there technical limitations to both CGH and aCGH, notable that they identify cases where the affected area of the chromosome is very small and that they have limited sensitivity for the detection of aberrations present in a low percentage of cells, respectively [14, 15]. Of note, when aCGH is employed in combination with iFISH, approximately 90% of the most common balanced rearrangements can be identified in pediatric ALL patients [10].

LOH

LOH is considered a tedious and time-consuming screening method in cases where there is no preliminary knowledge available. It cannot identify gains of chromosome material including hyperdiploid karyotypes, which have a prognostic significance in pediatric ALL cases [4].

Numerical Chromosomal Abnormalities

Numerical abnormalities may involve the whole chromosome set, resulting in ploidy changes, or the gain or loss of individual chromosomes (aneuploidy) [2]. It should be noted that ploidy is generally considered an imperative prognostic factor in childhood ALL [16].

High Hyperdiploidy

High hyperdiploidy (51-67 chromosomes or DNA index >1.16) is considered the largest cytogenetic subgroup in B-cell childhood ALL comprising 25-30% of pediatric B-cell ALL cases, whereas it is rarely seen in T-cell ALL [17-18]. Normally, these children have favorable outcome with an event free survival (EFS) of >80% at five years [19]. However, an inferior outcome has been related to the subgroup with 51-55 chromosomes with an EFS of 72% at five years, when compared to the subgroup with 56-67 chromosomes; EFS of 86% at 5 years [6].

The normal karyotypic feature of high hyperdiploidy is a non-random pattern of chromosomal gains, with chromosomes 4, 6, 10, 14, 17, 18, 21 and X resulting in certain trisomies or tetrasomies with specific prognosis [12, 20]. For instance, the gain of chromosomes 4 and 10 as well as 6 and 17 has been linked to a favorable prognosis, whereas the gain of chromosome 5 and isochromosome 17 has been associated with inferior prognosis in these patients [19]. Regarding trisomies and tetrasomies, they occur rarely at a prevalence of 1-1.5% of total pediatric ALL cases. Near-tetraploid patients frequently exhibit a T-cell phenotype and have been associated with an inferior prognosis, whereas the presence of certain trisomies and younger age (1-10 years) have been associated with a more favorable outcome [18, 20]. Moreover, approximately 50% of the high hyperdiploid ALL cases harbor structural chromosomal aberrations in addition to the chromosomal gains [17]. These patients tend to present several factors associated with favorable prognosis, including age between 2 and 10 years, leukocyte count <10 000 x 10^6/l, L1 morphology and an early pre-B phenotype (CD10$^+$) [22]. Conventional cytogenetics, CGH, FISH-based and SKY analyses provide reliable detection of high hyperdiploidy in childhood ALL cases [3,5,9].

Low hyperdiploidy is distinct from high hyperdiploidy both regarding the chromosome pattern and clinical features. Structural abnormalities occur in approximately 75% of cases pediatric ALL cases [5]. Low hyperdiploid ALL (47-50 chromosomes) is usually associated with older patient age and short survival times [23]. The iFISH technique is being used for the detection of low hypediploid cases [5].

Hypodiploidy

Karyotypes with <46 chromosomes are classified as hypodiploid and are found in approximately 7% of pediatric ALL cases [5, 22]. Children with hypodiploidy are associated with an inferior outcome. The vast majority of patients bear 45 chromosomes and are characterized by an intermediate outcome [5, 19]. However, this group of patients has a more favorable outcome compared to patients with fewer than 45 chromosomes, which is quite uncommon [6, 16]. More specifically, clones with 33-44 chromosomes occur rarely in childhood ALL accounting for <1% cases and are linked to an overall poorer prognosis [6]. The iFISH technique has proved valuable for the detection of hypodipolid clones [5].

Near Haploidy

Near haploidy defines a karyotype of 23-29 chromosomes. It is considered a rare hypodiploid subgroup in ALL with a prevalence of 0.7-2.4% [19]. Near haploidy is considered similar to high hyperdiploidy in that a specific pattern of numerical changes can be seen with the majority of cases retaining disomies for 14, 18, 21 and X/Y [24]. It is frequently associated with particularly dismal prognosis and a median survival of eleven months [18, 25]. Near haploidy is readily identified by conventional cytogenetics or iFISH [9].

Pseudodiploidy and Diploidy

Pseudodiploid ALL has a modal number of 46 chromosomes; however the leukemia cell has numeric and/or structural rearrangements. It has a reported incidence of 40% [26]. The clinical outcome is dependent on specific structural chromosomal abnormalities however it is normally associated with an intermediate prognosis [5, 26]. Both, FISH and SKY techniques have proved extremely informative and sensitive for the identification of this numerical chromosomal aberration [5].

Diploid ALL occurs in 10-15% of pediatric ALL cases and is associated with an intermediate prognosis. On average, in diploid ALL, no additional chromosomal abnormalities are apparent (26. Normally FISH studies using two different probes are employed to distinguish between diploid and aneuploid clones; nevertheless using automated four-color i-FISH allows the identification of additional clonal populations and high heterogeneity [27].

Structural Chromosomal Abnormalities

Structural abnormalities include translocations, deletions, insertions and inversions (Figure 1). They may be balanced or unbalanced in form with unbalanced rearrangements leading to changes in the copy number [2]. The most established chromosomal abnormalities are discussed.

BCR/ABL

A significant abnormality in childhood ALL is the reciprocal translocation between chromosomes 9 and 22, t(9;22)(q43;q11), which results in the formation of Philadelphia chromosome (Ph). This translocation gives rise to the *BCR/ABL* hybrid gene resulting from joining of 3' sequences of the tyrosine kinase *ABL* proto-oncogene on chromosome 9 to the 5' sequences of the *BCR* gene on chromosome 22 [6].

The Ph$^+$ occurs in children with an incidence <5%, which is slightly increased in adolescence and young adulthood [28] Due to the two different breakpoint cluster regions in the *BCR* gene, 'minor' (m-bcr) and 'major' (M-bcr), this fusion gene encodes p190kDa protein or p210 kDa protein, respectively [29]. The m-bcr occurs in over 90% of Ph positive pediatric ALL cases [5, 23], whereas M-bcr can be met in the minority of children with ALL [19].

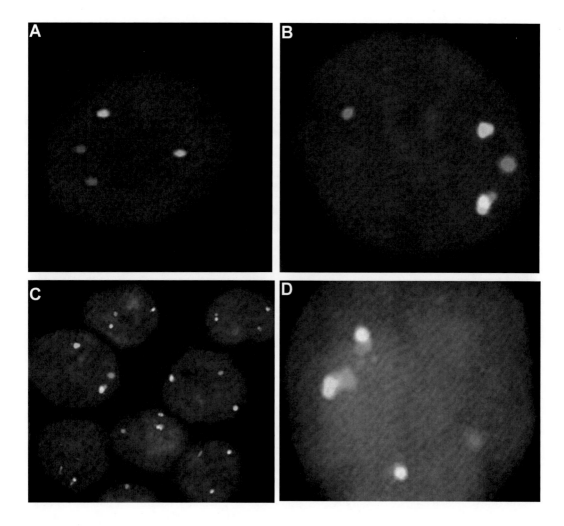

Figure 1. FISH studies representing A; Normal nuclei, B; *ETV6/RUNX1*, C; *MLL* gene rearrangement, D; *BCR/ABL*.

The Ph$^+$ exhibits predominantly an early B cell phenotype. Clinically, patients are older than 10 years, have elevated leukocyte counts and frequently suffer from central nervous system (CNS) disease [22]. Even in the era of intensive chemotherapy, the presence of Ph$^+$ chromosome has been linked to an inferior outcome in pediatric ALL, with EFS of 15% at five years and an elevated risk of relapse [6, 30, 31]. Allogeneic bone marrow transplantation is considered a curative therapy for this group of patients [19].

Approximately 95% of Ph positive ALL cases are detectable using chromosome banding, however due to the presence of potential cryptic rearrangements, which might be overlooked, iFISH, RT-PCR or RQ-PCR analyses can also be employed [1, 3, 7, 19]. Of note, when RT-PCR techniques are employed, the frequency of this rearrangement is higher than with conventional cytogenetic testing [32].

Mixed Lineage Leukemia (*MLL*) Gene Rearrangements

The gene is called *MLL* because it is altered in both myeloid and lymphoid leukemic cells and in an elevated proportion of mixed lineage leukemia, which suggests origin from a stem cell or early progenitor cell [5].

Infants much more frequently harbor rearrangements involving the *MLL* gene (chromosome 11q23), at a frequency of 40-50%. More specifically, detectable *MLL* gene rearrangements are more prevalent in younger infants; ~90% of infants <6 months old at diagnosis compared to 30-50% of infants aged 6-12 months [33]. This group of infants are usually characterized by a pro-B immunophenotype (CD19$^+$, CD10$^-$), an elevated number of leukocytes and CNS involvement [19]. *MLL* plays a key role in hematopoiesis by regulating the *HOX* group of genes, which sequentially influence hematopoietic stem cell renewal and leukemogenesis [30]. Prognosis of *MLL* rearranged ALL differs by age [18]. More specifically, infants harboring *MLL* rearrangements have been associated with a particularly inferior prognosis with long-term EFS rates of 10-30%, when compared to other children diagnosed with acute leukemia [18, 34]. The overall survival at five years remains 40-50% [34]. The type of partner gene fused to *MLL* does not influence the clinical outcome [30].

The *AF-4* gene at 4q21 is fused to *MLL* in [4;11]. The incidence of the *MLL/AF4* t(4;11)(q21;q23) fusion gene among pediatric ALL patients is approximately 2-6%, whereas in infants it is regarded as the most common translocation comprising 70% of *MLL* rearranged cases [29, 33]. Another abnormality seen at a frequency of ~15% of infant cases and in <1% of pediatric ALL cases is t(11;19)(q23;p13.3), which fuses *MLL* to *ENL* gene. Importantly, this abnormality is occurring in ~4% of infant cases [33]. There are additional well defined chromosomal abnormalities involving *MLL*, such as t(6;11)(q27;q23), in which *MLL* is fused to the *AF6* and t(10;11)(p12;q23), in which the *MLL* is fused to the *AF10* [19].

The subtle translocations including t(6;11) and t(11;19) or the rare and cryptic abnormalities may be difficult to be identified by cytogenetics alone [19]. The *MLL/AF4* fusion transcripts are detectable by RT-PCR, which is especially useful in tracking minimal residual disease (MRD) [3, 22, 33]. The majority of *MLL* gene rearrangements can be detected using Southern blotting, however, application of this technique with cytogenetics and iFISH in a complementary fashion, comprises the most sensitive approach for the accurate identification of the *MLL* status [3, 9, 19, 22, 33]. An alternative approach might comprise the uses of FISH for the rapid screening of *MLL* rearrangements and of Southern blotting for a definitive assessment of the *MLL* gene status [35].

ETV6/RUNX1

The *TEL/AML1* also known as *ETV6/RUNX1* is considered the most common translocation in childhood ALL with a prevalence of 20-25% [29]. The t(12;21)(p13;q22), involves the ETS type variant 6 (*ETV6*) or translocated ETS leukemia (*TEL*) gene on 12p13 and the *RUNX1* gene (*AML1;* acute myeloid leukaemia 1) on 21q22 [22, 36]. Patients harboring this translocation are usually between 1 to 10 years and have a B-cell phenotype, but no bad prognostic markers including high leukocyte counts, CNS involvement or hepatosplenomegaly [5]. In addition, *ETV6/RUNX1* is not found in patients with hyperdiploidy [18]. Nevertheless, it has been previously suggested that *ETV6/RUNX1* and hyperdiploid ALL share a lot in common [37]. In this context, at the mRNA level, overlapping gene expression profiles (*miR*-126/126, *miR*-151 and *miR*-545) can be detected supporting the above statement. Understanding miRNA expression levels in different genetic ALL subgroups may provide additional information regarding the biology of the underlying genetic abnormalities [38].

Regarding the prognostic significance of *TEL/AML1* fusion gene, several studies have provided divergent results. Prognostic outcome of patients' with *TEL/AML1* is regarded favourable, since 90% of children remain relapse free, though, there are reports suggesting that late relapses may occur [19, 29, 39-41].

This translocation is invisible with chromosome banding analysis [1, 7, 9, 19]. It is frequently identified using FISH, which shows the fusion of *ETV6* and *RUNX1*), RT-PCR, which detects *ETV6/RUNX1* transcripts, or RQ-PCR analyses [1, 3, 7, 9, 19, 36]. In addition, the SKY technique could be useful, since although it cannot identify specifically the der 21 of the *ETV6/RUNX1* translocation, it can still identify additional chromosomal changes [5].

TCF3/PBX1 or *E2A/PBX1*

The t(1;19)(q23;p13) characterizes 25% of pediatric precursor B-lineage ALL patients and can be either balanced t(1;19) or unbalanced der(19)t(1;19)(q23;p13) with two normal chromosomes [1, 23]. Of note, occasional cases with co-existing t(1;19) and der(19) positive clones have been previously described and have been associated with inferior prognosis [19, 24]. The more frequent form met in children is the unbalanced form, which has been linked to a significantly more favorable outcome [19].

Translocation (1;19) results in fusion of the *TCF3* (or *E2A*) gene at 19p13 with the *PBX1* gene at 1q23, As a result of the *TCF3/PBX1* or *E2A/PBX1* fusion, a chimeric transcription factor is produced [5]. The *TCF3/PBX1* fusion causes abnormal activation and truncation of the *PBX*1 (homeobox gene), leads to trans-activation of several genes and generates a malignant cell phenotype [42]. This fusion is detected in children 10 years or older and in B-

ALL. Regarding outcome, the prognosis still remains controversial and unclear, however is substantially improved with intensive therapeutic regimens [5, 29]. Reliable identification of both balanced and unbalanced forms of t(1;19) and additional rearrangements involving *TCF3* can be succeeded by RT-PCR and FISH methods [19].

Additional Recurrent Cytogenetic Abnormalities

HOX11L2

A cryptic t(5;14)(q35;q32) is prevalent is approximately 20-30% of children and adolescents with T-ALL [23]. This translocation leads to the ectopic expression of HOX11Like2, an orphan homeobox gene, *HOX11L2* (5q35), as a consequence of the abnormal control of the gene by *CPT12*, which is located at 14q32 and is highly expressed during T-lymphoid differentiation. The finding of this translocation has confirmed Hox11 family member activation as an imperative pathway in T-ALL leukemogenesis [19]. Translocation (5;14) and/or *HOX11L2* ectopic expression have been associated with inferior outcome in pediatric patients with T-ALL [43]. The M-FISH has been successfully used as a diagnostic tool of this rearrangement [12].

NUP98-RAP1GDS1

The translocation (4;11)(q21;p15.5) is a rare abnormality frequently associated with del(12p) and specific for a subset of T-ALL originating from an early progenitor, which has the potential to express T-cell antigens [44]. The rearrangement fuses the nucleoporin 98 (*NUP98*) gene at 11p15 with *RAP1GDS1* gene at 4q21 to encode the *NUP98-RAP1GDS1* fusion transcript abbreviated as NRG. It has been associated with worse clinical outcomes [23, 45].

6q Deletions

Abnormalities of the long arm of chromosome 6 (6q) have been identified in 11% of pediatric ALL cases, with the vast majority of them being deletions from 6q15 to 6q21 and comprising 4-13% of children with ALL [22, 46]. Importantly, approximately 5% of high hyperdiploid cases harbor deletions involving the long arm of chromosome 6 [17]. The clinical outcome of this particular abnormality is similar to all other ALL pediatric cases. Regarding diagnostic methods, conventional cytogenetics is not considered sensitive to detect the frequency and region of small interstitial deletions. Alternatively, LOH analysis with microsatellite markers on chromosome 6 using PCR has proved valuable [46-47].

9p Abnormalities

Cytogenetic abnormalities of the short arm of the chromosome 9 (9p) are observed in approximately 7-12% of childhood ALL cases [22]. Most of the 9p abnormalities result in a deletion of this arm, which usually includes cell cycle regulatory genes, mainly the p16 *INK4* [19]. LOH of 9p have been found in 40% of patients, whereas deletions of *CDKN2/INK4A/p16* gene in approximately 75% of T-ALL and 15% of pre-B ALL [46]. FISH affords the reliable method of choice in approximately 80% of childhood T-ALL and 20% of pre-B ALL.

Conclusion

Cytogenetic analyses have been extensively performed for the identification of recurrent chromosomal translocations and deletions. Both structural and numerical cytogenetic abnormalities have proved exceptionally reliable diagnostic and prognostic parameters highly associated with individualized therapeutic advances. Nonetheless, the prognostic significance of less frequent recurrent aberrations in pediatric ALL remains to be established. Consequently, there is a constant need for high throughput complementing molecular-cytogenetic strategies to define conclusively the impact of pediatric ALL-relevant chromosomal aberrations on patients' remission rates and survival.

References

[1] Bacher U, Schnittger S, Haferlach C, et al. Molecular diagnostics in acute leukemias. *Clin Chem Lab Med.* 2009;47:1333-1341.
[2] Harrison CJ. Cytogenetics of paediatric and adolescent acute lymphoblastic leukaemia.*Br J Haematol.* 2009 Jan;144:147-156.
[3] Avet-Loiseau H. Fish analysis at diagnosis in acute lymphoblastic leukemia. *Leuk Lymphoma.* 1999;33:441-449.
[4] Scholz I, Popp S, Granzow M. et al. Comparative genomic hybridization in childhood acute lymphoblastic leukemia: correlation with interphase cytogenetics and loss of heterozygosity analysis. *Cancer Genet Cytogenet.* 2001;124:89-97.
[5] Nordgren A. Hidden aberrations diagnosed by interphase fluorescence in situ hybridisation and spectral karyotyping in childhood acute lymphoblastic leukaemia.*Leuk Lymphoma.* 2003; 44:2039-2053.
[6] Harrison CJ. The detection and significance of chromosomal abnormalities in childhood acute lymphoblastic leukaemia.Blood Rev. 2001; 15:49-59.
[7] Olde Nordkamp L, Mellink C, van der Schoot E, et al. Karyotyping, FISH, and PCR in acute lymphoblastic leukemia: competing or complementary diagnostics? J Pediatr Hematol Oncol. 2009; 31:930-935.
[8] Kuchinskaya E, Heyman M, Nordgren A, et al. Interphase fluorescent in situ hybridization deletion analysis of the 9p21 region and prognosis in childhood acute

lymphoblastic leukaemia (ALL): results from a prospective analysis of 519 Nordic patients treated according to the NOPHO-ALL 2000 protocol. *Br J Haematol.* 2011;152:615-622

[9] Kearney L. Molecular Cytogenetics. *Best Pract Res Clin Haematol.* 2001;14:645-669.

[10] Kuchinskaya E, Heyman M, Nordgren A, et al. Array-CGH reveals hidden gene dose changes in children with acute lymphoblastic leukaemia and a normal or failed karyotype by G-banding. *Br J Haematol.* 2008;140:572-577.

[11] Hélias C, Leymarie V, Entz-Werle N, et al. Translocation t(5;14)(q35;q32) in three cases of childhood T cell acute lymphoblastic leukemia: a new recurring and cryptic abnormality. *Leukemia.* 2002 J;16:7-12.

[12] Kearney L, Horsley SW. Molecular cytogenetics in haematological malignancy: current technology and future prospects. *Chromosoma.* 2005; 114: 286-294.

[13] Inazawa J, Inoue J, Imoto I. Comparative genomic hybridization (CGH)-arrays pave the way for identification of novel cancer-related genes.*Cancer Sci.* 2004; 95: 559-563.

[14] Hanlon K, Ellard S, Rudin CE, et al. Evaluation of 13q14 status in patients with chronic lymphocytic leukemia using single nucleotide polymorphism-based techniques. *J Mol Diagn.* 2009 ;11:298-305.

[15] Hanlon K, Harries LW, Ellard S, Rudin CE. Evaluation of 13q14 status in multiple myeloma by digital single nucleotide polymorphism technology. *J Mol Diagn.* 2009;11: 450-457.

[16] Nachman JB, Heerema NA, Sather H, et al. Outcome of treatment in children with hypodiploid acute lymphoblastic leukemia. *Blood.* 2007;110:1112-1115.

[17] Paulsson K, Johansson B. High hyperdiploid childhood acute lymphoblastic leukemia. *Genes Chromosomes Cancer.* 2009; 48:637-660.

[18] Vrooman LM, Silverman LB. Childhood acute lymphoblastic leukemia: update on prognostic factors. *Curr Opin Pediatr.* 2009; 21:1-8.

[19] Harrison CJ, Foroni L. Cytogenetics and molecular genetics of acute lymphoblastic leukemia. *Rev Clin Exp Hematol.* 2002; 6: 91-113.

[20] Paulsson K, Horvat A, Strömbeck B, et al. Mutations of FLT3, NRAS, KRAS, and PTPN11 are frequent and possibly mutually exclusive in high hyperdiploid childhood acute lymphoblastic leukemia. *Genes Chromosomes Cancer.* 2008;47:26-33.

[21] Oláh E, Balogh E, Kajtár P, et al. Diagnostic and prognostic significance of chromosome abnormalities in childhood acute lymphoblastic leukemia. *Ann N Y Acad Sci.* 1997; 824:8-27.

[22] Martinez-Climent JA. Molecular cytogenetics of childhood hematological malignancies. *Leukemia.* 1997;11:1999-2021.

[23] Mrózek K, Heerema NA, Bloomfield CD. Cytogenetics in acute leukemia. *Blood Rev.* 2004 ;18: 115-36.

[24] Paulsson K, Horvat A, Fioretos T, et al. Formation of der(19)t(1;19)(q23;p13) in acute lymphoblastic leukemia. *Genes Chromosomes Cancer.* 2005 ;42:144-148.

[25] Gibbons B, MacCallum P, Watts E. et al. Near haploid acute lymphoblastic leukemia: seven new cases and a review of the literature. *Leukemia.* 1991; 5:738-743.

[26] Mandrell BN. The genetic profile and monitoring of acute lymphoblastic leukemia in children and adolescents. *J Pediatr Nurs.* 2009; 24:173-178.

[27] Talamo A, Chalandon Y, Marazzi A, et al. Clonal heterogeneity and chromosomal instability at disease presentation in high hyperdiploid acute lymphoblastic leukemia. *Cancer Genet Cytogenet.* 2010;203:209-214.
[28] Ravandi F, Kebriaei P. Philadelphia chromosome-positive acute lymphoblastic leukemia. *Hematol Oncol Clin North Am.* 2009 ;23:1043-63
[29] Lazic J, Tosic N, Dokmanovic L, et al. Clinical features of the most common fusion genes in childhood acute lymphoblastic leukemia. *Med Oncol.* 2010;27:449-453.
[30] Bhojwani D, Howard SC, Pui CH. High-risk childhood acute lymphoblastic leukemia. *Clin Lymphoma Myeloma.* 2009;9 Suppl 3:S222-30.
[31] Katsibardi K., Braoudaki M., Papadhimitriou S.I, et al. Duplication of Philadelphia chromosome and trisomy in a case of childhood acute lymphoblastic leukemia. *Medical Oncology* 2010 (Epub ahead of print)
[32] Milone JH, Enrico A. Treatment of Philadelphia chromosome-positive acute lymphoblastic leukemia. *Leuk Lymphoma.* 2009 ;50 Suppl 2:9-15.
[33] Silverman LB. Acute lymphoblastic leukemia in infancy. *Pediatr Blood Cancer.* 2007; 49 (7 Suppl):1070-1073.
[34] Emerenciano M, Koifman S, Pombo-de-Oliveira MS. Acute leukemia in early childhood. *Braz J Med Biol Res.* 2007; 47:749-760.
[35] Mathew S, Behm F, Dalton J, et al. Comparison of cytogenetics, Southern blotting, and fluorescence in situ hybridization as methods for detecting MLL gene rearrangements in children with acute leukemia and with 11q23 abnormalities. *Leukemia.* 1999;13:1713-1720.
[36] Alvarez Y, Gaitán S, Perez A. et al. ETV6/RUNX1 rearrangement in childhood B-precursor acute lymphoblastic leukemia with normal karyotypes or without cytogenetic results. *Cancer Genet Cytogenet.* 2004 1;152:77-80.
[37] Den Boer ML, van Slegtenhorst M, De Menezes RX. et al. A subtype of childhood acute lymphoblastic leukaemia with poor treatment outcome: a genome-wide classification study. *Lancet Oncol.* 2009 ;10:125-134.
[38] Schotte D, De Menezes RX, Moqadam FA, et al. MicroRNA characterize genetic diversity and drug resistance in pediatric acute lymphoblastic leukemia. *Haematologica.* 2011;96:703-711.
[39] Harbott J, Viehmann S, Borkhardt A, et al. Incidence of TEL/AML1 fusion gene analyzed consecutively in children with acute lymphoblastic leukemia in relapse.B*lood* 1997;90: 4933-4937.
[40] Woo HY, Kim DW, Park H, et al. Molecular cytogenetic analysis of gene rearrangements in childhood acute lymphoblastic leukemia. *J Korean Med Sci* 2005; 20: 36-41.
[41] Loh ML, Goldwasser MA, Silverman LB, et al. Prospective analysis of TEL/AML1-positive patients treated on Dana-Farber Cancer Institute Consortium Protocol 95-01. *Blood* 2006; 107: 4508-4513.
[42] Burmeister T, Gökbuget N, Schwartz S, et al. Clinical features and prognostic implications of TCF3-PBX1 and ETV6-RUNX1 in adult acute lymphoblastic leukemia. *Haematologica.* 2010; 95:241-246.

[43] Cavé H, Suciu S, Preudhomme C, et al. Clinical significance of HOX11L2 expression linked to t(5;14)(q35;q32), of HOX11 expression, and of SIL-TAL fusion in childhood T-cell malignancies: results of EORTC studies 58881 and 58951. *Blood.* 2004;103:442-450.

[44] Mecucci C, La Starza R, Negrini M, et al. t(4;11)(q21;p15) translocation involving NUP98 and RAP1GDS1 genes: characterization of a new subset of T acute lymphoblastic leukaemia. *Br J Haematol.* 2000;109:788-793.

[45] Hussey DJ, Nicola M, Moore S, et al. The (4;11)(q21;p15) translocation fuses the NUP98 and RAP1GDS1 genes and is recurrent in T-cell acute lymphocytic leukemia. *Blood.* 1999; 94:2072-2079.

[46] Takeuchi S, Koike M, Seriu T, et al. Frequent loss of heterozygosity on the long arm of chromosome 6: identification of two distinct regions of deletion in childhood acute lymphoblastic leukemia. *Cancer Res.* 1998 ;58:2618-2623.

[47] Merup M, Moreno TC, Heyman M, et al. 6q deletions in acute lymphoblastic leukemia and non-Hodgkin's lymphomas. *Blood.* 1998;91:3397-3400.

In: Acute Lymphoblastic Leukemia
Editors: Severo Vecchione and Luigi Tedesco

ISBN: 978-1-61470-872-8
©2012 Nova Science Publishers, Inc.

Chapter IX

Maintenance Therapy in Ph Negative Adult Acute Lymphoblastic Leukemia

Michael Doubek[*] *and Jiří Mayer*
Department of Internal Medicine – Hematology/Oncology
University Hospital, Jihlavska 20, 62500 Brno, Czechia

Standard Maintenance

Maintenance therapy means long-term administration of low-dose chemotherapy or other drugs. Despite extensive study involving many types of leukemia, maintenance therapy has clinically proven efficacy for only two diseases: acute lymphoblastic leukemia (ALL) and acute promyelocytic leukemia (APL).

This section focuses on maintenance therapy in Ph negative ALL. Maintenance therapy in Ph positive ALL is discussed in a separate section.

Current Practice

With the exception of patients with mature B-cell ALL, long-term maintenance therapy, adapted from its successful use in pediatric ALL, is generally given in adult ALL for one to three years, with a backbone of daily 6-mercaptopurine (MP) and weekly methothrexate (MTX). The use of maintenance therapy primarily in pediatric ALL dates back to the 1970's. [1,2] Unlike other components of therapy for adult ALL, no randomized study demonstrating the benefits of maintenance therapy exists; however, attempts at omitting maintenance therapy have often resulted in an inferior outcome with leukemia-free survival (LFS) rates of

---

[*] E-mail: mdoubek@fnbrno.cz.

18-28% when compared to historical controls. [3,4,5] It is possible that long-term drug exposure of the host immune system is needed to kill residual, slowly dividing leukemic cells (minimal residual disease, MRD), to suppress their growth, allowing programmed cell death to occur, or to induce leukemia progenitor differentiation. [6]

Drugs for Maintenance Therapy

As mentioned before, MP given orally and MTX given intravenously (I.V.), intramuscularly (I.M.) or orally (P.O.) are the main drugs used in maintenance therapy. Nevertheless, some groups include anthracyclines and additional medication (Table 1). The POMP regimen (MP, MTX, prednisone [P], vincristine [V] in various P.O. or I.V. schemes) is the most common combination. [7,8,9,10] There is no clear evidence that either I.V. or oral administration of MTX is to be preferred although the intravenous route may overcome compliance problems and could be better than oral MTX. [11] Attempts for intensification by I.V. application of higher doses of MP did not increase efficacy in adults. [12] In childhood ALL, several randomized studies have shown that thioguanine (TG) offers no advantage over MP in maintenance. [13] Although TG confers a significantly lower risk of isolated CNS relapse than MP, the benefit is offset by an increased risk of death in remission, mainly due to infections during continuing therapy and veno-occlusive disease of the liver. [14] For unknown reasons, MP is more effective in children when administered in the evening than in the morning. It should not be given with milk or milk products that contain xanthine oxidase, which can degrade the drug. [15] The preliminary results of MP liver toxicity do not prove but suggest that MTHFR 677C/T and RFC1 80G/A polymorphisms may serve as predictors of increased toxicity during maintenance chemotherapy with MP. [16]

Role of Intensification of Maintenance

Some groups prolong maintenance therapy beyond conventional 2 years of the total treatment duration. In children, a meta-analysis of 42 trials showed that both prolonged maintenance therapy (3 years versus 2 years), as well as the use of pulses with vincristine and glucocorticoid, result in increased rates of death in remission but also in lower relapse rates. [17] On the other hand, although shortening maintenance therapy in children to 12 months increases the relapse rates, it still allows cure in two thirds of patients. Unfortunately, it is currently not clear how to identify those patients for whom the shortened maintenance therapy would be sufficient. [18] The most important factor reducing relapses and improving survival was the use of reinduction course at the start of maintenance. When such an intensive reinduction course is given before the start of maintenance, neither a longer maintenance nor the use of vincristine/glucocorticoid pulses contribute significantly to a better overall survival in pediatric patients. [18]

In children, randomized trials failed to demonstrate any advantage of intensified maintenance with high-dose cycles. [3,17] However, only a few patients actually received these regimens as scheduled; adults often show poor compliance to intensive maintenance due to toxicities and for social reasons. [3,19] A randomized trial failed to prove any effect of maintenance therapy with increased intensity on disease-free survival compared to the conventional POMP maintenance. [19] The use of dexamethasone instead of P in maintenance therapy may lead to an increased incidence of infectious deaths. [20] Therefore, maintenance with less intensive reinforcements may be more feasible. It is still open whether and to what extent maintenance therapy is necessary in ALL subgroups. Patients with mature B-ALL do not require maintenance. In T-ALL with relapses up to 2½ years, it may be less important than in B-precursor ALL, with relapses up to 5 years. [21]

Table 1. Types of maintenance therapy in adult ALL treatment and long-term outcomes of therapy

Group	N (patients)	Maintenance	LFS
PETHEMA ALL-89 [8]	108	MP, MTX (V, P, Mi, A, C, VM, AC)	41% at 4y
CALGB 9111 [7]	198	MP, MTX, V, P	36% at 3y
MRC/ECOG E2993 [27]	920	MP, MTX, V, P	-
MDACC [9]	204	MP, MTX, V, P	38% at 5y
GMALL 05/93 [28]	1163	MP, MTX	42% at 5y
GIMEMA 0288 [19]	794 (*Arm I:* 201; *Arm II:* 187)	*Arm I:* MP, MTX, V, P *Arm II:* MP, MTX, V, P (C, AC, DNR, VM, Mi)	*Arm I:* 38% at 8y *Arm II:* 37% at 8y (p=0.171)
JALSG-ALL93 [29]	263 (maintenance in 127)	MP, MTX (P, V, DOX, E, AC, ASP, Mi)	30% at 6y
EORTC ALL3 [10]	340 (67 in chemotherapy arm)	MP, MTX, V, P	37% at 6y
LALA94 [30]	922 (59 high-risk patients in chemotherapy arm)	MP, MTX	30% at 5y
PETHEMA ALL-93 [31]	222 (48 in chemotherapy arm)	MP, MTX	50% at 5y
MRC XII/ECOG [32]	1929 (227 in chemotherapy arm)	Unspecified	46% at 5y

A study of large groups for adult ALL for the last 10 years. LFS – leukemia free survival. A - asparaginase; AC - cytarabine; ASP – L-asparaginase; C - cyclophosphamide; DNR - daunorubicine; DOX - doxorubicine; DX - dexamethasone; E - etoposide; Mi - mitoxantrone; MP – 6-mercaptopurine; MTX - methothrexate; P - prednisone; V - vincristine; VM – teniposide.

Table 2. Recommendations for maintenance therapy in Ph negative acute lymphoblastic leukemia (ALL)

	Recommendation	Level of evidence	Comment
Maintenance therapy	Recommended	A II	No randomized trial maintenance vs. no maintenance in adults. Maintenance not necessary after allogeneic HSCT and in mature B ALL.
Maintenance therapy after autologous HSCT	Recommended	B II-III	
Intensity of maintenance	Low intensity maintenance is comparable with high intensity maintenance	B I	MP and MTX (event. plus V and P) are main drugs for maintenance
Length of maintenance	2 years of total treatment duration comparable with longer administration	B II	Studies in children
MRD evaluation during maintenance	Recommended	B II	Conversion to MRD positivity during maintenance therapy is predictive of subsequent hematologic relapse

HSCT – hematopoietic stem cell transplantation; MP – 6-mercaptopurine; MRD – minimal residual disease; MTX – methothrexate.

Strength of recommendations:
- A – Strong evidence for efficacy and substantial clinical benefit. Strongly recommended.
- B – Strong or moderate evidence for efficacy, but only limited clinical benefit. Generally recommended.
- C – Insufficient evidence for efficacy, or efficacy does not outweigh possible adverse consequences (for example drug toxicity). Optional.
- D – Moderate evidence against efficacy of for adverse outcome. Generally not recommended.
- E – Strong evidence against efficacy or of adverse outcome. Never recommended.

Quality of evidence:
- I – Evidence from at least one well-executed randomized trial.
- II – Evidence from at least one well-designed clinical trial without randomization, cohort or case controlled analytic studies, or dramatic results from uncontrolled experiments.
- III – Evidence from opinions of respected authorities based on clinical experience, descriptive studies, or reports from expert committees.

Maintenance Therapy after Autologous Hematopoietic Stem Cell Transplantation (autoHSCT)

Although the role of maintenance therapy after autoHSCT has not been studied in any randomized trial, studies describing a positive effect of maintenance (MP + MTX or POMP administered for 2 years) after autoHSCT have been published. This method can provide 7-year probabilities of disease-free survival and overall survival up to 45% and 48%, respectively. [22,23,24,25] However, other groups so far have not confirmed these results. Other medication, such as interleukin-2, does not seem to have any positive effect after autoHSCT. [3]

MRD-evaluation for Decision Making

According to the majority of current European protocols only patients who are MRD negative after induction-consolidation therapy are referred for maintenance, while the remaining ones used to be offered HSCT. However, even for patients with undetectable MRD before start of the maintenance, the risk of subsequent relapse is as high as 30%. [26] As demonstrated by Raff et al. conversion to MRD positivity during maintenance therapy is highly predictive of hematologic relapse and the median interval between the two events is 9.5 months. Therefore it appears that patients treated with maintenance should regularly be monitored the level of MRD and introduced more intensive therapy, possibly HSCT, in case of MRD-positivity. The time-points at which MRD should be monitored in the course of maintenance remain to be established.

Recommendation for Maintenance in Ph- ALL

Recommendations are summarized in Table 2.

References

[1] Willemze R, Hillen H, Hartgrink-Groeneveld CA, Haanen C. Treatment of acute lymphoblastic leukemia in adolescents and adults: A retrospective study of 41 patients (1970-1973). *Blood.* 1975;46:823-834.

[2] Seshadri R, Turner DR. Is maintenance therapy necessary for acute lymphoblastic leukaemia? *Lancet.* 1986;2(8504):452-453.

[3] Hoelzer D, Gökbuget N. New approaches in acute lymphoblastic leukemia in adults. Where do we go? *Semin Oncol.* 2000;27:540-559.

[4] Ellison RR, Mick R, Cuttner J, et al. The effects of postinduction intensification treatment with cytarabine and daunorubicin in adult acute lymphocytic leukemia: a prospective randomized clinical trial by Cancer and Leukemia Group B. *J Clin Oncol.* 1991;9:2002-2015.

[5] Dekker AW, van't Veer MB, Sizoo W, et al. Intensive postremission chemotherapy without maintenance therapy in adults with acute lymphoblastic leukemia. *J Clin Oncol.* 1997;15:476-482.

[6] Lin TL, Vala MS, Barber JP, et al. Induction of acute lymphocytic leukemia differentiation by maintenance therapy. *Leukemia.* 2007;21:1915-1920.

[7] Larson RA, Dodge RK, Linker CA, et al. A randomized controlled trial of filgrastim during remission induction and consolidation chemotherapy for adults with acute lymphoblastic leukemia. CALGB study 9111. *Blood.* 1998;92:1556-1564.

[8] Ribera JM, Ortega JJ, Oriol A, et al. Late intensification chemotherapy has not improved the results of intensive chemotherapy in adult acute lymphoblastic leukemia. Results of a prospective multicenter randomized trial (PETHEMA ALL-89). *Haematologica.* 1998;83:222-230.

[9] Kantarjian HM, O´Brien S, Smith TL, et al. Results of treatment with hyper-CVAD, a dose-intensive regimen, in adult acute lymphocytic leukemia. *J Clin Oncol.* 2000;18:547-561.

[10] Labar B, Suciu S, Zittoun R, et al. Allogeneic stem cell transplantation in acute lymphoblastic leukemia and non-Hodgkin's lymphoma for patients ≤ 50 years old in first complete remission: results of the EORTC ALL-3 trial. *Haematologica.* 2004;89:809-817.

[11] Matloub Y, Bruce C, Bostrom MD, et al. Escalating Dose Intravenous Methotrexate without Leucovorin Rescue during Interim Maintenance Is Superior to Oral Methotrexate for Children with Standard Risk Acute Lymphoblastic Leukemia (SR-ALL): Children's Oncology Group Study 1991. *Blood.* 2008:112:Abstract #9.

[12] Kantarjian H, Thomas D, O'Brien S, et al. Long-term follow-up results of hyperfractionated cyclophosphamide, vincristine, doxorubicin, and dexamethasone (Hyper-CVAD), a dose-intensive regimen, in adult acute lymphocytic leukemia. *Cancer.* 2004;101:2788-2801.

[13] Harms DO, Göbel U, Spaar HJ, et al. Thioguanine offers no advantage over mercaptopurine in maintenance treatment of childhood ALL: results of the randomized trial COALL-92. *Blood.* 2003;102:2736-2740.

[14] Vora A, Mitchell CD, Lennard L, et al. Toxicity and efficacy of 6-thioguanine versus 6-mercaptopurine in childhood lymphoblastic leukaemia: a randomized trial. *Lancet.* 2006;368:1339-1348.

[15] Pui CH, Evans WE. Treatment of acute lymphoblastic leukemia. *N Engl J Med.* 2006;354:166-178.

[16] Shimasaki N, Mori T, Torii C, et al. Influence of MTHFR and RFC1 Polymorphisms on toxicities during maintenance chemotherapy for childhood acute lymphoblastic leukemia or lymphoma. *J Pediatr Hematol Oncol.* 2008;30:347-352.

[17] Richards S, Gray R, Peto R, et al. Duration and intensity of maintenance chemotherapy in acute lymphoblastic leukemia: overview of 42 trials involving 12000 randomized children. *Lancet.* 1996;347:1783-1788.

[18] Toyoda Y, Manabe A, Tsuchida M, et al. Six months of maintenance chemotherapy after intensified treatment for acute lymphoblastic leukemia of childhood. *J Clin Oncol.* 2000;18:1508-1516.

[19] Annino L, Vegna ML, Camera A, et al. Treatment of adult acute lymphoblastic leukemia (ALL): long-term follow-up of the GIMEMA ALL 0288 randomized study. *Blood.* 2002;99:863-871.

[20] Te Poele EM, de Bont ES, Marike Boezen H, et al. Dexamethasone in the maintenance phase of acute lymphoblastic leukaemia treatment: is the risk of lethal infections too high? *Eur J Cancer.* 2007;43:2532-2536.

[21] Gökbuget N, Hoelzer D. Treatment of adult acute lymphoblastic leukemia. *Hematology Am Soc Hematol Educ Program.* 2006:133–141.

[22] Bassan R, Lerede T, DiBona E, et al. Induction-consolidation with idarubicin-containing regimen, unpurged marrow autograft, and post-graft chemotherapy in adult acute lymphoblastic leukaemia. *Br J Haematol.* 1999;104:755-762.

[23] Mehta J, Powles R, Sirohi B, et al. High-dose melphalan and autotransplantation followed by post transplant maintenance chemotherapy for acute lymphoblastic leukemia in first remission. *Bone Marrow Transplant.* 2004;33:1107-1114.

[24] Sirohi B, Powles R, Treleaven J, et al. The role of maintenance chemotherapy after autotransplantation for acute lymphoblastic leukemia in first remission: single-center experience of 100 patients. *Bone Marrow Transplant.* 2008;42:105-112.

[25] Doubek M, Folber F, Koristek Z, et al. Autologous hematopoietic stem cell transplantation in adult acute lymphoblastic leukemia: still not out of fashion. *Ann Hematol.* 2009;88:881-887.

[26] Raff T, Gökbuget N, Lüschen S, et al. Molecular relapse in adult standard-risk ALL patients detected by prospective MRD monitoring during and after maintenance treatment: data from the GMALL 06/99 and 07/03 trials. *Blood.* 2007;109:910-915.

[27] Rowe JM, Richards S, Wiernik PH, et al. Allogeneic bone marrow transplantation (BMT) for adults with acute lymphoblastic leukemia (ALL) in first complete remission (CR): *Early results from the international ALL trial* (MRC UKALL/ECOG E2993). Blood. 1999;94:732a.

[28] Gökbuget N, Arnold R, Buechner T, et al. Intensification of induction and consolidation improves only subgroups of adult ALL: analysis of 1200 patients in GMALL study 05/93. *Blood.* 2001;98:802a.

[29] Takeuchi J, Kyo T, Naito K, et al. Induction therapy by frequent administration of doxorubicin with four other drugs, followed by intensive consolidation and maintenance therapy for adult acute lymphoblastic leukemia: The JALSGALL93 Study. *Leukemia.* 2002;16:1259-1266.

[30] Thomas X, Boiron J-M, Huguet F, et al. Outcome of Treatment in Adults With Acute Lymphoblastic Leukemia: Analysis of the LALA-94 Trial. *J Clin Oncol.* 2004; 22:4075-4086.

[31] Ribera JM, Oriol A, Bethencourt C, et al. Comparison of intensive chemotherapy, allogeneic or autologous stem cell transplantation as post-remission treatment for adult patients with high-risk acute lymphoblastic leukemia. Results of the PETHEMA ALL-93 trial. Haematologica/*Hematol J.* 2005;90:1346-1356.
[32] Goldstone AH, Richards SM, Lazarus HM, et al. In adults with standard-risk acute lymphoblastic leukemia, the greatest benefit is achieved from a matched sibling allogeneic transplantation in first complete remission, and an autologous transplantation is less effective than conventional consolidation/maintenance chemotherapy in all patients: final results of the International ALL Trial (MRC UKALL XII/ECOG E2993). *Blood.* 2008;111:1827-1833.

In: Acute Lymphoblastic Leukemia
Editors: Severo Vecchione and Luigi Tedesco

ISBN: 978-1-61470-872-8
©2012 Nova Science Publishers, Inc.

Chapter X

The Role of Innate and Adaptive Immunity in Childhood Acute Lymphoblastic Leukemia

*Maria Hatzistilianou**
Aristotle University of Thessaloniki, Thessaloniki, Greece

Introduction

Acute lymphoblastic leukemia (ALL) accounts for about 30–50 new cases per million children and represents 25–30% of all childhood malignancies (Hodgson et al., 2007, Gallucci et al., 2001). ALL is the most common subtype of leukemia in childhood (approximately 80%) (Hodgson et al., 2007, Matzinger, 1997, Petridou et al., 2002,).

The pathogenesis of ALL is unknown. The development of leukemias requires the concerted action of different agents (Belson et al., 2007, *Dockerty,* 2009, *MacArthur* et al., 2008, Zeller et al., 2007). Patients with ALL demonstrate alteration of normal immune function. Several investigators have demonstrated poor *in vivo* anti-leukemia immune responses in ALL patients, even in the bone marrow as the primary site of disease (Malmberg et al., 2006, Michael et al., 2009, Nash et al., 1993, Pui et al., 2008). The central problem is to determine the effector mechanisms responsible for resistance of the host against tumor growth.

ALL arises from genetic aberrations and environmental agents that impair the normal differentiation of lymphatic cells either at the stem cell or at an early lymphocyte precursor stage (Le Viseur et al., 2008, Malmberg et al., 2006, Michael et al., 2009, Pui et al., 2008). Abnormal immune response to infection may cause greater cell proliferation after common infections and, as a result, increased risk of childhood ALL (Gallucci et al., 2001, Kim et al.,

---

* Mailing address: Dr. Maria Hatzistilianou, Paediatrician-Immunologist, Professor, Medical School, Aristotle University of Thessaloniki, Agiou Ioannou 23, Kalamaria, 551 32 Thessaloniki, GREECE, Tel: ++3031 0994807 , Fax: ++3031 0996143, Email: nontas@topo.auth.gr

2007, *MacArthur* et al., 2008). Also, genetic variation of the immune system needs to be considered to elucidate the molecular and cellular mechanisms mediating infection, immune response, and childhood leukemia (Brown et al., 2008, Han et al., 2010, Hodgson et al., 2007, Michael, 2009, Mullighan, 2009).

The key to developing an effective antitumor response is to understand why the immune system is initially unable to detect transformed cells and subsequently is tolerant of lymphoblast growth.

A complete description of the immune response is beyond the scope of this article. We will briefly provide a general overview of our current understanding of the immune system and we will highlight areas relevant to ALL Immunology. Especially, we focus on concepts in ALL Immunology, followed by a discussion of how these concepts are being utilized in the clinical practice.

The Innate Immune System in ALL

In general, the immune system can be divided into the innate immune system, which allows rapid, nonspecific protection, and the adaptive immune system, which develops more slowly but provides specific recognition of antigens via expression of carefully rearranged receptors (Medzhitov et al., 2000).

The characteristics of the innate immune system include: a) a broad-spectrum response (non-specific) which is phylogenetically ancient b) no memory and c) limited repertoire of recognition molecules (Matzinger, 1998).

The malignant cells are recognized by the innate and the adaptive immune system, which play an important and fundamental role in host defense (Redaelli et al., 2005). Ineffective antigen presentation limits the response of the adaptive immune system; however, we are now learning that the innate immune system of the host may first fail to recognize the blast cells as posing a danger (Ribera et al., 2009). Thus, the innate immune system not only provides the first line of defense against microorganisms but also the biological context, "the danger signal", that instructs the adaptive immune system to mount a response (Gallucci et al., 2001, Leung et al., 2010, Medzhitov et al., 2000).

The vast majority of potential microorganisms, which are encountered routinely are destroyed within minutes or hours by innate defenses. The innate immune system, which includes skin and epithelial barriers, circulating effector proteins (complement, collectins, pentraxins), leukocytes, natural killer cells (NK cells), chemokines, cytokines (e.g. TNF, IL-1, IL-2, type I IFNs, and IFN-γ, IL-8 and others), plays a primary role in the defense mechanisms against infectious agents and malignant cells (Elmaagacli, 2006, Matzinger, 1998, Medzhitov et al., 2000, Park et al., 2006).

Skin is the physical barrier and its involvement can be the initial symptom of ALL in children. In these children specific cutaneous lesions can be observed which result from infiltration of the skin by the lymphoblasts. These lesions are cutaneous signs of infection or hemorrhage resulting from the bone marrow dysfunction induced by the malignant process. Also, there are lesions, macules or papules, which may be scattered all over the body surface and represent collections of mast cells in the dermis, resulting in hyperpigmentation of the overlying epidermis (Athanassiadou et al., 2000, Millot et al., 1997, Taijanovic, 2004).

Mast cells originate from pluripotent bone marrow cells and disseminate as unrecognized progenitors for tissue-specific proliferation and maturation. We have reported a case of a baby with congenital urticaria pigmentosa who developed ALL (Athanassiadou et al., 2000). Skin biopsy from a representative lesion showed dermal infiltration, with round and oval cells, which, when stained with toluidine blue, revealed metachromatic granules. This finding confirmed the clinical diagnosis of urticaria pigmentosa (Athanassiadou et al., 2000).

There is no association between skin lesions and prognosis because cutaneous involvement can be observed not only among high risk ALL patients but can also be observed among low risk patients. The skin lesion could disappear within 15 days after the cytotoxic therapy and complete remission could be obtained after induction therapy. We would like to highlight that a small growing cutaneous lesion or urticaria pigmentosa could be the presenting manifestation of ALL (Athanassiadou et al., 2000, Taijanovic, 2004).

After skin, mucosal surfaces are the largest area of host pathogen interaction in the human immune system. The mucous membrane that covers the digestive and urogenital tracts, the respiratory canal, the eye conjunctiva, the inner ear, and layers of most of the exocrine glands, is a strong component of the immune system, with very specialized mechanical and chemical barriers that either prevent the entry of foreign bodies or facilitate their degradation through a series of chemical processes, most of which are yet to be fully clarified (Marcotte et al., 1998).

Specialized epithelial and intraepithelial cells also form a part of the mucosa, and maintain a balance by self-renewal, as well as maintain a balance between the colonies residing in the mucosa.

Patients with ALL will first consult a dentist because of the oral manifestations of their underlying disease. The oral manifestations include, pallor, gingivitis, gingival hyperplasia, petechiae, mucosal bleeding and ulceration (Hahn et al., 2007, *Ou-Yang* et al., 2010, Patrick et al., 2007). Thus, dentists must be aware of these manifestations due to ALL in order to avoid the potentially catastrophic post-surgical complications of oral hemorrhage, tissue necrosis, and infection (De Morales et al., 2007, Sepulveda et al., 2005).

Oral mucous includes saliva. The salivary constituents in ALL patients have been analyzed and reported that the mean values for amylase activity and total protein concentrations were significantly higher in these subjects. Also, these patients had significantly higher peroxidase and amylase activity and elevated concentration of salivary total protein at the time of diagnosis (Patrick et al., 2007, Wahlin et al., 2007). The children receiving induction chemotherapy had significantly lower values of salivary flow rate and sIgA concentration. It has been suggested that chemotherapy alters the quality and quantity of saliva, which may be a contributing factor to oral complications. Thus it becomes apparent to establish an oral preventive intervention. Also, it has been found that in children with ALL the prevalence of oral colonization with Candida albicans is higher than those in healthy children (Patrick et al., 2007, Wahlin et al., 2007).

Vascular endothelium is currently being regarded not as a passive barrier between flowing blood and the vascular wall, but as a highly specialized metabolically active tissue (Betzing, 2001, *Mengarelli* et al., 2001, Victor et al., 2010). The most important changes that occur during the activation of endothelial cells, under the stimulatory influence of various factors, consist of an increased expression of adhesion molecules.

Adhesion molecules play a central role in the functions of the immune system (Hatzistilianou et al., 1997, Hatzistilianou et al., 1999, Victor et al., 2010). Cell adhesion molecules are cell surface receptors involved in leukocyte homing, adhesion and migration. Circulating leukocytes use several adhesion molecules to bind to the vascular endothelium before they leave the bloodstream and migrate into tissues (Hatzistilianou et al., 1997, Hatzistilianou et al., 1999). The fate of hematopoietic stem cells is largely regulated by interactions with the bone marrow environment.

Adhesive interactions between haemopoietic cells and a specialized microenvironment within the bone marrow play a critical role in regulating normal haemopoiesis and the egress of mature blood cells into the circulation. Adhesion molecules are expressed by stroma cells, extracellular matrix, hematopoietic stem cells and committed hematopoietic progenitors and play a pivotal role in the distribution of hematopoietic stem cells in the bone marrow and in the regulation of the immune response. It is hypothesized that an altered expression or function of adhesion molecules on leukemic blasts could contribute to the evolution and biological behavior of acute leukemias, and determine the egress of blasts into peripheral blood and the homing of others to extramedullary sites (Christiansen et al., 1994, Victor et al., 2010).

Intercellular adhesion molecule-1 (ICAM- 1; CD54) serves as a ligand for leukocyte integrin adhesion. Through intercellular interactions, it mediates granulocyte extravasation, inflammatory processes, and immunologic response. The increased expression leads to the rolling, activation, and firm adhesion of leukocytes to the endothelium (Olejnik et al 1999, Daĝdemir 1998).

It has been hypothesized that ICAM-1 (CD54) expression by leukaemic blasts could increase their susceptibility to lysis by non-HLA-restricted cytotoxic cells such as natural killer (NK) (Daĝdemir et al., 1998, Hatzistilianou et al., 1997, Olejnik et al., 1999). Hence, down-regulation of CD54 could enable tumour cells to escape from host immunosurveillance. An inverse correlation has been reported between CD54 expression and WBC in childhood ALL at the time of diagnosis (Hatzistilianou et al., 1997, Hatzistilianou et al., 1999).

Although the adhesion molecules are usually membrane-bound, soluble forms exist and are generated by shedding of the extracellular portions from the cell surface through proteolytic cleavage (Rothlein et al., 1991).

The functional role of cellular and soluble adhesion molecules in patients with malignancy is unclear. It is not known whether increased serum soluble adhesion molecule levels such as sICAM- I result from shedding by normal host cells (because of the immune response to tumor, inflammation, or tissue damage) or by lymphoblast. The higher levels in patients with more advanced malignancy may represent increased host immune response to malignant cells or may simply reflect a larger tumor burden (Hatzistilianou et al., 1997).

The concentration of soluble adhesion molecules may be dependent on different factors such as the rate of synthesis of the receptor by cells, the rate of shedding from cells and their capacity to bind ligands expressed on cells and vascular endothelium (Hatzistilianou et al., 1999).

In one of our studies we have demonstrated increased circulating concentrations of sICAM-1, sVCAM-1 and sE-selectin in children with ALL. The presence of soluble adhesion molecules in the sera of patients with ALL may be of diagnostic importance because in our study all of our patients presented, at the onset of the disease. In these patients the soluble adhesion molecule levels were higher than the corresponding mean levels of the control group. Not only the expression of ICAM-1 on tumour cells has demonstrated prognostic significance, but also the level of the soluble form as measured in patients' sera (Hatzistilianou et al., 1997).

In our study a strong linear correlation was found in ALL patients between sE-selectin, sVCAM-1 and sICAM-1 levels and the clinical course of ALL. This finding points to the possibility of using any one of these adhesion molecules as a different alternative parameter for monitoring the activity of the disease. Normal range levels were observed in patients in complete remission and after the end of treatment and high levels in patients with leukemia relapse. Thus, monitoring the above soluble adhesion molecule levels was helpful for the early diagnosis of leukemia relapse in patients with ALL (Hatzistilianou et al., 1997).

In the same study, the patients with the highest levels of soluble adhesion molecules at the onset of the disease may serve to indicate possible trends to later relapse and thus separate a subgroup of patients with higher risk of relapse that will need closer monitoring. In particular, patients with sICAM-1 >800 ng/ml, sVCAM-1 > 3000 ng/ml and sE-selectin concentration >200 ng/ml relapsed. The above high values of soluble adhesion molecules may provide a marker for the severity of the disease.

The adhesion molecule system and the cytokine network are intercellular signal pathways. Innate immunity cells release inflammatory cytokines that subsequently activate the components of the adaptive immune system.

NK cells are innate immune lymphocytes critical to host defense against invading infectious pathogens and malignant transformation through elaboration of cytokines and cytolytic activity (Jarosz et al., 2009).

NK cells are key members of the innate immune system, which each single individual possesses, and are of fundamental importance to limit or eradicate pathogens during the early phases of a primary infection, i.e. before T and B cells can mount efficient responses (Jarosz et al., 2009). NK cells have direct or natural cytotoxic activity against some virus-infected, leukemic, and other tumor cells, and they also mediate antibody dependent cellular cytotoxicity (ADCC) of targets through FcRIII (CD16), a receptor that binds the Fc portion of antibody. Functionally, NK cells are an important source of innate immunoregulatory cytokines (eg, IFN), tumor necrosis factor (TNF), granulocyte macrophage colony-stimulating factor [GM-CSF]) that coorchestrate the early immune response and contribute to the delayed T-cell response following infection or malignancy (Athanassiadou et al., 1999, Betzing et al., 2001, Catriou et al., 1998).

Dendritic cells (DC) represent another group of cells, which are the key initiators of immune responses *in vivo*. Dendritic cells play a critical role in the generation of antitumor immunity. Recently, some investigators showed reduced DC in a group of adult and pediatric patients with B-cell precursor ALL. Numerical defects as well as functional abnormalities of DC in patients with ALL may impact on poor antileukemia immune responses in childhood with ALL (Maecker et al., 2006).

The quantitative and/or qualitative aberrations in DC might reflect impaired immunity in children with ALL, in particular acute leukemias.

Decreased numbers of DC could not be explained by mere bone marrow dysfunction owing to infiltration of leukemic blast cells, as it was unable to document a correlation between DC numbers and other myeloid cell numbers such as neutrophils and monocytes (Mami et al., 2004).

Among functional defects, there is decreased expression of MHC or co-stimulatory molecules, insufficient T-cell stimulatory capacity and accumulation of immature DC in leukemic patients (Gabrilovich et al., 2004).

The Adaptive Immune Response in ALL

The development of leukemia itself is evidence that there has been a failure in the immune system. The host immune response to foreign challenge requires the coordinated action of both innate and adaptive arms of the immune system. The adaptive specific immune response comes into play only if the defenses of the innate immune system are breached (Chang et al., 2010).

Adaptive immunity displays four characteristic attributes: (a) antigenic specificity, (b) diversity (c) immunologic memory and (d) Self/nonself recognition.

The immune responses can be divided into humoral and cell-mediated responses (Soonie et al., 2007, Zhang et al., 2000).

The humoral branch of the immune system is at work in the interaction of B cells with antigen and their subsequent proliferation and differentiation into antibody-secreting plasma cells. The antibody functions as the effector of the humoral response by binding to antigen and neutralizing it or facilitating its elimination (Soonie et al., 2007).

Cell mediated immunity is the arm of the adaptive immune response. This type of immunity is mediated by T lymphocytes. Thus, effector T cells generated in response to antigen are responsible for this type of immunity. The response of T lymphocytes to cell-associated antigens consists of a series of sequential steps. Naïve T lymphocytes constantly recirculate through peripheral lymphoid organs. To perform its function the naïve T cells have to be stimulated to differentiate into effector cells and this process is initiated by antigen recognition (Zhang et al., 2000, Zou et al., 2006).

Humoral immunity was found to be defective in children with ALL during the initial diagnosis (Hatzistilianou et al., 1996).

In one of our studies we have studied Ig concentration of patients with ALL at initial diagnosis and through disease's evolution (Hatzistilianou et al., 1996). It was observed that at leukemia's onset and during chemotherapy Ig concentration was lower in patients than those of the control group. Age related data might show an even greater discrepancy. Furthermore, total IgG concentrations were significantly reduced in children with ALL, suggesting that the reduction in a specific antibody was a reflection of the total immunoglobulin concentrations (Hatzistilianou et al., 1996). Our results are in agreement with those of other investigators of the immune status of children with ALL who have reported low concentrations of immunoglobulins after treatment has started (MacArthur et al., 2008, *Lindblom* et al., 2008, Hatzistilianou et al., 1998).

In the same study the children with ALL were treated with IVIG every 15 days for 3 months during the induction chemotherapy (six cycles IVIG treatment). This treatment with IVIG prevented the patients from sepsis during induction chemotherapy. Thus, the first 6 months after the start of chemotherapy only 25% of children with ALL had more than one episode of neutropenia with fever and bacterial infection and 28% of them presented with sepsis. On the contrary, when this IVIG treatment was not used, during the first 6 months after the start of chemotherapy 76% of children with ALL had more than one episode of neutropenia with fever and bacterial infections and 61.5% of them presented with sepsis (Hatzistilianou et al., 1996).

The conclusion of our study was that the children with ALL at the onset of the disease present humoral deficiency and the IVIG treatment during induction chemotherapy protects the patients during neutropenia period from infections and sepsis.

In our series there are no significant differences in Ig's concentration evolution between patients with ALL-B and those with ALL-T. Our study demonstrated that in patients with a favourable evolution of their ALL, the Ig concentration was normalized 6-12 months after the end of treatment.

There are investigators who suggest that there is a significant decrease in all Ig concentration at relapse and that the persistent IgM deficit is correlated with a higher risk of relapse and death (Jackson et al., 1990, Reid et al., 1981)

The B and T lymphocytes as well as antigen presenting cells secrete different cytokines. Cytokines are soluble proteins that mediate immune and inflammatory reactions and are responsible for communications between leukocytes and between leukocytes and other cells.

The cytokine network is important for proliferation and cytokine secretion by acute leukemia blasts, and membrane-bound adhesion molecules are important for blast interactions with neighboring cells of the *in vivo* microenvironment. The cytokine effects are modulated *in vivo* by soluble cytokine antagonists, whereas the cell-to-cell contact mediated by adhesion molecules and their ligands may be blocked by the soluble forms of the adhesion molecules (Roman et al., 2007).

The release of cytokines such as interferon gamma (IFN-γ), interleukin-1 (IL-1), and tumor necrosis factor (TNF) at sites of inflammation and immune response augments cellular expression of ICAM-1 by normal cells (Shams et al., 200). IFN is crucial for initiating the innate immune response and for the generation of the adaptive response (Beyer et al., 2006, Catriu et al., 1998, Betzing et al., 2001, Katz, 1987).

Cytokines seem to play a major role in malignancies. Cellular proliferation of malignant B and T cells is believed to be regulated by a network of cytokines with autocrine, paracrine and pleiotropic activities. Patients with ALL demonstrate alteration of normal immune function. Investigators have studied the immune activity against human ALL cells (Catriu et al., 1998, Ma et al., 2009, Park et al., 2006, Yin HQ et al., 2006). They found that the death of leukemia cells *in vivo* was correlated with the production of IFN-α, IFN-γ and IL-12 by the host. They detected also an elevated level of serum IFN-γ in ALL children and that their peripheral blood mononuclear cells were continuously exposed to this cytokine. A rise in helper T lymphocytes has been demonstrated producing IFN-γ (Th1), T cell activation and

Th2 predominance at the time of diagnosis, which confirm the involvement of cellular immunity in the leukemic process and can be used in immune therapy in leukemia.

Inflammatory cytokines TNF, IL-1, IL-6 and IL-8 are produced by cells of the immune system after immunologic stimuli and are vital to normal immunity. It has been suggested that these cytokines act in a network of factors directing both immune and malignancy responses (Yin et al., 2006).

The immunologic basis for the appearance of TNF-α, IL-1β, IL-6 and IL-8 in ALL is unknown. In one of our studies we found that serum TNF-α, IL-1β, IL-6 and IL-8 levels were significantly higher in children with ALL at initial diagnosis and during relapse than in those in complete remission and in healthy children (Catriu et al., 1998). Also, our results show that TNF-α may be considered as a prognostic indicator for monitoring the course of ALL disease. TNF-α has been suggested to have a pro-inflammatory role in *in vivo* antitumor activities. It is a cytokine released in acute leukemia in an autocrine and paracrine way. However, results of studies about its effects on malignant/normal lymphoid cells are controversial. Studies of *in vitro* cytokine production from cell cultures may provide important information but this information is irrelevant *in vivo* and it cannot take into account the influence of multiple cytokines and other mediator combinations.

In our study, regression analysis showed a significant correlation between IL-6 and IL-1β and a weaker correlation between IL-6 and TNF-α. It is unknown whether the production of these cytokines is directly interlinked, or whether this correlation exists because IL-1 induces IL-6 (Catriu et al., 1998).

The Dysfunction of Immune Response in ALL

The dysfunction of innate and adaptive immunity in ALL is another problem for the patients with ALL. In this case the patients cannot fight the different microorganisms and these patients suffer from infections. Systemic infections represent the most important cause of morbidity and mortality in children suffering from ALL before and during chemotherapy.

Regarding the immune system, it is important to remember that patients with leukemia have a wide variety of defects, which affect both cellular and humoral immunity. One of the most obvious defects is the fact that the blast cells have grown without an appropriate immune response to stop them. On the other hand, treatment also contributes to immunodeficiency in these patients, raising their susceptibility to infections. ALL-directed chemotherapy leads to considerable B-cell depletion in the bone marrow and peripheral blood, often accompanied by transient hypogammaglobulinemia. After chemotherapy, B-cells seem to recover within months, whereas the amount of CD4 T-helper cells remains low for longer periods of time, but T-cell memory seems to be spared.

Immune disorders associated with leukemia are varied and quantitative; qualitative changes have been described as well. Among the quantitative ones the following stand out: decrease of lymphocytes number, decrease of delayed hypersensitivity, decrease of mitogen responses, decrease of immunoglobulins (Ig) synthesis, decrease of monocyte oxidative responses, decrease of cytokine responses, and increase of monocyte suppressor activity. Regarding qualitative changes, the deficiencies in chemotaxis, phagocytosis and bactericidal activity stand out. Thus, viral, fungal and bacterial infections are an important cause of morbidity and mortality in patients with leukemia (Athanassiadou et al., 1997 Athanassiadou et al., 2003, Malmberg et al., 2006).

Identifying patients with bacterial infection and sepsis is a major challenge for physicians.

Neutropenia as a state of immunosuppression is probably the major problem in children with ALL at initial diagnosis and undergoing intensive chemotherapy. During neutropenia, the morbidity and mortality rates due to bacterial infections are high. Early diagnosis of febrile neutropenic patients at high risk for severe infections would be helpful in management decisions regarding antimicrobial therapy and hospitalization. There is no consensus so far regarding the diagnostic approach to infection, its differentiation into bacterial, viral, or fungal, and the requisite treatment during the first critical 24-hour period of neutropenia with fever.

Thus, the early diagnosis of bacterial infections must be accurate. In the majority of neutropenic fever episodes, causative infectious agents cannot be identified (Hatzistilianou et al., 2010). Discrimination between serious infections and harmless fever episodes in febrile patients with neutropenia is difficult. However, this discrimination is very difficult because the typical clinical features of bacterial infections, and routine laboratory tests used to diagnose bacterial infection and sepsis (e.g., CRP, neopterin, white blood cell, cytokines, chemokines, lactate etc), lack diagnostic accuracy and can be misleading.

Neutropenic ALL children with infection may or may not have a fever. However, in these patients, fever may be due to other causes than infections, such as the underlying disorder, or the administration of drugs or blood products (Hatzistilianou, 2008).

Therefore, specific, rapid, and cost-efficient markers indicating early bacterial infection, ongoing infection, or deterioration during the febrile neutropenic period would be highly warranted (Hatzistilianou et al., 2007).

Some of these markers are C-reactive protein (CRP), ADA, cytokines, chemokines, WBC and others (Hitoglou et al., 1998, Hitoglou-Hatzi et al., 2005, Hatzistilianou et al., 1996, Hatzistilianou et al., 2002).

CRP is an acute-phase protein released by the liver after the onset of inflammation or tissue damage. The measurement of CRP has enjoyed periodic emphasis over the years as a measure of general illness and as an adjunct to physical examination and other laboratory data. It has been studied as a screening device for occult inflammation, as a marker of disease activity, and as a diagnostic tool.

Also, this protein is used frequently to differentiate between viral and bacterial infections. However, CRP is neither highly specific nor sensitive for bacterial infection. There are a great deal of conflicting data regarding the use of CRP for diagnostic purposes since it can remain at low concentrations in bacterial infections and can increase significantly in viral infections. Some argue that as a nonspecific indicator of inflammation, CRP, by definition, cannot accurately differentiate among the many sources of potential tissue destruction; but the CRP monitoring may be useful to distinguish between causes of fever.

In addition, other disadvantages for use of CRP are: (a) its late response to inflammation and to fever onset and (b) the high variety of serum levels related with the amount of tissue injury. Recently, more rapid and precise methods of quantifying CRP have led to a renewed interest in its value in clinical medicine. Unfortunately, the nonspecific nature of the acute phase response prevents CRP from being a useful discriminatory diagnostic test. Based on the literature, it has been concluded that CRP has a limited role in ALL.

Enzymes involved in purine metabolism may be used to map acute leukemias.

Adenosine deaminase (ADA; EC 3.5.4.4) participates in the degradation of purines by catalyzing the conversion of adenosine to inosine and deoxyadenosine to deoxyinosine. Two isoenzymes of ADA, ADA1 and ADA2 have been described that have different molecular weights and are coded by different gene loci. ADA is present in serum and in most tissues, particularly lymphoid tissues, and is essential for the maturation and function of lymphocytes, especially those of T lineage and is required for the maturation of human blood monocytes to macrophages (Gougoustamou D et al., 1999). Measurements of total ADA (tADA) and its isoenzymes ADA1 and ADA2 activity in various body fluids have been used to diagnose infectious diseases. In one of our studies we found significant high levels of ADA in febrile ALL neutropenic patients with infection when compared to afebrile ALL neutropenic patients without infection (Hitoglou et al., 1998). A possible explanation of these results is that adenosine-mediated signaling may play a role in the hypothalamic mechanisms controlling the degree of body temperature increase during fever.

In the same study, according to its results, tADA activity as well as ADA2 levels were higher in ALL neutropenic patients with microbial infection when compared to those with viral infections. The source of elevated serum tADA and ADA2 are the macrophages and monocytes that are the predominant cells in inflammation. These results are in agreement with those of other studies, which have demonstrated elevated ADA activity and ADA2 during inflammatory responses and in septic conditions.

At the time of diagnosis and during eventual relapse ADA levels were increased in children with ALL while during remission and after the end of the treatment ADA levels were as in normal children without ALL.

However, the effects of chemotherapeutic agents on the enzyme activities of ADA are unknown. Thus, in the same study, the decrease of ADA activity, which we observed during chemotherapeutic agent treatment in afebrile neutropenic patients, may be explained in several ways. Firstly, chemotherapeutic agents might have a direct inhibiting effect on ADA and secondly, ADA may be inhibited indirectly to compensate for the decrease of adenosine during chemotherapeutic agent treatment, caused by inhibition of purine *de novo* synthesis and homocysteine remethylation. Theoretically, decrease of ADA would lead to an increment of adenosine and subsequent anti-inflammatory effects.

Among the known markers, CRP, ADA, cytokines, chemokines and others, which indicate the infection there is a new and innovative marker, the procalcitonin (PCT).

In 1993, PCT was described as a new and innovative parameter of infection (Chesney et al., 1983). Procalcitonin is a 116-amino-acid residue peptide with a molecular weight of about 13 kDa and is governed by the calcitonin I (CALC-I) gene on chromosome 11p15.2-p15.1 (Le Moullec et al., 1984, Assicot et al., 1993).

During microbial infection, there is an increase of CALC-I gene expression that causes release of PCT from all parenchymal tissues and from differentiated cell types throughout the body (Becker et al., 2001, Muller et al., 2001). The inflammatory release of PCT can be induced in two main ways: one (direct way) is due to toxins or lipopolysaccharides released by microbes and the other (indirect way) is through cell-mediated host response mediated by inflammatory cytokines (e.g., IL-1b, IL-6, TNF-α). Moreover, PCT plays a significant role in the diagnosis of infections in immunosuppressed patients.

In one of our studies that included children with ALL undergoing intensive chemotherapy, the level of PCT in serum increases significantly during an infection of bacterial origin (Hatzistilianou et al., 2010). Today, PCT is considered to be one of the earliest and most specific markers of bacterial infections.

However, PCT is not only a specific marker of infection, but is also useful in monitoring the host response to the infection and to the treatment (Hatzistilianou, 2008, Hatzistilianou, 2010). Thus, PCT must be determined serially. If PCT levels decrease by more than 30% of the initial value after the first 24 h from the onset of antibacterial treatment, it indicates that the treatment is the appropriate one and the infection is under control. If PCT levels increase, it means that the antimicrobial treatment must be changed. If PCT levels continuously increase, the host response to infection is very poor and the host immune system must be reinforced (Hatzistilianou, 2008, Hatzistilianou, 2010).

Also, we pointed out that, based on a cutoff level of 2 ng/ml PCT, groups with bacterial infections showed a sensitivity and specificity of 94% and 96.5%, respectively, for predicting bacteremia (Hatzistilianou et al., 2008, Hatzistilianou, 2010). In comparison with other markers, such as CRP, IL-6, IL-8, IL-1b, sTNFRII, TNF-α, and soluble adhesion molecules, PCT was a better marker, in any case, taking into account its specificity and sensitivity. The discriminatory power of PCT and the above markers in neutropenic patients was evaluated in terms of the area under the receiver operating characteristic (ROC) curve (AUC). PCT was the best discriminator for bacterial infections (Hatzistilianou, 2008, Hatzistilianou et al., 2010, Hatzistilianou, 2010).

Another reason that PCT is a valuable marker of bacterial infection is the fact that PCT may be determined easily and quickly by any doctor at the patient's bedside and without any special equipment except a simple centrifuge. This determination is done by the semi-quantitative method called PCT-Q at the onset of infection. If PCT-Q is positive, it must be continued by serial quantitative determination of PCT levels by classical methods (Athanassiadou et al., 2001).

Conclusion

The malignant cells in ALL are recognized by the innate and the adaptive immune system, which play an important and fundamental role in host defense. On the other hand, the dysfunction of innate and adaptive immunity in ALL is another problem for the patients with ALL.

The pathogenesis of ALL is still unknown. However, functional defects or disorders in cells, molecules and proteins of the innate and adaptive immunity have been found to be associated with the onset of ALL. Although their specific roles have not been determined yet, some of them can be utilized for the prognosis of the course of the disease. Notably, the role of adhesion molecules is discussed in this chapter. Definitely, more research is needed both *in vitro* and *in vivo* for the understanding of ALL pathogeny.

Although the action mechanism of cells, molecules and genetic agents of the innate as well as the adaptive immunity has not been clarified so far, many of these agents have been established as prognostic factors for the course of ALL. This fact is of great significance in clinical practice because children with ALL are particularly vulnerable to serious microbial infections threatening their lives. Therefore, the timely diagnosis and therapeutic management of these infections is very important. For this purpose a number of markers, reviewed in this chapter, have been presented and discussed in the literature.

In particular PCT has been found to present certain advantages as a diagnostic and prognostic factor in comparison to other established markers. The use of PCT in combination with other factors has also been considered in this chapter.

References

Assicot M, Gendrel D, Carsin H, Raymond J, Guilbaud J, Bohuon C. (1993). High serum procalcitonin concentrations in patients with sepsis and infection. *Lancet* 341:515–8.

Athanassiadou F, Catriu D, Hatzistilianou M, Papageorgiou Th, Fidani S. (1999) Effect of GM-CSF on TNF-a, IL-3 and IL-7 levels in vitro and in vivo in children with acute Lymphoblastic leukemia (ALL). *Haema*, 2(3) 139-144.

Athanassiadou F, Fidani L, Papageorgiou Th, Hatzistilianou M, Catriu D. (2000). Acute lymphoblastic leukemia and urticaria pigmentosa in an infant. *Med Ped Onc.* 34: 368-369.

Athanassiadou F, Hatzistilianou M, Catriu D, Papageorgiou T. (1997) Fungal infection in a patient with T cell lymphoma. *Med J Infect Parasit Dis*. 12(3): 132-133.

Athanassiadou F, Hatzistilianou M, Kourti M, Benos A, Papageorgiou T, Stamou M, Katriu D. (2003). Evaluation of treatment in childhood acute lymphoblastic leukaemia based on prognostic factors. *Heama*, 6(3):328-335.

Athanassiadou F, Hatzistilianou M, Rekliti A, Catriu D. (2001). Comparative study of two methods for the determination of procalcitonin. *Proceed.of the 2nd Balkan Conference of Microbiology, Thessaloniki*, pp 383.

Becker K, Móller B, Nylen E, Cohen R, Silva O, Snider R. Calcitonin gene family of peptides. In: *Principles and Practice of Endocrinology and Metabolism* (2001). Becker K, ed. Philadelphia: J.B. Lippincott, p. 520–34.

Belson M, Kingsley B, Holmes A (2007). Risk Factors for Acute Leukemia in Children: A Review. *Envir Health Persp* 115 (1):35-39.

Betzing CK, Körner G, Badiali L, Buchwald D, Möricke A, Korte A, Köchling J, Wu S, Kappelmeier D, Oettel K, Henze G, Seeger K. (2001) Characterization of cytokine, growth factor receptor, costimulatory and adhesion molecule expression patterns of bone marrow blasts in relapsed childhood B cell precursor ALL. *Cytokine*,13(1):39-50.

Beyer M, Schultze JL. (2006). Regulatory T cells in cancer. *Blood*, 108(3):804–11.

Brown VI, Seif AE, Reid GSD, Teachey DT, Grupp SA. (2008) Novel molecular and cellular therapeutic targets in acute lymphoblastic leukemia and lymphoproliferative disease *Immunol Res*. 42(1-3): 84–105. doi:10.1007/s12026-008-8038-9.

Catriu D, Hatzistilianou M., Agguridaki C, Athanassiadou F. (1998). Clinical correlations of serum TNF- α, IL-1β, IL-6 and IL-8 in ALL in children. *Haema*, 1(4):177-183.

Chang JS, Wiemels JL, Chokkalingam AP, Metayer C, Barcellos LF, Hansen HM, et al (2010). Genetic Polymorphisms in Adaptive Immunity Genes and Childhood Acute Lymphoblastic Leukemia. *Cancer Epid Biomark.* 19: 2152

Chesney RW, McCarron DM, Haddad JG, Hawker CD, DiBella FP, Chesney JP, David JP (1983). Pathogenic mechanism of the hypocalcemia of the staphylococcal toxic-shock syndrome. *J Lab Clin Med* 101:576–585.

Christiansen I, Gidlof C, Wallgren AC, Simonsson B, Totterman TH (1994). Serum levels of soluble intercellular adhesion molecule 1 areincreased in chronic B-lymphocytic leukemia and correlate with clinical stage and prognostic markers. *Blood*, 84:3010-3016 .

Dağdemir A, Ertem U, Duru F, Kirazli Serafettcn (1998). Soluble L-Selectin Increases in the Cerebrospinal Fluid Prior to Meningeal Involvement in Children with Acute Lymphoblastic Leukemia. *Leuk. Lymph.* 28(3-4):391-398.
(doi:10.3109/10428199809092695).

De Morales RT, Navas R, Viera N, Álvarez CJ, Chaparro N, Griman D (2007). pH and salivary sodium bicarbonate during the administration protocol for methotrexate in children with leukemia. *Med Oral Pathol Oral Cir Bucal.* 12(6):E435-9.

Dockerty JD (2009). Epidemiology of childhood leukemia in New Zealand: studies of infectious hypotheses. *Blood Cel Mol Dis.* 42(2):113-6.

Elmaagacli AH, Koldehoff M, Hindahl H, Steckel NK, Trenschel R, Peceny R, et al (2006). Mutations in innate immune system NOD2/CARD 15 and TLR-4 (Thr399Ile) genes influence the risk for severe acute graft-versus-host disease in patients who underwent an allogeneic transplantation. *Transplantation*, 81:247–254.

Gabrilovich D. (2004) Mechanisms and functional significance of tumour-induced dendritic-cell defects. *Nat Rev Immunol*, 4: 941–952.

Gallucci S, Matzinger P (2001). Danger signals: SOS to the immune system. *Curr Opin Immunol*, 13:114–9.

Gougoustamou D., Hitoglou S., Hatzistilianou M., Kotsis A., Athanasiadou F., Catriu D. (1999) Adenosine Deaminase and 5´-Nucleotidase activities in acute lymphoblastic leukemia. *Biochem Biophys Newslet.* 45:69-70.

Hahn CL, Liewehr FR. (2007). Innate immune responses of the dental pulp to caries. *J Endod,* 33:643–651.

Han S, Lan Q, Kyung Park A, Lee KM, Park S, Ahn H S, Shin HY, Kang HJ, et al (2010). Polymorphisms in innate immunity genes and risk of childhood leukemia. *Hum. Immunol.* 71: 727–730.

Hatzistilianou M. (2008). The Role of Procalcitonin in Febrile Neutropenic Children with Hematological Malignancies. *US Pediatrics*, 77-79.

Hatzistilianou M. (2010). Diagnostic and Prognostic Role of Procalcitonin in Infections. *TheScientificWorldJOURNAL*, 10:1941–1946.

Hatzistilianou M, Agguridaki C, Athanassiadou F, Catriu D. (1999). Serum sCD4, sCD14 and sICAM-1 under the effect of rhG-CSF in children with ALL. *Haema*, 2(1): 18-21.

Hatzistilianou M, Athanassiadou F, Agguridaki C, Catriu D. (1997). Circulating soluble adhesion molecule levels in children with ALL. *Europ J Ped.* 156(7): 537-540.

Hatzistilianou M, Catriu D, Athanassiadou F, Aggouridaki C, Aktseli K, Papageorgiou Th. (1996) Humoral immunity of children with ALL after IVIG administration. *Proccedings, of VIII Meeting of the European Society for Immunodeficiencies, ESID,* Goteburg, pp.118.

Hatzistilianou M, Papaeconomou A, Hitoglou S, Athanassiadou F, Catriu D, Makedou A. (1996). Prognostic significance of Adenosine Deaminase in children with malignancies. *Ped Hemat Onc.* 13(4):339-347.

Hatzistilianou M, Rekleity A, Athanassiadou F, Catriu D. (2007). Significance of serial Procalcitonin responses in infection of children with secondary immunodeficiency. *Clinic Investig Med.* 30(2): 75-85.

Hatzistilianou M., Reklity A., Athanassiadou F., Aggouridaki Ch., Catriu D. (2002). *Procalcitonin and inflammatory cytokine mRNA in children with secondary immunodeficiency Proceed of 10º Meeting of ESID Weimar,* pp 1-2.

Hatzistilianou M., Rekliti A, Athanassiadou F, Catriu D. (2010). Procalcitonin as an early marker of bacterial infection in neutropenic febrile children with acute lymphoblastic leukemia. *Inflam Res.* 59 (5):339-347.

Hatzistilianou M, Souliou E, Catriu D, Alexiou S, Papageorgiou Th, Rekliti A, Athanassiadou F (1998). Immunity to diphtheria, tetanus, pertussis, measles, mumps and rubella in children with acute lymphoblastic leukemia. *Mol Immunol.* 35(11-12):757.

Hitoglou-Hatzi S, Hatzistilianou M, Gougoustamou D, Rekliti A, Agguridaki C, Athanassiadou F, Frydas S, Kotsis A, Catriu D. (2005) Serum adenosine deaminase and procalcitonin concentrations in neutropenic febrile children with acute lymphoblastic leukaemia. *Clin Exper Med.* 5(2):60-65.

S. Hitoglou, M. Hatzistilianou, D. Gougoustamou, F. Athanassiadou, A. Kotsis, D. Catriu (1998). Adenosine deaminase activity and isozyme levels in serum and peripheral blood lymphocytes in childhood acute lymphoblastic leukemia. *Mol Immunol.* 35(11-12):754.

Hodgson S, Foulkes W, Eng C, Maher E. (2007) *A practical guide to human cancer genetics.* 3rd Ed. New York: Cambridge University Press.

Jackson SK, Parton J, Shortland G, Stark JM, Thompson EN. (1990). Serum immuneglobulins to endotoxin core glycolipid: establishment of normal concentrations. *Arch Dis Child.* 65:768-70.

Jarosz M, Hak Ł, Więckiewicz J, Balcerska A, Myśliwska J. (2009). Clinical immunology NK cells in children with acute lymphoblastic leukemia and non-Hodgkin lymphoma after cessation of intensive chemotherapy. *Centr Eur J Immunol.* 34 (2): 94-99.

Katz J, Walter BN, Bennetts GA (1987). Abnormal cellular and humoral immunity in childhood acute lymphoblastic leukemia in long-term remission. *West J Med.* 146:179-187.

Kim R, Emi M, Tanabe K. (2007) Cancer immunoediting from immune surveillance to immune escape. *Immunology,* 121(1):1–14.

Le Moullec J.M. (1984). The complete sequence of human procalcitonin. // *FEBS Lett.,* 167 (1): 93-97.

Leung W, Neale G, Behm F, Iyengar R, Finkelstein D, Michael B. K, Pui CH (2010) Deficient innate immunity, thymopoiesis, and gene expression response to radiation in survivors of childhood acute lymphoblastic leukemia. *Cancer Epidem* 34: 303–308.

Le Viseur C, Hotfilder M, Bomken S, Wilson K, et al (2008). In Childhood Acute Lymphoblastic Leukemia Blasts at Different Stages of Immunophenotypic Maturation Have Stem Cell Properties. *Canc Cell* 14: 47–58.

Lindblom A, Heyman M, Gustafsson I, Norbeck O, Kaldensjö T, Vernby A, Henter JI, Tolfvenstam T, Broliden K Parvovirus (2008). B19 infection in children with acute lymphoblastic leukemia is associated with cytopenia resulting in prolonged interruptions of chemotherapy. *Clin Infect Dis.* 46(4):528-36.

Ma X, Urayama K, Chang J, Wiemels JL, Buffler PA (2009). Infection and pediatric acute lymphoblastic leukemia. *Blood Cells, Molecules, and Diseases* 42:117–120.

MacArthur AC, McBride ML, Spinelli JJ, Tamaro S, Gallagher RP, Theriault GP (2008). Risk of childhood leukemia associated with vaccination, infection, and medication use in childhood: the Cross-Canada Childhood Leukemia Study. *Am J Epidemiol.* 167(5):598-606.

Maecker B, Mougiakakos D, Zimmermann M, Behrens M, Hollander S, Schrauder A, Schrappe M, Welte K, Klein C (2006). Dendritic cell deficiencies in pediatric acute lymphoblastic leukemia patients. *Leukemia* 20: 645–649.

Malmberg KJ, Ljunggren HG. (2006) Escape from immune- and nonimmune-mediated tumor surveillance. Semin Cancer Biol, 16(1):16–31.

Mami NB, Mohty M, Chambost H, Gaugler B, Olive D. (2004) Blood dendritic cells in patients with acute lymphoblastic leukaemia. Br J Haematol; 126: 77–80.

Marcotte H, Lavoie MC (1998). Oral Microbial Ecology and the Role of Salivary Immunoglobulin A. Microb Molec Biology Rev. 62(1): 71–109

Matzinger P. (1998) An innate sense of danger. Semin Immunol. 10:399–415.

Medzhitov R, Janeway C. (2000). Innate immunity. N Engl J Med. 343:338–44.

Mengarelli A, Zarcone D, Caruso R, Tenca C, Rana I, Pinto RM, Grossi CE, De Rossi G. (2001). Adhesion molecule expression, clinical features and therapy outcome in childhood acute lymphoblastic leukemia. Leuk Lymph. 40(5-6):625-30.

Millot F, Robert A, Bertrant Y (1997). Cutaneous involvement in children with acute lymphoblastic leukemia or lymphoblastic lymphoma. Pediatrics, 100:60-4.

Muller B, White JC, Nylen E, Snider RH, Becker KL, Habener JF. (2001). Ubiquitous expression of the calcitonin-1 gene in multiple tissues in response to sepsis. J Clin Endocrinol Metab, 86: 396–404.

Mullighan CG (2009) Genomic analysis of acute leukemia. Int. Jnl. Lab. Hem., 31, 384–397.

Nash KA, Mohammed G, Nandapalan N, Kernaham J, Scott R, Craft AW, Toms GL (1993). T cell function in children with acute lymphoblastic leukemia. Br J Haematol 83(3):419-427.

Olejnik, I. (1999). Serum soluble L-selectin in childhood acute lymphoblastic leukemia. Pediat Internat. 41: 246–248. doi: 10.1046/j.1442-200x.1999.01062.x

Ou-Yang LW, Chang PC, Tsai AI, Jaing TH, Lin SY. (2010). Salivary microbial counts and buffer capacity in children with acute lymphoblastic leukemia. Pediatr Dent. 32(3):218-22.

Park HH, Kim M, Lee BH, Kim Y, Lee EJ, Min WS, Kang CS, Kim WI, Shim SI, Han K (2006). Intracellular IL-4, IL-10 and IFN-gamma levels of leukemic cells and bone marrow T cells in acute leukemia. Ann Clin Lab Sci 36(1):7-15.

Petridou E, Trichopoulos D. Leukemias (2002). In: Textbook of cancer epidemiology Adami HO, Hunter D, Trichopoulos D, editors. New York: Oxford University Press; p. 556-72.

Preedy VR (2010). Adhesion Molecules Adhesion Molecules in Normal Hematopoiesis and Leukemia. Science 359–373, ISBN: 978-1-57808-671-9 eBook ISBN: 978-1-4398-4060-3 DOI: 10.1201/b10167-25

Pui CH, Robison LL, Look AT. (2008). Acute lymphoblastic leukaemia. Lancet. 22(371): 1030-43.

Redaelli BL, Laskin JM, Stephens MF, Botteman CL, Pashos (2005). A systematic literature review of the clinical and epidemiological burden of acute lymphoblastic leukaemia (ALL). *Eur J Canc Care*, 14(1): 53–62.

Reid MM, Craft AW, Cox JR. (1981) Immunoglobulin concentrations in children receiving treatment for acute lymphoblastic leukaemia. *J Clin Pathol.* 34:479-82.

Ribera JM, Oriol A. (2009). Acute lymphoblastic leukemia in adolescents and young adults. *Hematol Oncol Clin North Am*. 23(5):1033-42, vi.

Roman E, Simpson J, Ansell P, Kinsey S, Mitchell CD, McKinney PA, Birch JM, Greaves M, Eden T. (2007) Childhood Acute Lymphoblastic Leukemia and Infections in the First Year of Life: A Report from the United Kingdom Childhood Cancer Study. *Am. J. Epid.* 165 (5): 496-504.

Sepulveda E, Brethauer U, Rojas J, Fernandez E, Le Fort P. (2005) Oral ulcers in children under chemotherapy: clinical characteristics and their relation with Herpes Simplex Virus type 1 and Candida albicans. *Med Oral Pathol Oral Cir Bucal* 10: E1-8.

Shams M, Kholoussi M, Faten S Bayoumi, Hala El-Nady (2008) Estimation of serum interferon-gamma level in childhood acute lymphoblastic leukemia patients. *J Med Sci* 8(1):68-72.

Soonie R. Patel,1 Miguel Ortı´n,1 Bernard J. Cohen,2 Ray Borrow,5 Diane Irving,3 Joanne Sheldon,3 and Paul T. (2007). Heath4 Revaccination of Children after Completion of Standard Chemotherapy for Acute Leukemia Revaccination of Children. *CID*, 44: 635

Taijanovic MS, Hulett RL, Graham AR, Graham ML, Hunter TB (2004) Acute lymphoblastic leukemia of the skin and subcutaneous tissues; the first manifestation of disease in a 6-month-old infant: a case report with literature review. *Emerg Rad*. 11(1):60-64.

Teitell MA, Pandolfi PP (2009). Molecular Genetics of Acute Lymphoblastic Leukemia. *Annual Review of Pathology: Mechanisms of Disease* 4: 175-198.

Thompson PA, Murry DJ, Rosner GL, Lunagomez S, Blaney SM, Berg SL, Camitta BM, Dreyer ZE, Bomgaars LR (2007). Methotrexate pharmacokinetics in infants with acute lymphoblastic leukemia. *Canc Chemoth Pharmac*. 59(6): 847-853

Wahlin BY, Matsson L (2007). Oral mucosal lesions in patients with acute leukemia and related disorders during cytotoxic therapy. *Eur J Oral Sci*. DOI: 10.1111/j.1600-0722.1988.tb01419.x

Whicher J, Bienvenu J, Monneret G. (2001). Procalcitonin as an acute phase marker. *Ann Clin Biochem*. 38:483–93.

Yin HQ, Qiao ZH, Zhu L, Zhang L, Su LP, Lu YJ (2006) *Levels of intracellular IL-6 and IFN-gamma in children with acute lymphoblastic leukemia*. 8(6):461-463

Zeller JL, Lynm C, Class RM (2007). Acute lymphoblastic leukemia . *JAMA* 297 (11):1278.

Zhang XL, Komada Y, Chipeta J, Li QS, Inaba H, Azuma E, Yamamoto H, Sakurai M (2000). Intracellular cytokine profile of T cells from children with acute lymphoblastic leukemia. *Cancer Immunol Immunother* 49(3):165-172.

Zou W. (2006). Regulatory T cells, tumour immunity and immunotherapy. *Nat Rev Immunol,* 6(4):295–307.

Index

#

10q23, 24
10q24, 117
21st century, 121

A

access, 19, 138
accessibility, 5, 60, 65
accounting, 90, 104, 188
acetylation, 138, 140, 142, 143, 144, 145, 150
acid, 5, 10, 12, 13, 19, 22, 26, 33, 45, 136, 138, 139, 140, 141, 143, 145, 146, 147, 148, 149, 150, 151, 157, 214
activation complex, 15
acute leukemia, 8, 12, 13, 30, 32, 37, 38, 40, 41, 43, 48, 49, 50, 86, 88, 89, 90, 91, 100, 102, 113, 115, 118, 126, 130, 132, 141, 145, 148, 149, 179, 180, 190, 193, 194, 195, 208, 210, 211, 212, 214, 219, 220
acute lymphoblastic leukemia, vii, viii, ix, x, xi, 2, 3, 34, 35, 36, 40, 41, 42, 43, 44, 45, 46, 47, 48, 49, 50, 55, 73, 74, 83, 85, 87, 88, 91, 94, 105, 107, 108, 110, 112, 113, 114, 115, 116, 117, 118, 130, 131, 132, 133, 136, 150, 155, 169, 170, 172, 174, 176, 179, 180, 181, 184, 193, 194, 195, 196, 197, 200, 201, 202, 203, 204, 216, 217, 218, 219, 220, 221
acute myelogenous leukemia, 39, 45, 46, 132, 147, 149
acute myeloid leukemia, 32, 36, 39, 40, 44, 45, 49, 50, 88, 133, 147, 149
acute promyelocytic leukemia, xi, 11, 38, 138, 151, 197
ADA, 213, 214
adaptation, 122
adenocarcinoma, 168
adenosine, 214, 218
adhesion, 47, 103, 208, 209, 211, 215, 216, 217
adolescents, 165, 192, 194, 201, 220
adult T-cell, 44, 89
adulthood, 4, 189
adults, ix, 6, 9, 30, 44, 50, 55, 99, 103, 106, 132, 136, 146, 148, 153, 154, 198, 200, 201, 202, 203, 204
adverse effects, 24
adverse event, 145, 163, 165
aetiology, 113
afebrile, 214
age, vii, viii, 6, 12, 14, 18, 21, 26, 28, 32, 42, 53, 55, 57, 58, 75, 85, 86, 88, 89, 90, 94, 95, 96, 100, 102, 103, 104, 106, 107, 116, 123, 130, 132, 154, 170, 171, 187, 190
aggregation, 62
agonist, 137, 157, 160
alkaloids, 136
ALL pathogenesis, vii, 1, 26, 33
ALL therapy, vii, 1
allele, 12, 13, 20, 33, 62, 100, 105, 112, 175, 177
allelic exclusion, 61, 62, 74, 77, 78, 79
alters, 66, 99, 207
amino, 5, 7, 11, 12, 13, 14, 19, 23, 25, 33, 100, 138, 214
amino acid, 5, 7, 11, 12, 13, 14, 19, 23, 25, 100
amino groups, 138
amylase, 207
analgesic, 163, 165
aneuploid, 188
aneuploidy, 187
angiogenesis, 138, 162, 166
annotation, 130
anorexia, 145

Index

antibody, viii, 53, 58, 61, 67, 68, 77, 78, 81, 137, 209, 210
anticancer activity, 83, 139, 141
anticancer drug, 137, 140, 149, 163
anticonvulsant, 147
antigen, 54, 57, 58, 61, 66, 67, 68, 72, 76, 79, 90, 106, 143, 170, 171, 174, 175, 178, 180, 206, 210, 211
antimicrobial therapy, 213
antisense, 60
antitumor, x, 44, 143, 147, 154, 155, 159, 163, 164, 166, 167, 168, 206, 209, 212
antitumor agent, 147, 154
aorta, 124
APC, 29
APL, xi, 197
apoptosis, viii, x, 4, 8, 10, 14, 16, 24, 25, 27, 30, 39, 47, 54, 64, 66, 69, 71, 83, 94, 97, 103, 111, 138, 140, 141, 142, 143, 147, 148, 149, 150, 151, 153, 155, 158, 159, 162, 163, 167, 168
arginine, 22
Aristotle, 205
arrest, 4, 17, 24, 56, 64, 69, 71, 72, 75, 77, 141, 142, 143
arsenic, 89
aspartic acid, 12
assessment, 46, 50, 131, 170, 171, 172, 174, 180, 186, 191
astrocytoma, 155, 165, 166
asymptomatic, 143
ataxia, 88, 108
ATP, 128
attribution, ix, 119
authorities, 200
autoantibodies, 66
autoimmunity, 125
autosomal recessive, 55, 88
avoidance, 122

B

B19 infection, 219
bacteremia, 215
bacteria, 138
bacterial infection, 211, 213, 215, 218
barriers, 206, 207
base, 13, 21
base pair, 13
BCAP, 63
B-cell lineage, vii, 53, 55, 90

BCR-ABL translocation, viii, 53, 56
beneficial effect, 165
benefits, 197
benign, 155
benzene, 89, 125, 132
bicarbonate, 217
bimodal distribution, viii, 85, 86
biochemistry, 121
biological behavior, 208
biological processes, 64
biological sciences, ix, 119, 121
biological systems, ix, 119, 129
biopsy, 207
birds, 131
blacks, 112
bleeding, 207
blood, 3, 20, 31, 38, 50, 88, 100, 107, 123, 124, 136, 155, 157, 162, 163, 171, 173, 207, 208, 213, 214
blood flow, 162
blood monocytes, 214
blood stream, 157, 208
blood vessels, 162, 163
blood-brain barrier, 162
body fluid, 214
bone, vii, viii, x, xi, 4, 7, 8, 9, 14, 15, 22, 26, 31, 32, 36, 37, 38, 41, 45, 47, 53, 56, 66, 67, 75, 78, 81, 85, 86, 88, 101, 104, 123, 136, 145, 157, 158, 168, 169, 170, 171, 177, 178, 179, 181, 184, 185, 190, 203, 205, 206, 207, 208, 210, 212, 216, 219
bone marrow, vii, viii, x, xi, 5, 7, 8, 9, 14, 15, 22, 26, 31, 32, 36, 37, 38, 41, 45, 47, 53, 56, 66, 67, 75, 78, 81, 85, 86, 88, 101, 104, 123, 136, 145, 157, 158, 168, 169, 170, 171, 177, 178, 179, 181, 184, 185, 190, 203, 205, 206, 207, 208, 210, 212, 216, 219
bone marrow transplant, 137, 184, 190, 203
Brazil, 135, 146
breast cancer, 30, 49, 148, 157, 168
breastfeeding, 89
Britain, 132
Brno, 197

C

cadmium, 89
calcitonin, 214, 219
calcium, 62, 82, 157
cancer, vii, ix, x, 1, 14, 25, 29, 43, 46, 49, 72, 83, 84, 86, 99, 122, 124, 125, 126, 127, 128, 130, 131, 132, 133, 135, 136, 138, 147, 149, 153, 154, 155,

Index

157, 158, 159, 162, 163, 165, 167, 168, 184, 194, 216, 218, 220
cancer cells, x, 122, 127, 128, 147, 153, 154, 155, 158, 160, 162
cancer pediatric patients, vii, 1
cancer progression, 157, 162
candidates, 29, 126, 160, 184
capillary, 154
carcinogenesis, 122, 124, 125, 128, 129, 130, 132
carcinoma, 156, 157, 158
caries, 217
catalytic activity, 74
CDK inhibitor, 98
cDNA, 9, 156, 174
cell culture, 171, 212
cell cycle, vii, viii, 1, 7, 17, 24, 35, 43, 54, 55, 58, 65, 69, 72, 74, 105, 110, 111, 138, 193
cell cycle regulation, vii, 1, 111
cell death, x, 16, 70, 83, 103, 128, 140, 141, 142, 146, 147, 154, 160, 163, 198
cell differentiation, viii, 4, 6, 12, 14, 18, 26, 30, 34, 53, 56, 61, 65, 70, 138
cell division, 58, 72, 103
cell fate, 14, 58, 66, 75, 138
cell line, vii, 5, 9, 11, 14, 16, 17, 18, 19, 20, 21, 24, 25, 30, 37, 38, 39, 42, 43, 47, 48, 53, 55, 57, 58, 75, 80, 90, 140, 141, 142, 143, 149, 150, 154, 155, 156, 157, 158, 159, 161, 163, 166, 167, 168, 172
cell movement, 162
cell signaling, 74, 79
cell surface, 29, 57, 58, 61, 62, 65, 66, 72, 90, 157, 208
cellular immunity, 212
cellular signaling pathway, 164
central nervous system (CNS), 22, 96, 100, 102, 103, 104, 106, 115, 123, 170, 190, 191, 198
chaos, 127
charge coupled device, 186
charge density, 138
chemical, 89, 120, 138, 139, 207
chemical reactions, 121
chemicals, 89, 121, 125
chemokines, 206, 213, 214
chemotaxis, 212
chemotherapeutic agent, 140, 154, 214
chemotherapy, xi, 11, 31, 33, 50, 100, 102, 103, 104, 123, 137, 164, 165, 168, 171, 180, 190, 197, 198, 199, 202, 203, 204, 207, 210, 211, 212, 213, 215, 218, 219, 220

childhood, vii, viii, x, xi, 1, 4, 11, 12, 25, 27, 29, 30, 32, 35, 39, 40, 41, 44, 45, 46, 47, 48, 49, 50, 53, 55, 56, 74, 85, 86, 87, 88, 89, 90, 91, 93, 94, 96, 97, 100, 102, 104, 105, 106, 107, 108, 109, 110, 111, 112, 113, 114, 115, 116, 117, 118, 120, 122, 123, 127, 131, 132, 133, 150, 154, 167, 169, 170, 173, 175, 176, 177, 178, 179, 180, 181, 184, 187, 188, 189, 191, 193, 194, 195, 196, 198, 202, 203, 205, 208, 209, 216, 217, 218, 219, 220
children, vii, viii, ix, x, xi, 3, 5, 13, 27, 32, 35, 36, 38, 40, 49, 50, 85, 86, 88, 89, 90, 94, 95, 99, 100, 102, 103, 104, 105, 106, 107, 108, 109, 110, 111, 112, 114, 115, 117, 119, 120, 122, 131, 132, 136, 145, 153, 154, 162, 165, 169, 171, 173, 177, 179, 180, 181, 184, 187, 189, 190, 191, 192, 194, 195, 198, 200, 203, 205, 206, 207, 209, 210, 211, 212, 213, 214, 215, 216, 217, 218, 219, 220, 221
China, 132
chloroform, 89
chondroitin sulfate, 100
chromatid, 59, 76
chromosomal abnormalities, viii, x, 54, 86, 88, 108, 170, 183, 184, 186, 188, 190, 193
chromosomal instability, 195
chromosomal translocations, vii, 41, 53, 54, 55, 58, 68, 73, 82, 97, 106, 108, 110, 193
chromosome, x, 22, 24, 30, 34, 59, 60, 69, 76, 77, 81, 88, 93, 94, 95, 97, 99, 100, 101, 102, 103, 105, 108, 109, 110, 111, 115, 116, 141, 142, 169, 174, 183, 184, 186, 187, 189, 190, 191, 192, 193, 194, 195, 196, 214
chromosome 10, 24
chronic lymphocytic leukemia, 73, 84, 147, 194
chronic myelogenous, 30, 35, 40, 74, 136, 147, 149
circulation, 208
classes, 41
classical methods, 215
classification, 90, 111, 112, 113, 117, 127, 170, 178, 179, 181, 195
cleavage, 15, 18, 24, 143, 208
clinical application, 17, 170
clinical diagnosis, 207
clinical trials, ix, 13, 107, 122, 135, 139, 140, 143, 145, 146, 150, 164, 177
clonality, 175, 181
clone, 33, 90, 97, 112, 127, 170, 171, 173
clusters, 8, 108
coding, 5, 10, 59
codon, 23, 26, 27, 33, 45
cognitive impairment, 138

collaboration, 43
colon, 25, 48, 69, 156, 158, 160
colon cancer, 48
colonization, 207
color, 101, 104, 179, 186, 188
combined effect, 142
comparative genome hybridization (CGH), xi, 183, 184
competition, 160
complement, 206
complementarity, 61
complementary DNA, 174
complexity, 54, 122
compliance, 198
complications, 207
composition, 4, 146, 171, 175
compounds, 107, 138, 154, 159, 163
computer, 120
concordance, 88, 107, 126
condensation, 162
configuration, 12, 56
conjunctiva, 207
consensus, 213
conservation, 37, 128
consolidation, 177, 201, 202, 203, 204
constituents, 207
contamination, 50, 89, 174, 176
contraceptives, 89
control group, 31, 209, 210
controversial, 24, 62, 192, 212
convergence, 71
COOH, 5, 19
cooperation, 18, 63
correlation, 6, 21, 22, 27, 31, 39, 50, 193, 208, 209, 210, 212
correlations, viii, 86, 217
cortical neurons, 147
cost, 73, 213
covering, 185
CRP, 213, 214, 215
CSCs, 126
CSF, 9, 30, 209, 216, 217
culture, 159, 162
cure, 128, 129, 154, 184, 198
cycles, 144, 145, 198, 211
cycling, viii, 15, 54, 58, 65, 71
cyclophosphamide, 137, 142, 199, 202
cytogenetics, xi, 39, 90, 99, 100, 109, 116, 126, 183, 184, 185, 187, 188, 190, 192, 193, 194, 195
cytokines, 206, 209, 211, 212, 213, 214, 215

cytometry, x, 50, 144, 169, 172, 173, 176, 177, 178, 179, 180
cytoplasm, 4, 5, 7, 90, 157, 158
cytostatic drugs, 154
cytotoxicity, 149, 209

D

danger, 11, 206, 219
database, 73, 122, 130
deacetylation, 138, 144
deaths, 199
defects, vii, 4, 12, 34, 53, 55, 69, 124, 131, 209, 210, 212, 215, 217
defense mechanisms, 206
deficiencies, 9, 38, 75, 212, 219
deficiency, viii, 42, 53, 55, 56, 64, 69, 81, 211
deficit, 211
degenerate, 186
degradation, 16, 17, 19, 21, 40, 42, 83, 140, 149, 174, 176, 207, 214
Delta, 14, 131
dendritic cell, 4, 34, 219
dentist, 207
deprivation, 70
depth, vii, 53, 54, 126, 164
deregulation, 36, 69, 104
derivatives, 125, 147
dermis, 207
destruction, 29, 213
detectable, 31, 178, 190
detection, x, 11, 30, 32, 34, 39, 49, 50, 170, 171, 172, 173, 175, 177, 178, 180, 181, 183, 184, 185, 186, 187, 188, 193
determinism, 128
diacylglycerol, 64
diarrhea, 144, 145
dicentric chromosome, 106
digestion, 70
dimerization, 5, 9, 10
diploid, 188
discrimination, 172, 213
disease activity, 213
diseases, xi, 46, 88, 125, 197, 214
disorder, vii, viii, 26, 45, 85, 86, 88, 106, 213
displacement, 20
disposition, 146
dissociation, 19
distribution, viii, 60, 85, 86, 130, 208
diversification, 67, 68, 81

diversity, viii, 7, 53, 58, 59, 68, 85, 175, 180, 210
DNA, viii, ix, 3, 5, 6, 7, 9, 10, 12, 17, 19, 20, 28, 30, 32, 35, 41, 54, 55, 58, 59, 62, 67, 69, 70, 71, 73, 75, 76, 81, 88, 97, 99, 102, 109, 111, 130, 135, 136, 138, 140, 142, 144, 146, 149, 150, 165, 174, 175, 185, 186, 187
DNA damage, viii, 12, 54, 70, 71, 76, 142, 150, 165
DNA polymerase, 136
DNA repair, 12, 28, 55, 58, 76, 88, 97
DNA sequencing, 28, 33
DOI, 166, 220
dominance, 37
donors, 31, 32
dosing, 143
down syndrome, 88, 109, 111, 112, 173, 180
down-regulation, 4, 84, 142, 143, 147, 150, 208
drosophila, 14, 99
drug resistance, 83, 172, 195
drug targets, 24
drug toxicity, 200
drugs, ix, x, xi, 7, 24, 70, 94, 122, 135, 136, 137, 139, 140, 143, 146, 147, 150, 154, 159, 160, 163, 164, 165, 166, 171, 197, 198, 200, 203, 213
dyes, 185
dysplasia, 131

E

editors, 220
elaboration, 209
electromagnetic, 125
electromagnetic fields, 125
elongation, 10
elucidation, 129
embryogenesis, 30, 124
employability, 174
employment, 170, 173
encephalopathy, 144
encoding, 7, 8, 22, 37, 54, 55, 57, 58, 65, 97, 104, 111, 175
endocrine, 70, 157
endonuclease, 59
endothelial cells, 154, 168, 208
endothelium, 207, 208
energy, 122, 128, 129
energy transfer, 129
engineering, 83, 121
entropy, 128, 129
environment, 27, 208
environmental change, 122

environmental factors, viii, 85, 120, 123, 125
enzyme, 62, 81, 138, 145, 214
enzymes, 24, 138
epidemiology, 220
epidermis, 207
epigenetic silencing, 138
epigenetics, 146
Epstein-Barr virus, 89
equipment, 215
erythropoietin, 9
ethnicity, viii, 85, 180
etiology, vii, viii, x, 1, 29, 85, 86, 119, 122, 124, 125, 126, 183
eukaryotic, 58, 138
eukaryotic cell, 58, 138
Europe, 180
evidence, ix, x, 8, 9, 30, 69, 88, 89, 100, 107, 110, 113, 122, 124, 127, 135, 143, 170, 198, 200, 210
evolution, 8, 122, 125, 176, 177, 208, 210, 211
exaggeration, ix, 119
excision, 68
excitability, 157
exclusion, 62, 78
execution, 141
exons, 3, 6, 7, 8, 9, 19, 21, 28, 33, 56, 100
exonuclease, 50
expertise, 176
exposure, 10, 88, 89, 107, 122, 125, 131, 140, 157, 171, 186, 198
extracellular matrix, 208
extracellular signal regulated kinases, 64
extravasation, 208

F

facilitators, 42
false negative, 171
false positive, 174, 176
families, 59, 60, 126, 138
family history, 88
fatty acids, 138, 139
FDA, 146
fermentation, 122
fetal development, 4, 88
fever, 211, 213, 214
fibroblasts, 46, 47
fibrosis, 9, 38
flank, 58
flavopiridol, 150
flow cytometry (FC), x, 169

fluctuations, 171
fluid, 129
fluorescence, x, xi, 74, 100, 169, 171, 174, 183, 184, 185, 193, 195
fluorescence in situ hybridization (FISH), x, xi, 169, 171, 174, 183, 184
folate, 24
follicle, 66
formation, 12, 29, 62, 68, 69, 78, 81, 97, 106, 141, 162, 189
fragments, 28, 120
frameshift mutation, 33
fungi, 138
fusion, viii, x, 8, 11, 20, 53, 55, 56, 72, 88, 93, 97, 99, 100, 101, 102, 104, 107, 109, 110, 114, 115, 123, 126, 132, 169, 170, 171, 173, 174, 177, 178, 180, 183, 184, 189, 190, 191, 192, 195, 196

G

gait, 145
gastrulation, 124
GDP, 2, 25, 26, 46
gene expression, 8, 36, 42, 49, 50, 51, 65, 92, 100, 102, 111, 115, 118, 125, 126, 128, 138, 139, 142, 191, 214, 218
gene mutations, vii, 1, 3, 25, 34, 39, 45, 51, 92
gene promoter, 47
gene regulation, 124, 128
gene targeting, 17
gene therapy, 163
gene transfer, 45
genes, x, 3, 6, 7, 8, 11, 14, 15, 16, 22, 25, 28, 29, 30, 31, 36, 37, 46, 47, 48, 54, 55, 56, 58, 59, 60, 63, 64, 65, 68, 71, 72, 75, 76, 77, 78, 84, 88, 92, 97, 98, 99, 103, 105, 108, 110, 111, 117, 120, 124, 125, 126, 130, 131, 141, 142, 150, 160, 169, 170, 171, 173, 174, 175, 178, 181, 183, 184, 186, 190, 191, 193, 194, 195, 196, 217
genetic abnormalities, vii, viii, 53, 55, 73, 85, 107, 110, 173, 184, 185, 191
genetic alteration, 6, 11, 13, 27, 54, 73, 92, 97, 107, 111, 140
genetic background, 29
genetic defect, 105
genetic diversity, 195
genetic marker, 3
genetic mutations, 122
genetic predisposition, 88
genetic syndromes, 88

genetic traits, 170
genetics, viii, 85, 115, 116, 133, 194, 218
genome, vii, viii, xi, 1, 7, 26, 54, 55, 58, 68, 73, 81, 85, 110, 111, 117, 129, 183, 184, 185, 186, 195
genomic instability, 15, 72
genomic regions, 185
genomics, 118
genotype, 102
germ line, 21
Germany, 180
germline mutations, 26
gingival, 207
gingivitis, 207
glioblastoma, 30, 48, 155
glioma, 156, 158, 160, 166, 167, 168
glucocorticoid receptor, 16
glucose, 122, 128
glutamic acid, 15
glutamine, 15
glycine, 13
glycogen, 29
glycolysis, 122
glycoproteins, 29, 66
glycosylation, 62, 78
grades, 145
granules, 207
gravitational force, 120, 129
Greece, 1, 119, 131, 169, 183
growth, ix, x, 9, 10, 13, 16, 18, 21, 24, 26, 29, 30, 36, 37, 38, 39, 43, 44, 47, 48, 55, 64, 69, 86, 100, 124, 131, 138, 139, 140, 142, 143, 146, 154, 157, 160, 161, 162, 163, 166, 168, 184, 198, 206, 216
growth arrest, 17, 139, 140, 142
growth factor, 9, 30, 36, 38, 47, 48, 64, 216
growth rate, 13
GTPases, 25
guanine, 67
guardian, 75
guidelines, 180

H

haemopoiesis, 208
hairpins, 59
hairy cell leukemia, 31
half-life, 19, 144, 145
haploid, 95, 114, 194
HDAC, 138, 140, 143, 145, 146, 148, 150
headache, 163
heat shock protein, 140, 149, 150

height, 120
hematologic neoplasms, 132
hematology, 179
hematopoietic stem cells, 8, 16, 25, 26, 45, 46, 126, 127, 132, 208
hematopoietic system, 30
hemorrhage, 206, 207
hepatosplenomegaly, 104, 106, 191
heterochromatin, 34, 62
heterogeneity, 38, 122, 130, 188, 195
hispanics, 112
histone, vii, ix, 15, 62, 78, 83, 109, 111, 136, 138, 139, 142, 143, 144, 145, 146, 147, 148, 149, 150, 151
histone deacetylase, vii, ix, 83, 109, 111, 136, 138, 139, 145, 146, 147, 148, 149, 150, 151
Histone deacetylase inhibitors (HDIs), ix, 135
histones, 138
history, 125
HLA, 88, 90, 96, 100, 106, 113, 208
homeostasis, 26
homocysteine, 214
hospitalization, 213
host, xi, 165, 198, 205, 206, 207, 208, 209, 210, 211, 215, 217
hotspots, 18
house, 113
HSCT, 200, 201
human, x, 4, 8, 15, 16, 21, 24, 25, 29, 34, 35, 36, 37, 38, 40, 41, 42, 43, 44, 45, 47, 48, 49, 50, 54, 69, 70, 72, 73, 77, 79, 82, 83, 89, 100, 124, 126, 131, 132, 133, 140, 141, 142, 143, 147, 148, 149, 150, 151, 153, 155, 156, 157, 158, 159, 160, 161, 163, 164, 165, 166, 167, 168, 180, 186, 207, 211, 214, 218
human brain, 167
human genome, 124, 163
human leukemia cells, 38, 47, 141, 142, 148, 149, 150
humoral immunity, 212, 218
Hunter, 220
hybrid, 99, 102, 103, 189
hybridization, xi, 55, 72, 110, 174, 183, 184, 186, 193, 194
hypermethylation, 105
hyperplasia, 207
hypersensitivity, 18, 212
hypogammaglobulinemia, 212
hypokalemia, 144, 146
hypophosphatemia, 143

hypothesis, 15, 54, 88, 122, 124, 126, 130

I

ICAM, 208, 209, 211
identical twins, 107
identification, vii, viii, 6, 28, 34, 36, 39, 53, 55, 73, 85, 92, 115, 171, 175, 176, 177, 178, 184, 185, 186, 188, 191, 192, 193, 194, 196
identity, 75, 121
IFN, 206, 209, 211, 219, 220
Ig H chain, viii, 53, 55, 58, 59, 60, 61, 62, 67, 68, 69
Ig L chain recombination, viii, 53, 63, 65, 70
IL-17, 64
IL-8, 206, 212, 215, 217
image, 186
imbalances, 186
immune function, xi, 205, 211
immune memory, 81
immune response, xi, 66, 205, 206, 208, 209, 210, 211, 212, 217
immune system, 54, 78, 80, 198, 206, 207, 208, 209, 210, 212, 215, 217
immunity, 61, 73, 209, 210, 212, 215, 216, 218, 219, 221
immunodeficiency, 55, 88, 212, 218
immunofluorescence, 31
immunoglobulin, viii, x, 9, 53, 56, 68, 75, 76, 77, 78, 79, 80, 82, 90, 97, 102, 103, 104, 169, 170, 171, 173, 175, 177, 178, 180, 181, 210
immunoglobulins, 81, 90, 211, 212, 218
immunoreactivity, 168
immunosuppression, 213
immunosurveillance, 208
immunotherapy, 49, 221
improvements, 92, 110, 138, 184
in situ hybridization, x, xi, 93, 99, 100, 101, 104, 108, 110, 169, 171, 174, 183, 184, 193, 195
in utero, 88, 89, 100, 107, 128
in vitro, 8, 13, 17, 24, 36, 37, 38, 64, 140, 141, 161, 164, 184, 212, 215, 216
in vivo, xi, 8, 15, 17, 36, 65, 81, 127, 129, 143, 145, 146, 164, 166, 168, 205, 209, 211, 212, 215, 216
incidence, viii, ix, 11, 13, 21, 26, 27, 36, 54, 56, 69, 70, 72, 82, 85, 86, 89, 106, 114, 117, 132, 135, 178, 188, 189, 190, 199
individuals, 62, 140, 171
induction, 11, 17, 32, 42, 47, 63, 65, 69, 71, 141, 142, 143, 145, 150, 157, 159, 162, 177, 178, 181, 201, 202, 203, 207, 211

induction chemotherapy, 11, 207, 211
industrialization, 122
infants, 5, 13, 35, 86, 89, 96, 99, 100, 102, 106, 107, 116, 121, 190, 195, 220
infection, 45, 89, 107, 113, 143, 205, 206, 207, 209, 213, 214, 215, 216, 218, 219
inflammation, 165, 208, 211, 213, 214
inflammatory responses, 214
influenza, 89
influenza a, 89
inhibition, x, 13, 14, 18, 21, 25, 41, 42, 43, 47, 69, 79, 83, 109, 111, 138, 140, 142, 143, 145, 146, 147, 149, 150, 154, 159, 160, 161, 162, 163, 166, 214
inhibitor, 6, 17, 43, 44, 80, 83, 136, 137, 140, 141, 142, 145, 146, 147, 148, 149, 150, 151, 160, 166
initiation, 11, 18, 27, 32, 43, 70, 88, 131
injury, 213
innate immunity, 217, 218
inner ear, 207
inositol, 64, 157
insertion, 5, 10, 11, 12, 19, 21, 22, 27, 58, 175
insulin, 36, 47, 48, 62
integration, 8, 15, 17, 43, 121
integrin, 208
integrity, 77
intercellular adhesion molecule, 217
interferon, 57, 211, 220
interferon gamma, 211
internalization, 157, 166
interphase, 184, 193
intervention, 3, 24, 207
intravenously, 143, 144, 198
investment, 162
ionizing radiation, 89
isochromosome, 187
isozyme, 218
issues, 126
Italy, 179

J

Japan, 22, 39
joints, 59

K

karyotype, x, 6, 95, 107, 183, 188, 194
karyotyping, 108, 184, 193

kidney, 25, 30
kill, 198
killer cells, 2
kinase activity, 12, 43, 56, 62, 103, 160
kinetics, 21, 65
Kinsey, 113, 220
Kuwait, 85

L

labeling, 168, 184, 186
laboratory studies, 143, 144
laboratory tests, 213
lactate dehydrogenase, 96
laryngeal cancer, 165, 167
larynx, 156, 157, 158, 160
latency, 8, 126, 128
laws, 128
LDL, 29
lead, 10, 12, 20, 97, 112, 124, 125, 128, 129, 164, 176, 199, 214
learning, 206
lesions, vii, 1, 6, 35, 74, 97, 98, 110, 111, 166, 206, 207, 220
leukemogenesis, vii, ix, 1, 3, 4, 7, 13, 15, 18, 20, 24, 25, 26, 27, 29, 30, 33, 34, 35, 36, 42, 43, 46, 55, 69, 79, 119, 120, 125, 126, 128, 129, 132, 136, 184, 190, 192
leukocytosis, 38, 90
liberation, 18
life sciences, 121
ligand, 2, 9, 15, 18, 37, 38, 39, 62, 72, 78, 160, 208
light, viii, 53, 57, 59, 61, 65, 75, 78, 80
liquid chromatography, 2, 28
liver, 5, 9, 25, 66, 198, 213
localization, 5, 7, 62, 66, 166
loci, viii, x, 12, 53, 54, 55, 62, 65, 75, 77, 183, 214
locus, 3, 6, 12, 15, 17, 23, 26, 33, 47, 54, 59, 60, 62, 66, 68, 69, 75, 76, 77, 78, 79, 80, 82, 99, 108, 110, 177
LOH analysis, 192
loss of appetite, 144
low risk, 207
luciferase, 19
lung cancer, 48
Luo, 166
lymph, 31, 106
lymph node, 31
lymphadenopathy, 106
lymphoblast, 116, 123, 168, 206, 208

lymphocytes, ix, 4, 30, 34, 35, 61, 66, 76, 78, 79, 82, 119, 155, 175, 209, 210, 212, 214, 218
lymphoid, vii, viii, 1, 3, 4, 6, 8, 11, 14, 25, 27, 30, 31, 34, 36, 38, 42, 43, 45, 53, 54, 56, 58, 67, 73, 75, 82, 85, 86, 90, 99, 100, 106, 107, 111, 123, 137, 171, 175, 190, 192, 210, 212, 214
lymphoid development, vii, 1, 4, 6, 36, 55, 75
lymphoid organs, 67, 210
lymphoid tissue, 214
lymphoma, 2, 9, 14, 20, 26, 34, 37, 38, 41, 42, 43, 44, 46, 54, 69, 70, 73, 81, 82, 83, 86, 89, 90, 91, 104, 115, 116, 145, 146, 149, 202, 216, 218, 219
lysine, 138
lysis, 208
lysosome, 70

M

machinery, 5, 58, 138
macrophages, 214
magnetic field, 131, 132
major histocompatibility complex, 57
majority, viii, x, 7, 27, 42, 48, 59, 72, 85, 104, 117, 123, 143, 170, 172, 173, 175, 177, 178, 183, 184, 185, 187, 188, 190, 192, 201, 206, 213
malignancy, vii, viii, ix, 55, 82, 85, 86, 123, 138, 153, 154, 155, 158, 171, 175, 184, 194, 208, 209, 212
malignant cells, 104, 139, 175, 184, 206, 208, 215
malignant melanoma, 25, 158
malignant mesothelioma, 48
malignant tissues, 155
malignant tumors, 149
mammalian cells, 46
man, 130
management, 50, 213, 216
MAPK/ERK, 25, 137
mapping, 186
marriage, 121
marrow, 5, 8, 9, 14, 26, 31, 32, 136, 171, 178, 203, 208
mass, 90, 128
mast cells, 207
mathematics, ix, 119, 121
matter, 82, 120, 128, 129
measles, 218
measurement, 140, 181, 213
measurements, 32, 120
median, 22, 32, 95, 188, 201
medication, 136, 198, 201, 219

medicine, ix, 86, 112, 214
medulloblastoma, 131
MEK, 28, 45, 140
melanoma, 14, 30, 69, 156, 157, 158, 160, 166, 167
memory, 67, 206, 210, 212
mesoderm, 48, 124, 131
mesothelioma, 30, 48, 49
messenger RNA, 174
messengers, 64, 157
meta-analysis, 198
metabolism, 24, 64, 128, 132, 214
metaphase, 180, 184, 185, 186
metastasis, 154, 157, 163, 168
methodology, 171, 172, 178, 179
methylation, 29, 48, 78, 105, 108, 144
MHC, 210
mice, vii, 4, 8, 9, 16, 18, 21, 26, 27, 34, 38, 41, 42, 43, 45, 46, 55, 56, 57, 58, 62, 64, 65, 66, 69, 70, 72, 74, 76, 77, 79, 82, 83, 127, 131, 168
microorganisms, 206, 212
microRNA, 72, 84
microscope, 186
Middle East, 86
migration, 24, 64, 154, 162, 163, 208
Minimal residual disease (MRD), x, 169
mitochondria, 128
mitogen, 16, 37, 64, 155, 158, 160, 163, 166, 212
mitosis, 58
mitoxantrone, 136
model system, 55
models, vii, 4, 6, 9, 11, 15, 18, 21, 26, 27, 35, 44, 45, 53, 70, 78, 83, 122, 125, 145, 164
mole, 128
molecular biology, viii, 85, 92, 184
molecular weight, 58, 214
molecules, ix, 9, 10, 16, 24, 55, 57, 63, 64, 84, 120, 121, 128, 135, 137, 140, 146, 159, 160, 163, 172, 206, 208, 209, 210, 211, 215, 216
monosomy, 116
morbidity, 164, 212, 213
morphology, 90, 94, 95, 102, 104, 184, 187
mortality, vii, 1, 144, 164, 212, 213
mortality rate, 213
mother cell, 127
motif, 3
mRNA, x, 7, 11, 16, 31, 32, 33, 49, 50, 56, 57, 103, 142, 143, 154, 155, 163, 167, 173, 191, 218
mucosa, 207
mucous membrane, 207
multicellular organisms, 14

multiple myeloma, 9, 145, 194
multiples, 11
multiplication, 61
multivariate analysis, 32
mumps, 218
mutagenesis, 15, 17, 27, 43, 122
mutation, vii, 1, 4, 5, 9, 10, 11, 12, 13, 14, 19, 20, 22, 26, 27, 33, 34, 36, 40, 43, 44, 45, 46, 55, 68, 70, 72, 105, 108, 131, 140, 141, 147, 148, 180
mutational analysis, vii, 1, 28, 37
mutations, vii, 1, 3, 4, 6, 9, 11, 12, 13, 15, 16, 18, 20, 21, 24, 25, 27, 29, 30, 32, 34, 39, 40, 41, 44, 45, 46, 49, 51, 55, 67, 68, 71, 74, 80, 92, 109, 110, 111, 120, 122, 124, 125, 126, 127, 129, 141, 160
myelodysplasia, 9, 39
myelodysplastic syndromes, 4, 9, 30, 131, 133, 145, 149
myeloid cells, 63

N

NAD, 88, 112
natural killer cell, 206
natural science, ix, 119, 120, 121
nausea, 143, 144, 145, 165, 168
necrosis, 207
negativity, 107
neoangiogenesis, 154
neoplasm, 88, 120, 125
neovascularization, 162, 168
Nepal, 83
nerve, 157
nervous system, 157
Netherlands, 53, 73
neuroblastoma, 156, 157, 158, 160, 166, 167
neurokinin, ix, 153, 154, 165, 166, 167, 168
neuropeptides, 166
neurotransmitters, 166
neutropenia, 143, 146, 211, 213
neutrophils, 210
New England, 115
New Zealand, 217
NK cells, 2, 206, 209, 218
NK-1 receptor, x, 153, 154, 155, 156, 157, 158, 159, 160, 162, 163, 164, 165, 166, 167, 168
non-Hodgkin's lymphoma, 90, 202
nonsense mutation, 22, 32
normal children, 214
North Africa, 86
Northern blot, 11, 30, 31

notochord, 124
nuclei, 5, 189
nucleic acid, 171
nucleosome, 138
nucleotide sequencing, 5
nucleotides, 10, 11, 58, 175
nucleus, 4, 15, 18, 25, 29, 60, 93, 103, 158
null, 34
nutrient, 70

O

oncogenes, x, 3, 15, 25, 33, 54, 72, 110, 132, 183
oncogenesis, 8, 43, 105, 119, 120, 122
opportunities, 41
optical density, 159
organism, 124
organs, 9, 162
ovarian tumor, 48, 49
ovaries, 25

P

paclitaxel, 139, 147
pallor, 207
pancreas, 25, 158
pancreatic cancer, 146, 155, 157, 166, 167
parallel, 17, 32, 145, 175
parental smoking, 28
parotid, 158
parotid gland, 158
participants, 114
patents, 139
pathogenesis, vii, viii, x, xi, 1, 3, 6, 24, 26, 29, 33, 40, 86, 89, 110, 112, 114, 183, 205, 215
pathogens, 209
pathophysiology, 133
pathways, vii, 1, 13, 16, 21, 33, 35, 37, 39, 43, 58, 63, 67, 74, 124, 128, 160, 163, 209
PCT, 214, 215, 216
peptide, 5, 20, 24, 157, 159, 214
peptides, ix, 153, 154, 155, 216
peripheral blood, 9, 22, 31, 32, 49, 50, 104, 146, 208, 211, 212, 218
peripheral blood mononuclear cell, 146, 211
peripheral nervous system, 157
permission, 172
permit, 14
pertussis, 218

petechiae, 207
phagocytosis, 212
pharmacokinetics, 145, 149, 220
phenotype, 14, 56, 65, 90, 102, 103, 105, 106, 122, 126, 172, 187, 190, 191
phenotypes, x, 26, 31, 103, 129, 155, 171, 172, 176, 183
Philadelphia, 35, 101, 103, 115, 123, 141, 142, 189, 195, 216
phosphatidylcholine, 66
phosphorylation, 10, 12, 13, 37, 62, 64, 105, 122, 128, 142, 158, 160
physical chemistry, 121
physical laws, 129
physical phenomena, 120
physical theories, 120, 128
physicians, 213
physics, ix, 119, 121, 128
pilot study, 144
placebo, 163, 165
plants, 138
plasma cells, 67, 81, 210
plasma membrane, 25, 158, 165
plasticity, 127
platelets, 63
platform, 130
platinum, 136
ploidy, x, 95, 183, 187
point mutation, 12, 13, 19, 23, 26, 27, 33, 46, 68, 105
polarity, 124
pollutants, 125
polymerase, x, xi, 2, 45, 49, 169, 170, 180, 181, 183, 184
polymerase chain reaction (PCR), x, xi, 2, 5, 7, 10, 11, 19, 28, 30, 31, 32, 33, 50, 155, 169, 170, 171, 172, 173, 174, 175, 176, 177, 178, 180, 181, 183, 184, 185, 186, 190, 191, 192, 193
polymorphism, vii, 1, 28, 194
polymorphisms, vii, 1, 88, 113, 198
polyploid, 142
polyploidy, 92
pools, 27
population, ix, 27, 58, 66, 67, 95, 117, 120, 126, 127, 129, 132, 135, 170, 175, 177, 178
Portugal, 74
post-transcriptional regulation, 30
post-transplant, 26, 133
power lines, 131
power plants, 125

pre-B cell leukemia, viii, 53, 55, 56, 69, 72, 115
precursor cells, 107
prednisone, 21, 170, 198, 199
pregnancy, 28, 89, 131
prevention, 168
primary function, 61
primary tumor, 32, 123, 157
principles, ix, 119, 121
probability, 129
probe, 93, 99, 101, 104, 185
progenitor cells, 8, 26, 30, 37, 38, 48, 75, 102, 119, 126, 133
prognosis, vii, 1, 3, 6, 11, 12, 13, 21, 22, 28, 30, 31, 32, 33, 34, 35, 39, 40, 41, 46, 48, 94, 95, 97, 98, 102, 103, 104, 105, 106, 110, 113, 114, 116, 123, 160, 164, 177, 184, 187, 188, 190, 191, 192, 193, 207, 215
pro-inflammatory, 212
project, 163
proliferation, vii, viii, x, 8, 9, 13, 14, 17, 18, 24, 25, 27, 30, 37, 38, 39, 42, 47, 53, 55, 61, 63, 64, 67, 69, 72, 74, 78, 85, 86, 103, 105, 117, 123, 127, 128, 129, 140, 143, 150, 153, 154, 155, 157, 158, 159, 160, 162, 163, 164, 165, 166, 168, 172, 205, 207, 210,鸨211
proline, 15
promoter, 17, 45, 47, 48, 75, 97, 105, 108, 110, 138, 142, 143
propagation, 34, 127, 129
prophylaxis, 104
prostate cancer, 25
protection, 81, 89, 206
protein constituent, 168
protein kinases, 63
protein-protein interactions, 4
proteins, 2, 3, 9, 16, 21, 25, 29, 33, 42, 54, 55, 57, 58, 59, 60, 61, 62, 63, 64, 69, 71, 75, 76, 91, 99, 105, 111, 126, 132, 140, 141, 206, 211, 215
proteolysis, 14
proto-oncogene, 25, 47, 54, 69, 81, 103, 189
PTEN, 3, 17, 24, 25, 41, 44, 45, 55, 80
pulp, 217
purines, 214

Q

qualitative differences, 19
quality control, 180
quality of life, ix, 119

quantification, x, 30, 32, 33, 50, 169, 170, 176, 178, 180
quinacrine, 74
quinone, 88, 112

R

race, 96
racial differences, 86
radiation, 89, 125, 137, 218
radiation therapy, 137
radiotherapy, 154
reactions, 185, 211
reactive oxygen, 150
reactivity, 62
reading, 10, 12, 13, 56, 60, 77
real time, x, 31, 50, 169, 173
reality, 121, 146
receptors, x, 2, 9, 10, 12, 14, 20, 21, 25, 29, 30, 37, 55, 61, 63, 66, 67, 108, 124, 141, 153, 154, 155, 156, 157, 158, 159, 160, 162, 163, 166, 167, 168, 206, 208
reciprocal translocation, 8, 189
recognition, viii, 6, 58, 86, 90, 110, 171, 206, 210
recombination, viii, 15, 42, 53, 54, 57, 58, 59, 60, 62, 63, 64, 65, 66, 67, 68, 69, 70, 75, 76, 77, 78, 79, 80, 82, 175
recommendations, 200
recovery, 144
recurrence, 28, 30
regression, 16, 43, 212
regression analysis, 212
relapses, 123, 137, 191, 198, 199
relatives, 32
relevance, ix, xi, 50, 135, 183
reliability, 179
remission, ix, 11, 18, 27, 30, 31, 32, 33, 50, 110, 111, 135, 137, 143, 144, 170, 178, 181, 193, 198, 202, 203, 204, 207, 209, 212, 214, 218
renal cell carcinoma, 30, 48
repair, 54, 58, 73, 76, 88, 142
replication, 78, 136
repression, 4, 17, 41, 138
repressor, viii, 30, 54, 99
reprocessing, 132
requirements, 74
researchers, 4, 11, 17, 18, 22, 27, 31, 33, 111, 143, 163

residual disease, x, 2, 6, 11, 21, 30, 39, 48, 49, 50, 51, 133, 169, 170, 171, 172, 174, 176, 179, 180, 181, 190, 198, 200
residues, 9, 10, 13, 18, 22, 26, 67, 138
resistance, xi, 7, 21, 25, 27, 36, 44, 137, 138, 142, 205
resolution, 5, 6, 35, 74, 186
response, vii, x, 7, 17, 21, 28, 32, 33, 35, 38, 41, 47, 53, 54, 55, 64, 67, 69, 70, 71, 73, 76, 100, 103, 107, 111, 138, 142, 144, 145, 146, 150, 169, 170, 178, 180, 181, 206, 208, 209, 210, 211, 213, 215, 218, 219
restoration, 82
retina, 168
retinoblastoma, 122, 130, 156, 158, 160, 167, 168
retrovirus, 26
reverse transcriptase, 180, 184
ribonucleotide reductase, 136
risk, vii, viii, ix, x, 1, 6, 25, 27, 30, 32, 44, 85, 86, 88, 89, 95, 102, 106, 110, 111, 113, 115, 117, 125, 132, 133, 135, 167, 170, 173, 174, 177, 178, 179, 181, 184, 190, 195, 198, 199, 201, 203, 204, 205, 207, 209, 211, 213, 217
risk factors, 29, 89, 177
RNA, 7, 16, 30, 31, 84, 132, 160, 174, 176
rodents, 131
routes, 124
rubella, 218
rules, ix, 119, 123

S

safety, 145, 154, 163
SAHA, 83, 109, 111, 139, 140, 141, 143, 146, 149
saliva, 207
science, 120, 121
scope, 206
secrete, 67, 211
secretion, ix, 153, 155, 211
selectivity, 149
sensitivity, x, 24, 28, 94, 140, 169, 170, 171, 172, 173, 174, 175, 176, 185, 186, 215
sepsis, 211, 213, 216, 219
sequencing, 6, 7, 18, 120
serine, 13, 15, 24, 58, 64, 158
serum, 81, 208, 211, 212, 213, 214, 215, 216, 217, 218, 220
sex, 21, 90, 94, 100, 186
sex chromosome, 186
shape, viii, 53, 162, 163

shock, 217
showing, 21, 88, 93, 99, 100, 101, 104, 154
sibling, 204
side effects, 154, 163, 164
signal transduction, 10, 17, 18, 25
signaling pathway, viii, 16, 25, 42, 43, 54, 55, 64, 72, 111, 124, 137, 140
signalling, 9, 30, 42, 47, 78, 79, 166
signals, viii, 10, 13, 14, 15, 21, 43, 53, 55, 62, 64, 71, 72, 80, 93, 138, 154, 160, 165, 217
signs, 206
siRNA, 47, 142, 155, 156, 160
skeletal muscle, 25
skin, 25, 144, 206, 207, 220
smoking, 28
SNP, 33
sodium, 140, 144, 149, 150, 217
solid tumors, 48, 145, 146
solution, 121
somnolence, 144, 145
Southern blot, 184, 185, 190, 195
Spain, 153, 165
species, 150
specific surface, 104
spindle, 158
spleen, 9, 30, 66
splenomegaly, 103, 106
spontaneous abortion, 89
squamous cell, 150, 157, 158, 165
squamous cell carcinoma, 150, 157, 158, 165
stability, 19, 26, 71, 76, 145, 147, 181
standardization, 170, 173
state, ix, 15, 25, 29, 119, 128, 213
statistics, 168
status epilepticus, 145
stem cells, 2, 8, 9, 14, 15, 32, 34, 37, 50, 55, 124, 126, 127, 131, 133, 208
stimulus, 160
stochastic processes, 128
storage, 185
stratification, 34, 177, 178, 181, 184
stress, 40, 70, 71, 120, 122
striatum, 166
stroma, 78, 157, 208
stromal cells, 14, 72, 78
structural changes, x, 5, 93, 183
structure, 9, 18, 37, 63, 72, 73, 162
subcutaneous tissue, 220
subgroups, 36, 39, 96, 114, 115, 118, 191, 199, 203
substitutes, 61

substitution, 7, 12, 20
substitutions, 12, 19, 21, 22, 26, 33, 45
substrate, 62
substrates, 17, 21, 24, 37, 79
sulfate, 78
sulfonamide, 147
Sun, 4, 34, 35, 75, 131, 148
suppression, 7, 18, 41, 71, 72, 74, 79
surveillance, 82, 218, 219
survival, ix, 3, 6, 9, 12, 14, 17, 18, 21, 22, 24, 25, 27, 29, 30, 31, 35, 36, 45, 63, 64, 66, 67, 69, 70, 71, 72, 77, 80, 86, 95, 103, 107, 110, 112, 115, 123, 128, 135, 137, 144, 153, 154, 170, 178, 179, 187, 188, 190, 193, 197, 198, 199, 201
survival rate, ix, 3, 27, 110, 123, 135, 153, 154
survivors, 89, 218
susceptibility, viii, 12, 48, 85, 111, 113, 208, 212
symptoms, 143, 145
synapse, 78
syndrome, viii, 39, 40, 46, 85, 88, 123, 149, 217
synergistic effect, 24, 139, 140, 143, 147
synthesis, 9, 47, 150, 173, 208, 212, 214

T

T cell, 3, 4, 9, 14, 17, 18, 26, 34, 41, 42, 43, 44, 54, 62, 73, 76, 89, 103, 108, 180, 181, 194, 210, 211, 216, 219, 221
T lymphocytes, 4, 210, 211
tachykinin 1 (TAC1), x, 154
target, x, 11, 13, 15, 16, 17, 24, 30, 41, 43, 45, 54, 111, 126, 133, 139, 144, 149, 153, 162, 164, 167, 172, 174, 176, 178, 185
T-cell receptor, x, 97, 108, 117, 169, 170, 171, 175, 176, 181
TCR, 3, 4, 14, 15, 16, 42, 97, 108, 109, 110, 173, 175, 176, 177, 178, 180
technical assistance, 165
techniques, viii, x, xi, 85, 92, 99, 100, 112, 169, 170, 171, 173, 176, 177, 183, 184, 186, 188, 190, 194
technologies, 34
technology, 194
telangiectasia, 88, 108
temperature, 214
terminals, 157
termination codon, 19
testing, 107, 165, 172, 176, 190
testis, 25, 30
tetanus, 218
T-helper cell, 212

therapeutic agents, 159, 163, 164
therapeutic approaches, 7, 125
therapeutic effects, 164
therapeutic interventions, 111, 154, 184
therapeutic targets, ix, 86, 112, 126, 216
therapeutics, 127
therapy, vii, ix, xi, 1, 3, 21, 29, 32, 34, 46, 53, 54, 83, 86, 100, 102, 103, 107, 110, 123, 131, 133, 135, 137, 138, 139, 143, 144, 147, 149, 153, 154, 167, 178, 181, 184, 190, 197, 198, 199, 200, 201, 202, 203, 207, 212, 219, 220
thermodynamics, 128, 129
thoughts, 120, 128
threats, 122
threonine, 15, 24, 58, 64, 158
thrombocytopenia, 143, 144, 146
thymine, 23
thymus, 4, 9, 14, 25
thyroid, 25
tissue, 26, 58, 71, 77, 122, 124, 162, 185, 207, 208, 213
TLR, 67, 217
TLR2, 63
TLR4, 63
TNF-α, 212, 215
tobacco, 89
toxic side effect, 138
toxicity, 132, 138, 143, 144, 145, 198
traits, 124
transcription, 2, 3, 5, 7, 9, 15, 16, 21, 29, 30, 33, 34, 48, 49, 54, 55, 56, 60, 64, 65, 69, 70, 71, 75, 76, 78, 80, 83, 97, 99, 102, 103, 108, 111, 124, 125, 130, 138, 151, 174, 191
transcription factors, 3, 8, 16, 29, 55, 56, 64, 65, 70, 71, 80, 83, 97, 99, 108, 125, 130
transcripts, viii, x, 3, 24, 31, 32, 48, 49, 50, 53, 56, 60, 65, 99, 115, 169, 171, 173, 174, 176, 178, 180, 190, 191
transducer, 2, 9, 55, 61
transduction, 9, 10, 79, 97
transfection, 9, 10
transformation, vii, x, 4, 7, 8, 9, 15, 18, 26, 27, 29, 39, 40, 42, 44, 45, 53, 54, 56, 64, 69, 70, 71, 72, 79, 82, 83, 92, 105, 123, 126, 133, 183, 209
transforming growth factor (TGF), 30, 47
transgene, 16, 69
translocation, viii, 11, 12, 15, 18, 32, 36, 53, 54, 55, 56, 69, 72, 83, 88, 93, 94, 97, 99, 100, 101, 102, 103, 104, 105, 106, 109, 110, 114, 173, 189, 190, 191, 192, 196

transmembrane glycoprotein, 14
transmission, 58
transplant, 203
transplantation, 9, 50, 126, 171, 177, 200, 202, 203, 204, 217
treatment, vii, ix, x, xi, 1, 6, 13, 17, 21, 23, 24, 28, 29, 32, 34, 41, 53, 54, 55, 73, 86, 92, 95, 103, 104, 107, 110, 111, 113, 114, 115, 117, 118, 119, 123, 125, 135, 137, 139, 140, 141, 142, 143, 144, 145, 146, 149, 150, 153, 154, 155, 159, 162, 163, 164, 167,鸨169, 170, 172, 177, 178, 179, 180, 183, 184, 194, 195, 198, 199, 200, 202, 203, 204, 209, 211, 212, 213, 214, 215, 216, 220
trial, 22, 148, 168, 181, 199, 200, 201, 202, 203, 204
triggers, 71, 140
trisomy, 94, 102, 114, 195
tryptophan, 22, 159
tumor, viii, x, xi, 3, 7, 15, 16, 18, 21, 24, 25, 29, 30, 31, 32, 35, 43, 47, 48, 49, 50, 51, 54, 56, 64, 69, 70, 71, 72, 74, 79, 82, 83, 92, 105, 108, 110, 122, 123, 124, 127, 128, 129, 131, 139, 140, 144, 145, 146, 148, 153, 154, 155, 157, 158, 159, 162, 163, 164, 166, 168, 175, 205, 208, 209, 211, 219
tumor cells, x, 15, 31, 122, 124, 128, 129, 140, 153, 154, 155, 157, 158, 159, 162, 163, 209
tumor development, 70, 162, 163
tumor growth, xi, 17, 124, 154, 163, 166, 205
tumor necrosis factor (TNF), 148, 160, 206, 209, 211, 212, 215, 216, 217
tumorigenesis, 27, 40, 74, 80, 122, 127, 129
tumors, ix, 17, 21, 25, 46, 48, 69, 70, 72, 83, 104, 122, 124, 129, 153, 154, 155, 157, 158, 162, 163
tumour growth, 168
turnover, 15, 21, 104, 157
twins, 88, 107
tyrosine, viii, 2, 3, 6, 8, 10, 12, 13, 16, 25, 35, 37, 40, 54, 62, 64, 72, 74, 75, 79, 81, 91, 98, 103, 108, 109, 111, 140, 141, 142, 148, 189

U

uniform, 176
unique features, 18
united, 22, 154, 179, 220
United Kingdom, 22, 220
United States, 154, 179
urea, 19
urticaria, 207, 216
USA, 113, 166, 168

V

variations, 88, 111, 171
vascular wall, 207
vector, 45
velocity, 120
vertigo, 163
vessels, 154, 162
viral infection, 89, 213, 214
viruses, 25, 89, 132
visualization, 185
vitamin D, 30, 47
vomiting, 144, 145, 165, 168

W

Washington, 179
water, 89
web, 130
Western blot, 4, 155
white blood cell count, 95, 96, 102, 106
white blood cells, 46
wild type, 10
Wiskott-Aldrich syndrome, 88
withdrawal, 17
Wnt signaling, 29, 30, 47
World Health Organization (WHO), 90, 102, 104, 113

X

xenografts, 168

Y

yeast, 77, 138
yield, ix, 135
yolk, 124
young adults, 165, 220

Z

zinc, 3, 5, 30, 32, 58, 89